*Clinical Studies in
Behavior Therapy with
Children, Adolescents
and Their Families*

Clinical Studies in Behavior Therapy with Children, Adolescents and Their Families

By

JAMES M. STEDMAN, Ph.D.

Assistant Professor, University of Texas Medical School at San Antonio and Chief Psychologist, Community Guidance Center of Bexar County

WILLIAM F. PATTON, Ph.D.

Assistant Professor, University of Texas Medical School at San Antonio and Staff Psychologist, Community Guidance Center of Bexar County

KAY F. WALTON, M.S.

Associate School Psychologist, North East Independent School District, Pupil Appraisal Center

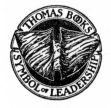

CHARLES C THOMAS • PUBLISHER
Springfield • Illinois • U.S.A.

Published and Distributed Throughout the World by
CHARLES C THOMAS · PUBLISHER

BANNERSTONE HOUSE

301-327 East Lawrence Avenue, Springfield, Illinois, U.S.A.

© *1973, by* CHARLES C THOMAS · PUBLISHER
ISBN-0-398-02736-6 (cloth)
ISBN-0-398-02763-3 (paper)
Library of Congress Catalog Card Number: 72-92179

With THOMAS BOOKS *careful attention is given to all details of manufacturing and design. It is the Publisher's desire to present books that are satisfactory as to their physical qualities and artistic possibilities and appropriate for their particular use.* THOMAS BOOKS *will be true to those laws of quality that assure a good name and good will.*

Printed in the United States of America
Y-2

Siebert Grant

PREFACE

O VER A DECADE AGO, Rachman (1962) reviewed the literature pertaining to behavior modification in the child-clinical field. At that time he found seventy-nine articles, some of which were only tangentially related to the subject at hand. However, he clearly foresaw that the principles of learning, adapted from the laboratory, held much promise for the treatment of disordered children and their families. This book of readings validates Rachman's vision. In the last ten years articles related to children, adolescents, and their families have proliferated.

Our labors in assembling this book of studies flowed from our own experience of the fertility of utilizing applied learning concepts and techniques in child clinical and family treatment. Daily experience in a large medical school, community mental health center, and public school district has taught us that a vast number of "disturbed" children, adolescents, and families can be quickly helped by these techniques. Hence, we chose readings on the basis of their ability to present the principles of applied learning, within the format of practical case material. Hopefully these readings will serve as guidelines, not only for psychology students and practitioners but also for our colleagues in psychiatry, social work, and other allied professions interested in the modification of the behavior of children and their families.

Perusal of the table of contents will indicate that the book is organized around issues familiar to practitioners in both inpatient and outpatient child-clinical work. There are two features of the book which are perhaps worth special mention. First, the lead article in Section I is intended to aid in coping with the sometimes confusing terminology and concepts of applied learning. As the reader will note, the definitions are presented in a general manner. However, in an effort to bridge the "terminology gap," there are references to the terms as used in practical case material. Secondly, an annotated bibliography is included and is designed to give the reader further references to quality articles which, because of their recency or other factors, could not be included in their entirety. We trust that these features will increase the reader's ability to learn and use behavior therapy concepts.

James M. Stedman
Kay F. Walton
William F. Patton

Rachman, S.: Learning Theory in Child Psychology: Therapeutic Possibilities. *Journal of Child Psychology and Psychiatry*, 3:149-163, 1962.

CONTENTS

vii

Section III

BEHAVIORAL CLASSROOM MANAGEMENT

Section IV

BEHAVIOR THERAPY WITH CHILD GROUPS

Section V

BEHAVIOR THERAPY WITH DELINQUENTS

Section VI

THERAPY BEHAVIOR WITH FAMILIES

Section VII

BEHAVIOR THERAPY WITH THE SEVERELY DISTURBED CHILD

Clinical Studies in Behavior Therapy with Children, Adolescents and Their Families

Section I

CONCEPTS AND ISSUES

SECTION I IS INTENDED TO INTRODUCE THE TERMINOLOGY OF AP-
PLIED LEARNING AND TO ORIENT READERS TO THE LOGIC OF BEHAVIOR
THERAPY AS APPLIED TO CHILD CLINICAL PROBLEMS. THE FIRST
CHAPTER DEFINES CONCEPTS AND TERMS. WHILE THE READING BY
KANFER AND SASLOW DOES NOT PERTAIN DIRECTLY TO CHILD, ADO-
LESCENT, OR FAMILY WORK, IT DOES PRESENT THE TRADITIONAL CON-
CEPTUAL MODEL OF PSYCHIATRIC DISORDER AS CONTRASTED WITH
THE MODEL PROPOSED BY ADVOCATES OF APPLIED LEARNING. FUR-
THER, IT SPECIFIES IMPLICATIONS FOR BOTH DIAGNOSIS AND TREAT-
MENT. THE FINAL ARTICLE FOCUSES ON CHILD CLINICAL PROBLEMS
PER SE AND DETAILS APPLICATION OF THE APPLIED LEARNING MODEL
TO THE ISSUE OF GOAL DIRECTED ASSESSMENT.

Chapter 1

THE LANGUAGE OF APPLIED LEARNING

T HE TERMS AND CONCEPTS of the psychology of learning, generated in the laboratory, seem to find their most precise definition
and use in that setting. As these concepts have become applied to
human problems, they often retain their original, precise laboratory
significance. However, at other times, their meanings seem disguised
or quite different, even to those practitioners with behavior science
backgrounds. To practitioners unfamiliar with the concepts and
methodology of learning psychology, the language of behavior modification often appears totally confusing and, frequently, leads to an
outright rejection of these principles as "not making any sense."

This chapter is designed to aid both the sophisticated and neophyte
in coping with the language of applied learning. Actually it represents a glossary and includes the majority of technical terms and concepts utilized in all the readings. In presenting it first, the authors
hope to give readers the opportunity to peruse the language of behavior modification before encountering it within the articles. Secondly, it should be noted that the terms are defined in a general, lab-
oratory-like manner. However, there are references to the various
articles, so that the reader can quickly refer to examples of the concepts in their applied settings. It should also be noted that, within
the limits of the subjective judgment of the authors, these references
are graded according to clarity of usage and the "goodness of fit" between the "laboratory" definition and the use of the concept in the
article(s). Thus, references qualified by (G) indicate the clearest

examples. Other references are to examples which, although appropriate, do not seem to be striking examples of clarity. Examples in the text appear in small cap type.

Definitions and References

1. AVERSIVE CONTROL—Behavior control techniques which rely on aversive (negative) stimuli, usually involving punishment and negative reinforcement techniques. Stuart (coercion) (G) 313; McAllister (G) 147; O'Leary 274.

2. AVOIDANCE RESPONSE—A response, performed under conditions of negative reinforcement, which allows the patient to avoid the onset of a negatively reinforcing stimulus. Simmons (G) 378; MacCulloch (G) 90.

3. AVERSIVE STIMULUS—Any stimulus, usually negative, which serves to reinforce a response leading to its removal or acts as a punishing stimulus when presented after a particular response. MacCulloch (shock) (G) 90.

4. BACKUP REINFORCERS—Any reinforcing stimulus, such as food, privileges, toys, etc., which is given in exchange for less reinforcing stimuli such as tokens. O'Leary (G) 269; Phillips (G) 229.

5. BASELINE—A procedure in which data regarding the frequency of occurrence of a particular response is collected under conditions of natural occurrence, prior to the introduction of behavior modification techniques. This data can then be compared to the frequency of occurrence of responses after the introduction of behavior modification techniques. McAllister (G) 146; Phillips (G) 232; Stedman 210; Miller 170.

6. BEHAVIOR CHAIN—A series of behaviors or responses in which the S-R units are conditioned separately and then linked together, via conditioning, to form a complex behavior unit. Ayllon (G) 67; Miller (G) 169; Stuart 316.

7. BEHAVIOR CONSEQUENCES—Usually this refers to any positive or negative stimulus which follows the occurrence of a response or which is removed following the occurrence of a response. Ayllon (G) 59.

8. BEHAVIORAL CONTRACT—A procedure in which the therapist arranges for the patient or patients to enter into a contractual ar-

rangement which specifies adaptive responses to be performed and the reinforcing consequences which will follow such responses. Stuart (G) 246; Cantrell (G) 131.

9. BEHAVIORAL DEFICIT—A class of responses described as problematic by the patient or an informant because it fails to occur with sufficient frequency, with adequate intensity, in appropriate form, or under socially expected conditions. Kanfer 24.

10. BEHAVIORAL EXCESS—A class of related behaviors described as problematic by the patient or an informant because of an excess in frequency, intensity, duration, or occurrence under conditions when it's socially sanctioned frequency approaches zero. Kanfer 24.

11. BEHAVIORAL REHEARSAL—A form of learning in which the therapist or others under the therapist's direction help the patient formulate prosocial, adaptive behavior by modeling these for the patient or by correcting and reinforcing the patient's own efforts to produce adaptive behaviors. Gittelman (G) 198.

12. CLASSICAL CONDITIONING—One of the two basic types of conditioning. In classical conditioning, the reinforcer is correlated with the stimulus. The reference experiment is one in which the neutral, conditioned stimulus is paired with the unconditioned stimulus, which itself evokes a particular response called the unconditioned response. Eventually, the conditioned stimulus acquires a capacity to evoke a conditioned response, often similar to the original unconditioned response. Kimmel 83.

13. CLASSES OF BEHAVIOR—Definably different patterns of behavior, such as deviant behavior, cooperative behavior, or isolate behavior. Individual responses performed by the patient can then be assigned within such categories. O'Leary (G) 267; Tate (SIB as a class) 352.

14. CONDITIONED RESPONSE (Classical Conditioning)—Any response which appears or is modified as a consequence of the occurrence of a conditioned stimulus in classical conditioning training. Kimmel (waking) (G) 84.

15. CONDITIONED STIMULUS (Classical Conditioning)—Any neutral stimulus which is presented together with a non-neutral stimulus (UCS) and acquires the ability to evoke a new conditioned response. Kimmel (bladder stimulation) 84.

16. CONTINGENCY (Operant Conditioning)—The temporal or spacial arrangement of a positive or negative consequence or the removal of either following a response. The particular contingency has a systematic effect on the response or class of responses. Simmons (G) 380; McAllister (G) 146; Miller (G) 170; Phillips (G) 230; Burchard (G) 219; Ryback 289; Engeln 280.

17. CONTINUOUS SCHEDULE—A schedule of reinforcement in which the reinforcing stimulus is presented upon each occurrence of the desired response. Brawley (G) 364; Holland 80; Engeln 280.

18. CUE—Any event having the properties of a stimulus. Brawley (G) 374.

19. CUMULATIVE RECORD—A method of recording data (number of responses produced by the patient) in which the number of responses is recorded along the vertical axis and time is recorded along the horizontal axis. Ryback (G) 296.

20. DELAY OF REINFORCEMENT—A procedure in which there is a temporal separation between the occurrence of the patient's response and the reinforcing stimulus. Generally speaking, the degree of control exercised by reinforcement decreases with increasing delay between response and reinforcer. However, if delay of reinforcement is introduced gradually, there may be a little loss of such control. O'Leary 270.

21. DIFFERENTIAL REINFORCEMENT—An operant conditioning procedure in which the reinforcer is made contingent upon the desired property of the patient's response. Eventually, the patient emits only the desired property of the reinforced response. Sulzbacher 346; Stedman 206; Simmons 380.

22. DISCRIMINATIVE STIMULUS—A stimulus which acquires a controlling function over a response or a class of responses by being consistently correlated with the occurrence or non-occurrence of a reinforcing or punishing stimulus. Holland (G) 79; Neale (example) (G) 98; MacCulloch (initial stimulus) (G) 90; Scrignar (example) (G) 116; Kimmel (example) 84.

23. DISCRIMINATION TRAINING—A type of conditioning in which responses or classes of responses are differentially reinforced in the presence of a stimulus with identifiable properties. This re-

sults in the response or class of responses being emitted in the presence of the positively discriminated stimulus. Neale (G) 110.

24. ESCAPE RESPONSE—A response, performed under conditions of negative reinforcement, which removes the patient from an ongoing, negative reinforcing stimulus. Simmons 378.

25. EXTINCTION—The decrease in response strength of a conditioned response under conditions of nonreinforcement. Stuart (G) 253; Brawley 371.

26. FADING (Stimulus)—The gradual shift of a discriminative stimulus originally controlling the patient's response to another discriminative stimulus, without disruption of the performance of the response. Eventually, the response comes under control of the new discriminative stimulus. Ayllon (example) (G) 66; Sulzbacher (example) (G) 333; Brawley (example) (G) 366; Stuart 321; Cantrell 138.

27. FINES (Punishment)—A technique in which the patient is "charged" some amount of a positive reinforcer, contingent upon the occurrence of an undesirable response. As a punishment technique, it reduces the probability of occurrence of that response. Phillips (G) 232.

28. FIXED RATIO SCHEDULE OF REINFORCEMENT—An intermittent reinforcement schedule in which the reinforcer is delivered after a standard number of responses, such as after every fifteenth trial. This schedule produces high rates of responding, often characterized by an initial pause, followed by a positively accelerated rate of responding which continues until reception of reinforcing stimulus. Ryback (G) 299; O'Leary (example) (G) 269; Miller (G) 169.

29. INCOMPATIBLE RESPONSES—Any two classes of responses, one of which is antagonistic to, or cannot be performed at the same time as the other. In behavior therapy, the incompatible response usually refers to a situation in which one response or a class of responses is maladaptive for the patient and the other response or class of responses is adaptive for the patient. The therapist attempts to establish adaptive responses in the patient's repertoire. Brawley (G) 375; Neisworth (G) 309; Sulzbacher 335; Gittelman 202.

30. INSTRUMENTAL CONDITIONING—One of the two basic types of conditioning in which the patient's responses are instrumental to the production of positive reinforcing stimuli or are effective in avoiding or escaping negatively reinforcing stimuli. Neale 99.

31. MALADAPTIVE APPROACH BEHAVIOR—Any behavior manifested by the patient which interferes with his effective living. Maladaptive approach behavior is one form of maladaptive behavior in which the patient engages in responses which interefere with life adjustment (e.g. delinquent seeking opportunities to steal). MacCulloch (G) 94.

32. MODELING—Learning in which the patient acquires responses by first observing another perform the responses. This can apply to prosocial behavior, such as modeled by a therapist, or deviant behavior, such as modeled by an adolescent gang. Brawley (G) 365; Sulzbacher (example) (G) 334.

33. OPERANT—Any behavior which can be controlled by its environmental consequences. Holland 79.

34. POSITIVE REINFORCER—Any stimulus which, when presented following a response, increases the probability of occurrence of that response. Stuart (G) 312; McAllister 153; Burchard 221.

35. PREMACK PRINCIPLE—The empirical rule, expressed by Premack, that any behavior with a high frequency of occurrence can be used as a reinforcer in conditioning a behavior with low probability of occurrence. Sulzbacher (G) 330; Stedman 161.

36. PRIMARY REINFORCER—A stimulus with reinforcing value which does not depend upon the fact of prior association with other reinforcing stimuli. Simmons (G) 384; Brawley (food) (G) 364.

37. PROMPT—A procedure in which the therapist, by word or example, instructs the patient to perform a component of the desired response. Ryback (G) 293; Brawley (example) (G) 365; Sulzbacher (G) 344.

38. PUNISHMENT—Any aversive stimulus which, when presented following a response, reduces the probability of or rate of occurrence of that response. Tate (G) 353; Burchard (G) 220; Ayllon 76; Simmons 379.

39. RECIPROCAL INHIBITION—A counter-conditioning technique in which the ability of a given stimulus to evoke anxiety is weak-

ened by pairing that stimulus with a response antagonistic to the occurrence of anxiety. This results in reduction of anxiety. Neale 99.

40. REINFORCEMENT SATIATION—The loss of power of a particular reinforcer to continue as a reinforcing event due to its too frequent use over a lengthy period of time. Stedman 161.

41. REINFORCER—Any stimulus which, when added as the consequence of a response (positive reinforcer) or removed as a consequence of a response (negative reinforcer), increases the probability of performance of that response. Miller 169.

42. REPERTOIRE OF BEHAVIOR—The patient's total available responses which have been learned under particular conditions and maintained by definable environmental and internal reinforcing stimuli. Kanfer (G) 24; Brawley 376; Sulzbacher 344.

43. RESISTANCE TO EXTINCTION—The continuation of a response under conditions of nonreinforcement. Resistance to extinction has been found to increase when learning occurs under intermittent conditions of reinforcement. Simmons (G) 384.

44. RESPONSE SUBSTITUTION—A procedure in which the patient replaces a maladaptive response with one which is less maladaptive or positively adaptive. Weiner (example) (G) 124.

45. REVERSAL—A procedure in which prosocial responses, previously established in the patient's repertoire by reinforcement, are placed on an extinction schedule. The usual result is a rapid decrease in emission of the prosocial responses. This procedure is used to demonstrate that the reinforcement contingencies have been effective in maintaining prosocial responses. Brawley (G) 368.

46. SCANNING—A process in which the patient evaluates assets or liabilities in others. If the patient is receiving abundant positive reinforcement from others, the "scan" is likely to be positive. If the patient receives no reinforcement, negative reinforcement, or punishment, the "scan" is likely to be negative. Stuart (G) 314.

47. SHAPING—A procedure in which responses, approximating the desired response, are systematically reinforced, such that closer and closer approximations to the desired response is obtained. Eventually the patient will produce the desired response. Can-

trell (example) (G) 136.

48. SOCIAL BANKRUPTCY—A condition in which one partner of at least a two-partner system (e.g., marital partners) cannot exercise control over the other partner's behavior through positive reinforcement strategies. Stuart (G) 312.

49. SOCIAL REINFORCER—A secondary reinforcing stimulus in which the reinforcement for a given response is some communication by another human being (e.g., therapist's praise for accomplishing desired behavior, etc.) Brawley (example) 364; Holland 81; Engeln 280.

50. STIMULUS CONTROL—See discriminative stimulus and references there.

51. STIMULUS GENERALIZATION—The behavioral fact that a conditioned response, formed to one stimulus, may be also elicited by other stimuli which have not entered into the original conditioning situation. The degree of generalization is inversely related to the distance (psychological or physical) of the stimuli from each other along some dimension. Brawley 363; Sulzbacher 332.

52. TARGET BEHAVIOR—That behavior, not present in the patient's repertoire, which the therapist wishes to establish or that behavior, present in the patient's repertoire, which the therapist wishes to eliminate. Phillips (G) 228; McAllister (G) 144; Stedman (G) 206; Sulzbacher (G) 329.

53. TIME OUT (Punishment)—A punishment procedure in which the patient is removed from a rewarding situation, usually contingent upon the occurrence of an undesirable response. The result is a decrease in the probability of occurrence of that response. Sulzbacher (G) 332; O'Leary (G) 270; Burchard (example) (G) 220; Tate 355.

54. TOKEN—Any tangible symbol (e.g., a poker chip, mark on a paper, washer, etc.) which can be exchanged later for a more desirable reinforcer, such as food, privileges, etc. O'Leary (checks) (G) 269; Stedman (G) 208; Phillips (G) 229.

55. TOKEN ECONOMY—A procedure in which tokens (any distinctive tangible stimulus, such as points, poker chips, etc.) are used as intermediate reinforcers in order to establish desirable, prosocial behavior in patients. Later these are exchanged for more desirable reinforcing stimuli, such as food, privileges, toys, etc.

Phillips (G) 241; Miller (G) 163; Stuart 317; Stedman 204.

56. UNCONDITIONED RESPONSE (Classical Conditioning) — Any measurable and regular response which is evoked in the presence of the unconditioned stimulus. Kimmel (elicited response) (G) 84.

57. UNCONDITIONED STIMULUS (Classical Conditioning—Any stimulus, which at the outset, evokes a regular and measurable response. Kimmel (G) 84.

58. VARIABLE RATIO SCHEDULE OF REINFORCEMENT—An intermittent schedule of reinforcement in which the reinforcing stimulus occurs after a number of responses which changes from one reinforcement period to another. A 15:1 schedule might be produced by reinforcing every fifth, tenth, fifteenth, twentieth, or twenty-fifth response. This schedule produces a uniform rate of responding. Engeln (G) 280.

59. WITHDRAWAL OF REINFORCEMENT (Punishment)—A punishment technique in which the reinforcing stimulus is removed, contingent upon the occurrence of some undesirable behavior. As a punishment technique, it reduces that probability of occurrence of that response. Holland (example) (G) 79; Engeln 280.

Chapter 2

BEHAVIORAL ANALYSIS*

An Alternative to Diagnostic Classification

FREDERICK H. KANFER, Ph.D. *and* GEORGE SASLOW, M.D.

D URING THE PAST DECADE attacks on conventional psychiatric diagnosis have been so widespread that many clinicians now use diagnostic labels sparingly and apologetically. The continued adherence to the nosological terms of the traditional classificatory scheme suggests some utility of the present categorization of behavior disorders, despite its apparently low reliability[1, 21]; its limited prognostic value[7, 26]; and its multiple feebly related assumptive supports. In a recent study of this problem, the symptom patterns of carefully diagnosed paranoid schizophrenics were compared. Katz et al[12] found considerable divergence among patients with the same diagnosis and concluded that "diagnostic systems which are more circumscribed in their intent, for example, based on manifest behavior alone, rather than systems which attempt to comprehend etiology, symptom patterns and prognosis, may be more directly applicable to current problems in psychiatric research." (p. 202).

We propose here to examine some sources of dissatisfaction with the present approach to diagnosis, to describe a framework for a behavioral analysis of individual patients which implies both suggestions for treatment and outcome criteria for the single case, and to indicate the conditions for collecting the data for such an analysis.

I. Problems in Current Diagnostic Systems

Numerous criticisms deal with the internal consistency, the ex-

*From the *Archives of General Psychiatry*, June 1965, 12, pp. 529-538. Reprinted by permission of the authors and the Journal.

plicitness, the precision, and the reliability of psychiatric classifications. It seems to us that the more important fault lies in our lack of sufficient knowledge to categorize behavior along those pertinent dimensions which permit prediction of responses to social stresses, life crises, or psychiatric treatment. This limitation obviates anything but a crude and tentative approximation to a taxonomy of effective individual behaviors.

Zigler and Phillips,[28] in discussing the requirement for an adequate system of classification, suggest that an etiologically-oriented closed system of diagnosis is premature. Instead, they believe that an empirical attack is needed, using "symptoms broadly defined as meaningful and discernible behaviors, as the basis of the classificatory system" (p. 616). But symptoms as a class of responses are defined after all only by their nuisance value to the patient's social environment or to himself as a social being. They are also notoriously unreliable in predicting the patient's particular etiological history or his response to treatment. An alternate approach lies in an attempt to identify classes of dependent variables in human behavior which would allow inferences about the particular controlling factors, the social stimuli, the physiological stimuli, and the reinforcing stimuli, of which they are a function. In the present early stage of the art of psychological prognostication, it appears most reasonable to develop a program of analysis which is closely related to subsequent treatment. A classification scheme which implies a program for behavioral change is one which has not only utility but the potential for experimental validation.

The task of assessment and prognosis can therefore be reduced to efforts which answer the following three questions: (*a*) which specific behavior patterns require change in their frequency of occurrence, their intensity, their duration or in the conditions under which they occur, (*b*) what are the best practical means which can produce the desired changes in this individual (manipulation of the environment, of the behavior, or the self-attitudes of the patient), and (*c*) what factors are currently maintaining it and what are the conditions under which this behavior was acquired. The investigation of the history of the problematic behavior is mainly of academic interest, except as it contributes information about the probable efficacy of a specific treatment method.

Expectations of Current Diagnostic Systems—In traditional medicine, a diagnostic statement about a patient has often been viewed as an essential prerequisite to treatment because a diagnosis suggests that the physician has some knowledge of the origin and future course of the illness. Further, in medicine, diagnosis frequently brings together the accumulated knowledge about the pathological process which leads to the manifestation of the symptoms, and the experiences which others have had in the past in treating patients with such a disease process. Modern medicine recognizes that any particular disease need not have a single cause or even a small number of antecedent conditions. Nevertheless, the diagnostic label attempts to define at least the necessary conditions which are most relevant in considering a treatment program. Some diagnostic classification system is also invaluable as a basis for many social decisions involving entire populations. For example, planning for treatment facilities, research efforts and educational programs take into account the distribution frequencies of specified syndromes in the general population.

Ledley and Lusted[14] give an excellent conception of the traditional model in medicine by their analysis of the reasoning underlying it. The authors differentiate between a disease complex and a symptom complex. While the former describes known pathological processes and their correlated signs, the latter represents particular signs present in a particular patient. The bridge between disease and symptom complexes is provided by available medical knowledge and the final diagnosis is tantamount to labeling the disease complex. However, the current gaps in medical knowledge necessitate the use of probability statements when relating disease to symptoms, admitting that there is some possibility for error in the diagnosis. Once the diagnosis is established, decisions about treatment still depend on many other factors including social, moral, and economic conditions. Ledley and Lusted[14] thus separate the clinical diagnosis into a two-step process. A statistical procedure is suggested to facilitate the primary or diagnostic labeling process. However, the choice of treatment depends not only on the diagnosis proper. Treatment decisions are also influenced by the moral, ethical, social, and economic conditions of the individual patient, his family and the society in which he lives. The proper assignment of the weight to be given to each of these values must in the last analysis be left to the physician's judgment (Ledley and Lusted[14]).

The Ledley and Lusted model presumes available methods for the observation of relevant behavior (the symptom complex), and some scientific knowledge relating it to known antecedents or correlates (the disease process). Contemporary theories of behavior pathology do not yet provide adequate guidelines for the observer to suggest what is to be observed. In fact, Szasz[25] has expressed the view that the medical model may be totally inadequate because psychiatry should be concerned with problems of living and not with diseases of the brain or other biological organs. Szasz[25] argues that "mental illness is a myth, whose function it is to disguise and thus render more potable the bitter pill of moral conflict in human relations." (p. 118).

The attack against use of the medical model in psychiatry comes from many quarters. Scheflen[23] describes a model of somatic psychiatry which is very similar to the traditional medical model of disease. A pathological process results in onset of an illness; the symptoms are correlated with a pathological state and represent our evidence of "mental disease." Treatment consists of removal of the pathogen, and the state of health is restored. Scheflen suggests that this traditional medical model is used in psychiatry not on the basis of its adequacy but because of its emotional appeal.

The limitations of the somatic model have been discussed even in some areas of medicine for which the model seems most appropriate. For example, in the nomenclature for diagnosis of disease of the heart and blood vessels, the criteria committee of the New York Heart Association[17] suggests the use of multiple criteria for cardiovascular diseases, including a statement of the patient's functional capacity. The committee suggests that the functional capacity be ". . . estimated by appraising the patient's ability to perform physical activity" (p. 80), and decided largely by inference from his history. Further,[17] ". . . (it) should not be influenced by the character of the structural lesion or by an opinion as to treatment or prognosis" (p. 81). This approach makes it clear that a comprehensive assessment of a patient, regardless of the physical disease which he suffers, must also take into account his social effectiveness and the particular ways in which physiological, anatomical, and psychological factors interact to produce a particular behavior pattern in an individual patient.

Multiple Diagnosis—A widely used practical solution and circumvention of the difficulty inherent in the application of the medical model to psychiatric diagnosis is offered by Noyes and Kolb.[18] They suggest that the clinician construct a diagnostic formulation consisting of three parts: (1) A *genetic* diagnosis incorporating the constitutional, somatic, and historical-traumatic factors representing the primary sources or determinants of the mental illness; (2) A *dynamic* diagnosis which describes the mechanisms and techniques unconsciously used by the individual to manage anxiety, enhance self esteem, ie, that traces the psychopathological processes; and (3) A *clinical* diagnosis which conveys useful connotations concerning the reaction syndrome, the probable course of the disorder, and the methods of treatment which will most probably prove beneficial. Noyes' and Kolb's multiple criteria[18] can be arranged along three simpler dimensions of diagnosis which may have some practical value to the clinician: (1) etiological, (2) behavioral, and (3) predictive. The kind of information which is conveyed by each type of diagnostic label is somewhat different and specifically adapted to the purpose for which the diagnosis is used. The triple-label approach attempts to counter the criticism aimed at use of any single classificatory system. Confusion in a single system is due in part to the fact that a diagnostic formulation intended to describe current behavior, for example, may be found useless in an attempt to predict that response to specific treatment, or to postdict the patient's personal history and development, or to permit collection of frequency data on hospital populations.

Classification by Etiology—The Kraepelinian system and portions of the 1952 APA classification emphasize etiological factors. They share the assumption that common etiological factors lead to similar symptoms and respond to similar treatment. This dimension of diagnosis is considerably more fruitful when dealing with behavior disorders which are mainly under control of some biological condition. When a patient is known to suffer from excessive intake of alcohol his hallucinatory behavior, lack of motor coordination, poor judgment, and other behavioral evidence disorganization can often be related directly to some antecedent condition such as the toxic effect of alcohol on the central nervous system, liver, etc. For these cases, classification by etiology also has some implications for prognosis and treatment. Acute hallucinations and other disorganized behavior due to alcohol usually clear up when the alcohol level in the blood stream falls. Similar examples can be drawn from any class of behavior disorders in which a change in behavior is associated primarily or exclusively with a single, *particular* antecedent factor. Under these conditions this factor can be called a pathogen and the situation closely approximates the condition described by the traditional medical model.

Utilization of this dimension as a basis for psychiatric diagnosis, however, has many problems apart from the rarity with which a specified condition can be shown to have a direct "causal" relationship to a pathogen. Among the current areas of ignorance in the fields of psychology and psychiatry, the etiology of most common disturbances probably takes first place. No specific family environment, no dramatic traumatic experience, or known constitutional abnormality has yet been found which results in the same pattern of disordered behavior. While current research efforts have aimed at investigating family patterns of schizophrenic patients, and several studies suggest a relationship between the mother's behavior and a schizophrenic process in the child,[10] it is not at all clear why the presence of these same factors in other families fails to yield a similar incidence of schizophrenia. Further, patients may exhibit behavior diagnosed as schizophrenic when there is no evidence of the postulated mother-child relationship.

In a recent paper Meehl[16] postulates schizophrenia as a neurological disease, with learned content and a dispositional basis. With this array of interactive etiological factors, it is clear that the etiological dimension for classification would at best result in an extremely cumbersome system, at worst in a useless one.

Classification by Symptoms—A clinical diagnosis often is a summarizing statement about the way in which a person behaves. On the assumption that a variety of behaviors are correlated and consistent in any given individual, it becomes more economical to assign the individual to a class of persons than to list and categorize all of his behaviors. The utility of such a system rests heavily on the availability of empirical evidence concerning correlations among various behaviors (response-response relationships), and the further assumption that the frequency of occurrence of such behaviors is relatively independent of specific stimulus conditions and of specific reinforcement. There are two major limitations to such a system. The first is that diagnosis by symptoms, as we have indicated in an earlier section, is often misleading because it implies common etiological factors. Freedman[7] gives an excellent illustration of the differences both in probable antecedent factors and subsequent treatment response among three cases diagnosed as schizophrenics. Freedman's patients were diagnosed by at least two psychiatrists, and one would expect that the traditional approach should result in whatever treatment of schizophrenia is practiced in the locale where the patients are seen. The first patient eventually gave increasing evidence of an endocrinopathy, and when this was recognized and treated, the psychotic symptoms went into remission. The second case had a definite history of seizures and appropriate anticonvulsant medication was effective in relieving his symptoms. In the third case, treatment directed at an uncovering analysis of the patient's adaptive techniques resulted in considerable improvement in the patient's behavior and subsequent relief from psychotic episodes. Freedman[7] suggests that schizophrenia is not a disease entity in the sense that it has a unique etiology, pathogenesis, etc, but that it represents the evocation of a final common pathway in the same sense as do headache, epilepsy, sore throat, or indeed any other symptom complex. It is further suggested that the term "schizophrenia has outlived its usefulness and should be discarded" (p.5). Opler[19, 20] has further shown the importance of cultural factors in the divergence of symptoms observed in patients collectively labeled as schizophrenic.

Descriptive classification is not always this deceptive, however. Assessment of intellectual performance sometimes results in a diagnostic statement which has predictive value for the patient's behavior in school or on a job. To date, there seem to be very few general statements about individual characteristics, which have as much predictive utility as the IQ.

A second limitation is that the current approach to diagnosis by symptoms tends to center on a group of behaviors which is often irrelevant with regard to the patient's total life pattern. These behaviors may be of interest only because they are popularly associated with deviancy and disorder. For example, occasional mild delusions interfere little or not at all with the social or occupational effectiveness of many ambulatory patients. Nevertheless, admission of their occurrence is often sufficient for a diagnosis of psychosis. Refinement of such an approach beyond current usage appears possible, as shown for example by Lorr et al[15] but this does not remove the above limitations.

Utilization of a symptom-descriptive approach frequently focuses attention on by-products of larger behavior patterns, and results in attempted treatment of behaviors (symptoms) which may be simple consequences of other important aspects of the patient's life. Emphasis on the patient's subjective complaints, moods and feelings tends to encourage use of a syndrome-oriented classification. It also results frequently in efforts to change the feelings, anxieties, and moods (or at least the patient's report about them), rather than to investigate the life conditions, interpersonal reactions, and environmental factors which produce and maintain these habitual response patterns.

Classification by Prognosis—To date, the least effort has been devoted to construction of a classification system which assigns patients to the same category on the basis of their similar response to specific treatments. The proper question raised for such a classification system consists of the manner in which a patient will react to treatments, regardless of his current behavior or his past history. The numerous studies attempting to establish prognostic signs from projective personality tests or somatic tests represent efforts to categorize the patients on this dimension.

Windle[26] has called attention to the low degree of predictability afforded by personality (projective) test scores, and has pointed out the difficulties encountered in evaluating research in this area due to the inadequate description of the population sampled and of the improvement criteria. In a later review Fulkerson and Barry[8] came to the similar conclusion that psychological test performance is a poor predictor of outcome in mental illness. They suggest that demographic variables such as severity, duration, acuteness of onset, degree of precipitating stress, etc, appear to have stronger relationships to outcome than test data. The lack of reliable relationships between diagnostic categories, test data, demographic variables, or other measures taken on the patient on the one hand, and duration of illness, response to specific treatment, or degree of recovery, on the other hand, precludes the construction of a simple empiric framework for a diagnostic-prognostic classification system based only on an array of symptoms.

None of the currently used dimensions for diagnosis is directly related to methods of modification of a patient's behavior, attitudes, response patterns, and interpersonal actions. Since the etiological model clearly stresses causative factors, it is much more compatible with a personality theory which strongly emphasizes genetic-developmental factors. The classification by symptoms facilitates social-administrative decisions about patients by providing some basis for judging the degree of deviation from social and ethical norms. Such a classification is compatible with a personality theory founded on the normal curve hypothesis and concerned with characterization by comparison with a fictitious average. The prognostic-predictive approach appears to have the most direct practical applicability. If continued research were to support certain early findings, it would be indeed comforting to be able to predict outcome of mental illness from a patient's premorbid social competence score,[28] or from the patient's score on an ego-strength scale,[4] or from many of the other signs and single variables which have been shown to have some predictive powers. It is unfortunate that these powers are frequently dissipated in cross validation. As Fulkerson and Barry have indicated,[8] single predictors have not yet shown much success.

II. A Functional (Behavioral-Analytic) Approach

The growing literature on behavior modification procedures derived from learning theory[3,6,11,13,27] suggests that an effective diagnostic procedure would be one in which the eventual therapeutic methods can be directly related to the information obtained from a continuing assessment of the patient's current behaviors and their controlling stimuli. Ferster[6] has said ". . . a functional analysis of behavior has the advantage that it specifies the causes of behavior in the form of explicit environmental events which can be objectively identified and which are potentially manipulable" (p.3). Such a diagnostic undertaking makes the assumption that a description of the problematic behavior, its controlling factors, and the means by which it can be changed are the most appropriate "explanations." It further makes the assumption that a diagnostic evaluation is never complete. It implies that additional information about the circumstances of the patient's life pattern, relationships among his behaviors, and controlling stimuli in his social milieu and his private experience is obtained continuously until it proves sufficient to effect a noticeable change in the patient's behavior, thus resolving "the problem." In a functional approach it is necessary to continue evaluation of the patient's life pattern and its controlling factors, concurrent with attempted manipulation of these variables by reinforcement, direct intervention, or other means until the resultant change in the patient's behavior permits restoration of more efficient life experiences.

The present approach shares with some psychological theories the assumption that psychotherapy is *not* an effort aimed at removal of intrapsychic conflicts, nor at a change in the personality structure by therapeutic interactions of intense nonverbal nature, (eg, transference, self-actualization, etc). We adopt the assumption instead that the job of psychological treatment involves the utilization of a variety of methods to devise a program which controls the patient's environment, his behavior, and the consequences of his behavior in such a way that the presenting problem is resolved. We hypothesize that the essential ingredients of a psychotherapeutic endeavor usually involve two separate stages: (1) a change in the perceptual discriminations of a patient, ie, in his approach to perceiving, classifying, and organizing sensory events, including perception of himself, and (2) changes in the response patterns which he has established in relation to social objects and to himself over the years.[11] In addition, the clinician's task may involve direct intervention in the patient's environmental circumstances, modification of the behavior of other people significant in his life, and control of reinforcing stimuli which are available either through self-administration, or by contingency upon the behavior of others. These latter procedures complement the verbal interactions of traditional psychotherapy. They require that the clinician, at the invitation of the patient or his family, participate more fully in planning the total life pattern of the patient outside the clinician's office.

It is necessary to indicate what the theoretical view here presented does *not* espouse in order to understand the differences from other procedures. It does *not* rest upon the assumption that (*a*) insight is a sine qua non of psychotherapy, (*b*) changes in thoughts or ideas inevitably lead to ultimate changes in actions, (*c*) verbal therapeutic sessions serve as replications of and equivalents for actual life situations, and (*d*) a symptom can be removed only by uprooting its cause or origin. In the absence of these assumptions it becomes unnecessary to conceptualize behavior disorder in etiological terms, in psychodynamic terms, or in terms of a specifiable disease process. While psychotherapy by verbal means may be sufficient in some instances, the combinations of behavior modification in life situations as well as in verbal interactions serves to extend the armamentarium of the therapist. Therefore verbal psychotherapy is seen as an *adjunct* in the implementation of therapeutic behavior changes in the patient's total life pattern, not as an end in itself, nor as the sole vehicle for increasing psychological effectiveness.

In embracing this view of behavior modification, there is a further commitment to a constant interplay between assessment and therapeutic strategies. An initial diagnostic formulation seeks to ascertain the major variables which can be directly controlled or modified during treatment. During successive treatment stages additional information is collected about the patient's BEHAVIOR REPERTOIRE, his reinforcement history, the pertinent controlling stimuli in his social and physical environment, and the sociological limitations within which both patient and therapist have to operate. Therefore, the initial formulation will constantly be enlarged or changed, resulting either in confirmation of the previous therapeutic strategy or in its change.

A Guide to a Functional Analysis of Individual Behavior—In order to help the clinician in the collection and organization of information for a behavioral analysis, we have constructed an outline which aims to provide a working model of the patient's behavior at a relatively low level of abstraction. A series of questions are so organized as to yield immediate implications for treatment. This outline has been found useful both in clinical practice and in teaching. Following is a brief summary of the categories in the outline.

    1. Analysis of a Problem Situation: *The patient's major complaints are categorized into classes of BEHAVIORAL EXCESSES AND DEFICITS. For each excess or deficit the dimensions of frequency, intensity, duration,

---

*For each patient a detailed analysis is required. For example, a list of behavioral excesses may include specific aggressive acts, hallucinatory behaviors, crying, submission to others in social situations, etc. It is recognized that some behaviors can be viewed as excesses or deficits depending on the vantage point from which the imbalance is observed. For instance, excessive withdrawal and deficient social responsiveness, or ex-

appropriateness of form, and stimulus conditions are described. In content, the response classes represent the major targets of the therapeutic intervention. As an additional indispensable feature, the behavioral assets of the patient are listed for utilization in a therapy program.

2. Clarification of the Problem Situation: Here we consider the people and circumstances which tend to maintain the problem behaviors, and the consequences of these behaviors to the patient and to others in his environment. Attention is given also to the consequences of changes in these behaviors which may result from psychiatric intervention.

3. Motivational Analysis: Since reinforcing stimuli are idiosyncratic and depend for their effect on a number of unique parameters for each person, a hierarchy of particular persons, events, and objects which serve as reinforcers is established for each patient. Included in this hierarchy are those reinforcing events which facilitate approach behaviors as well as those which, because of their aversiveness, prompt avoidance responses. This information has as its purpose to lay plans for utilization of various reinforcers in prescription of a specific behavior therapy program for the patient, and to permit utilization of appropriate reinforcing behaviors by the therapist and significant others in the patient's social environment.

4. Development Analysis: Questions are asked about the patient's biological equipment, his sociocultural experiences, and his characteristic behavioral development. They are phrased in such a way as (*a*) to evoke descriptions of his habitual behavior at various chronological stages of his life, (*b*) to relate specific new stimulus conditions to noticeable changes from his habitual behavior, and (*c*) to relate such altered behavior and other residuals of biological and sociocultural events to the present problem.

5. Analysis of Self-Control: This section examines both the methods and the degree of self-control exercised by the patient in his daily life. Persons, events, or institutions which have successfully reinforced self-controlling behaviors are considered. The deficits or excesses of self-control are evaluated in relation to their importance as therapeutic targets and to their utilization in a therapeutic program.

6. Analysis of Social Relationships: Examination of the patient's social network is carried out to evaluate the significance of people in the patient's environment who have some influence over the problematic behaviors, or who in turn are influenced by the patient for his

---

cessive social autonomy (nonconformity) and deficient self-inhibitory behavior may be complementary. The particular view taken is of consequence because of its impact on a treatment plan. Regarding certain behavior as excessively aggressive, to be reduced by constraints, clearly differs from regarding the same behavior as a deficit in self-control, subject to increase by training and treatment.

own satisfactions. These interpersonal relationships are reviewed in order to plan the potential participation of significant others in a treatment program, based on the principles of behavior modification. The review also helps the therapist to consider the range of actual social relationships in which the patient needs to function.

7. Analysis of the Social-Cultural-Physical Environment: In this section we add to the preceding analysis of the patient's behavior as an individual, consideration of the norms in his natural environment. Agreements and discrepancies between the patient's idiosyncratic life patterns and the norms in his environment are defined so that the importance of these factors can be decided in formulating treatment goals which allow as explicitly for the patient's needs as for the pressures of his social environment.

The preceding outline has as its purpose to achieve definition of a patient's problem in a manner which suggests specific treatment operations, or that none are feasible, and specific behaviors as targets for modification. Therefore, the formulation is *action oriented*. It can be used as a guide for the initial collection of information, as a device for organizing available data, or as a design for treatment.

The formulation of a treatment plan follows from this type of analysis because knowledge of the reinforcing conditions suggests the motivational controls at the disposal of the clinician for the modification of the patient's behavior. The analysis of specific problem behaviors also provides a series of goals for psychotherapy or other treatment, and for the evaluation of treatment progress. Knowledge of the patient's biological, social, and cultural conditions should help to determine what resources can be used, and what limitations must be considered in a treatment plan.

The various categories attempt to call attention to important variables affecting the patient's *current* behavior. Therefore, they aim to elicit descriptions of low-level abstraction. Answers to these specific questions are best phrased by describing classes of events reported by the patient, observed by others, or by critical incidents described by an informant. The analysis does not exclude description of the patient's habitual verbal-symbolic behaviors. However, in using verbal behaviors as the basis for this analysis, one should be cautious not to "explain" verbal processes in terms of postulated internal mechanisms without adequate supportive evidence, nor should inference be made about nonobserved processes or events without corroborative evidence. The analysis includes many items which are not known or not applicable for a given patient. Lack of information on some items does not necessarily indicate incompleteness of the analysis. These lacks must be noted nevertheless because they often contribute to the better understanding of what the patient needs to learn to become an autonomous person. Just as important is an inventory of his existing socially effective behavioral repertoire which can be put in the service of any treatment procedure.

This analysis is consistent with our earlier formulations of the principles of comprehensive medicine[9,22] which emphasized the joint operation of biological, social, and psychological factors in psychiatric disorders. The language and orientation of the proposed approach are rooted in contemporary learning theory. The conceptual framework is consonant with the view that the course of psychiatric disorders can be modified by systematic application of scientific principles from the fields of psychology and medicine to the patient's habitual mode of living.

This approach is not a substitute for assignment of the patient to traditional diagnostic categories. Such labeling may be desirable for statistical, administrative, or research purposes. But the current analysis is intended to replace other diagnostic formulations purporting to serve as a basis for making decisions about specific therapeutic interventions.

III. Methods of Data Collection for a Functional Analysis

Traditional diagnostic approaches have utilized as the main sources of information the patient's verbal report, his nonverbal behavior during an interview, and his performance on psychological tests. These observations are sufficient if one regards behavior problems only as a property of the patient's particular pattern of associations or his personality structure. A mental disorder would be expected to reveal itself by stylistic characteristics in the patient's behavior repertoire. However, if one views behavior disorders as sets of response patterns which are learned under particular conditions and maintained by definable environmental and internal stimuli, an assessment of the patient's behavior output is insufficient unless it also describes the conditions under which it occurs. This view requires an expansion of the clinician's sources of observations to include the stimulation fields in which the patient lives, and the variations of patient behavior as a function of exposure to these various stimulational variables. Therefore, the resourceful clinician need not limit himself to test findings, interview observations in the clinician's office, or referral histories alone in the formulation of the specific case. Nor need he regard himself as hopelessly handicapped when the patient has little observational or communicative skill in verbally reconstructing his life experience for the clinician. Regardless of the patient's communicative skills the data must consist of a description of the patient's behavior *in relationship* to varying environmental conditions.

A behavioral analysis excludes no data relating to a patient's past or present experiences as irrelevant. However, the relative merit of any information (as, e.g., growing up in a broken home or having had homosexual experiences) lies in its relation to the independent variables which can be identified as controlling the current problematic behavior. The observation that a patient has hallucinated on occasions may be important only if it has bearing on his present problem. If looked upon in isolation, a report about hallucinations may be misleading, resulting in emphasis on classification rather than treatment.

In the *psychiatric interview* a behavioral-analytic approach opposes acceptance of the content of the verbal self-report as equivalent to actual events or experiences. However, verbal reports provide information concerning the patient's verbal construction of his environment and of his person, his recall of past experiences, and his fantasies about them. While these self-descriptions do not represent data about events which actually occur internally, they do represent current behaviors of the patient and indicate the verbal chains and repertoires which the patient has built up. Therefore, the verbal behavior may be useful for description of a patient's thinking processes. To make the most of such an approach, variations on traditional interview procedures may be obtained by such techniques as role playing, discussion, and interpretation of current life events, or controlled free association. Since there is little experimental evidence of specific relationships between the patient's verbal statements and his nonverbal behavioral acts, the verbal report alone remains insufficient for a complete analysis and for prediction of his daily behavior. Further, it is well known that a person responds to environmental conditions and to internal cues which he cannot describe adequately. Therefore, any verbal report may miss or mask the most important aspects of a behavioral analysis, ie, the description of the relationship between antecedent conditions and subsequent behavior.

In addition to the use of the clinician's own person as a controlled stimulus object in interview situations, *observations of interaction with significant others* can be used for the analysis of variations in frequency of various behaviors as a function of the person with whom the patient interacts. For example, use of prescribed standard roles for nurses and attendants, utilization of members of the patient's family or his friends, may be made to obtain data relevant to the patient's habitual interpersonal response pattern. Such observations are especially useful if in a later interview the patient is asked to describe and discuss the observed sessions. Confrontations with tape recordings for comparisons between the patient's report and the actual session as witnessed by the observer may provide information about the patient's perception of himself and others as well as his habitual behavior toward peers, authority figures, and other significant people in his life.

Except in working with children or family units, insufficient use has been made of material obtained from *other informants* in interviews about the patient. These reports can aid the observer to recognize behavioral domains in which the patient's report deviates from or agrees with the descriptions provided by others. Such information is also useful for contrasting the patient's reports about his presumptive effects on another person with the stated effects by that person. If a patient's interpersonal problems extend to areas in which social contacts are not clearly defined, contributions by informants other than the patient are essential.

It must be noted that verbal reports by other informants may be no more congruent with actual events than the patient's own reports and need to be equally related to the informant's own credibility. If such crucial figures as parents, spouses, employers can be so interviewed, they also provide the clinician with some information about those people with whom the patient must interact repeatedly and with whom interpersonal problems may have developed.

Some observation of the patient's daily *work behavior* represents an excellent source of information, if it can be made available. Observation of the patient by the clinician or his staff may be preferable to descriptions by peers or supervisors. Work observations are especially important for patients whose complaints include difficulties in their daily work activity or who describe work situations as contributing factors to their problem. While freer use of this technique may be hampered by cultural attitudes toward psychiatric treatment in the marginally adjusted, such observations may be freely accessible in hospital situations or in sheltered work situations. With use of behavior rating scales or other simple measurement devices, brief samples of patient behaviors in work situations can be obtained by minimally trained observers.

The patient himself may be asked to provide samples of his own behavior by using tape recorders for the recording of segments of interactions in his family, at work, or in other situations during his everyday life. A television monitoring system for the patient's behavior is an excellent technique from a theoretical viewpoint but it is extremely cumbersome and expensive. Use of recordings for diagnostic and therapeutic purposes has been reported by some investigators.[2,5,24] Playback of the recordings and a recording of the patient's reactions to the playback can be used further in interviews to clarify the patient's behavior toward others and his reaction to himself as a social stimulus.

Psychological tests represent problems to be solved under specified interactional conditions. Between the highly standardized intelligence tests and the unstructured and ambiguous projective tests lies a dimension of structure along which more and more responsibility for providing appropriate responses falls on the patient. By comparison with interview procedures, most psychological tests provide a relatively greater standardization of stimulus conditions. But, in addition to the specific answers given on intelligence tests or on projective tests these tests also provide a behavioral sample of the patient's reaction to a problem situation in a relatively stressful interpersonal setting. Therefore, psychological tests can provide not only quantitative scores but they can also be treated as a miniature life experience, yielding information about the patient's interpersonal behavior and variations in his behavior as a function of the nature of the stimulus conditions.

In this section we have mentioned only some of the numerous life situations which can be evaluated in order to provide information about the patient. Criteria for their use lies in economy, accessibility to the clinician, and relevance to the patient's problem. While it is more convenient to gather data from a patient in an office, it may be necessary for the clinician to have first-hand information about the actual conditions under which the patient lives and works. Such familiarity may be obtained either by utilization of informants or by the clinician's entry into the home, the job situation, or the social environment in which the patient lives. Under all these conditions the clinician is effective only if it is possible for him to maintain a nonparticipating, objective, and observational role with no untoward consequences for the patient or the treatment relationship.

The methods of data collecting for a functional analysis described here differ from traditional psychiatric approaches only in that they require inclusion of the physical and social stimulus field in which the patient actually operates. Only a full appraisal of the patient's living and working conditions and his way of life allow a description of the actual problems which the patient faces and the specification of steps to be taken for altering the problematic situation.

Summary

Current psychiatric classification falls short of providing a satisfactory basis for the understanding and treatment of maladaptive behavior. Diagnostic schemas now in use are based on etiology, symptom description, or prognosis. While each of these approaches has a limited utility, no unified schema is available which permits prediction of response to treatment or future course of the disorder from the assignment of the patient to a specific category.

This paper suggests a behavior-analytic approach which is based on contemporary learning theory, as an alternative to assignment of the patient to a conventional diagnostic category. It includes the summary of an outline which can serve as a guide for the collection of information and formulation of the problem, including the biological, social, and behavioral conditions which are determining the patient's behavior. The outline aims toward integration of information about a patient for formulation of an action plan which would modify the patient's problematic behavior. Emphasis is given to the particular variables affecting the *individual* patient rather than determination of the similarity of the patient's history or his symptoms to known pathological groups.

The last section of the paper deals with methods useful for collection of information necessary to complete such a behavior analysis.

This paper was written in conjunction with Research grant MH 06921-03 from the National Institutes of Mental Health, United States Public Health Service.

References

1. Ash, P.: Reliability of Psychiatric Diagnosis, *J Abnorm Soc Psychol* 44:272-277, 1949.
2. Bach, G.: In Alexander, S.: Fight Promoter for Battle of Sexes, *Life* 54:102-108 (May 17) 1963.
3. Bandura, A.: Psychotherapy as Learning Process, *Psychol Bull* 58:143-159, 1961.
4. Barron, F.: Ego-Strength Scale Which Predicts Response to Psychotherapy, *J Consult Psychol* 17:235-241, 1953.
5. Cameron, D. E., *et al*: Automation of psychotherapy, *Compr Psychiat* 5:1-14, 1964.
6. Ferster, C. B.: Classification of Behavorial Pathology in Ullman, L. P. and Krasner, L. (eds.): Behavior Modification Research, New York: Holt, Rinehart & Winston, 1965.
7. Freedman, D. A.: Various Etiologies of Schizophrenic Syndrome, *Dis Nerv Syst* 19:1-6, 1958.
8. Fulkerson, S. E., and Barry, J. R.: Methodology and Research on Prognostic Use of Psychological Tests, *Psychol Bull* 58:177-204, 1961.
9. Guze, S. B.; Matarazzo, J. D.; and Saslow, G.: Formulation of Principles of Comprehensive Medicine With Special Reference to Learning Theory, *J Clin Psychol* 9:127-136, 1953.
10. Jackson, D. D. A.: Etiology of Schizophrenia, New York: Basic Books Inc., 1960.
11. Kanfer, F. H.: Comments on Learning in Psychotherapy, *Psychol Rep* 9:681-699, 1961.
12. Katz, M. M.; Cole, J. O.; and Lowery, H. A.: Nonspecificity of Diagnosis of Paranoid Schizophrenia, *Arch Gen Psychiat* 11:197-202, 1964.
13. Krasner, L.: "Therapist as Social Reinforcement Machine," in Strupp, H., and Luborsky, L. (eds.): Research in Psychotherapy, Washington, DC: American Psychological Association, 1962.
14. Ledley, R. S., and Lusted, L. B.: Reasoning Foundations of Medical Diagnosis, *Science* 130:9-21, 1959.
15. Lorr, M.; Klett, C. J.; and McNair, D. M.: Syndromes of Psychosis, New York: Macmillan Co., 1963.

16. Meehl, P. E.: Schizotaxia, Schizotypy, Schizophrenia, *Amer Psychol* *17*:827-838, 1962.
17. New York Heart Association: Nomenclature and Criteria for Diagnosis of Diseases of the Heart and Blood Vessels, New York: New York Heart Association, 1953.
18. Noyes A. P., and Kolb, L. C.: Modern Clinical Psychiatry, Philadelphia: W. B. Saunders & Co., 1963.
19. Opler, M. K.: Schizophrenia and Culture, *Sci Amer* *197*:103-112, 1957.
20. Opler, M. K.: Need for New Diagnostic Categories in Psychiatry, *J Nat Med Assoc* *55*:133-137, 1963.
21. Rotter, J. B.: Social Learning and Clinical Psychology, New York: Prentice-Hall, 1954.
22. Saslow, G.: On Concept of Comprehensive Medicine, *Bull Menninger Clin* *16*:57-65, 1952.
23. Scheflen, A. E.: Analysis of Thought Model Which Persists in Psychiatry, *Psychosom Med* *20*:235-241, 1958.
24. Slack, C. W.: Experimenter-Subject Psychotherapy—A New Method of Introducing Intensive Office Treatment for Unreachable Cases, *Ment Hyg* *44*:238-256, 1960.
25. Szasz, T. S.: Myth of Mental Illness, *Amer Psychol* *15*:113-118, 1960.
26. Windle, C.: Psychological Tests in Psychopathological Prognosis, *Psychol Bull* *49*:451-482, 1952.
27. Wolpe, J.: Psychotherapy in Reciprocal Inhibition, Stanford, Calif.: Stanford University Press, 1958.
28. Zigler, E., and Phillips, L.: Psychiatric Diagnosis: Critique, *J Abnorm Soc Psychol* *63*:607-618, 1961.

Chapter 3

THE ECOLOGICAL INTERVIEW: A FIRST STEP IN OUT-PATIENT CHILD BEHAVIOR THERAPY*

ROBERT G. WAHLER *and* WILLIAM H. CORMIER

D EVIANT CHILDREN display their problem behavior in a variety of environmental settings. A child referred for treatment because of unusual behavior may produce this kind of behavior in his home, his school classroom, his playground, and perhaps on the streets of his city. In addition, deviant child behavior may occur in several sub-settings within a particular setting. For example, the negativistic child may be negativistic at bedtime and at mealtime, but he may be quite cooperative at other times (of his day) at home. Also, the same child at school may be considered difficult to manage during the arithmetic lesson but no problem during the social studies lesson.

The above information is important to the clinician whose actions are guided by reinforcement theory (Bijou and Baer, 1961). According to this viewpoint, child behavior is to an important extent a function of its immediate environmental contingencies. Thus a child's problem behavior in his school classroom might be a reinforcement function of teacher and peer social attention; his problem behavior at home might be a similar function of parent and sibling

*From the *Journal of Behavior Therapy and Experimental Psychiatry*, 1970, 1, 279-289. Reprinted by permission of the author and Pergamon Press, Ltd.

social attention. The essence of the theory is that behavior is situation specific; it is controlled by stimuli dispensed by agents of the environmental setting in which the child behaves. This being the argument, one could contend that the child's actions in one particular setting are independent of his actions in another setting (Wahler, 1969a). If this assumption is valid, the adequately prepared clinician must be a skilled ecologist, as well as psychologist. In other words, the clinician's skill as an intervention agent might well be dependent on his skill in mapping the child in his social environment.

If social contingencies are to be therapeutically rearranged for the deviant child, one must know who provides these contingencies, in what behavioral form they are provided, for what child behaviors they are provided, and in what specific settings or sub-settings they are provided. Given this information, the clinician is in position to intervene—to train the significant "contingency dispensers" (e.g. parents and teachers) to modify their interactions with the child. The specific nature of the modifications is based not only on the above ecological information, but also on certain principles of reinforcement theory (see Bandura, 1969).

The Interview

Workers in child behavior therapy have typically emphasized direct observation as an indispensable part of the ecological assessment (see Bijou, Peterson and Ault, 1968). Observers, ranging from indigenous community members (Wahler and Erickson, 1969) to the child himself (Lovitt and Curtiss, 1969), have been utilized to obtain such data. However, before any observational system can be implemented, the observers must be told what to observe and where to observe it. In clinical situations, this kind of information is obtained by talking to members of the deviant child's social community (e.g. parents and teachers) and perhaps to the child himself. While an interview was undoubtedly involved in every reported child behavior therapy study over the past 10 years, it has never been reported in systematic fashion.* In view of the procedural rigor that usually defines behavior therapy, this state of affairs is truly amazing.

The ecological interview serves two important and often interde-

*Such is not the case for behavior therapy based on principles of respondent learning (e.g., Wolpe, Salter and Reyna, 1964) where investigators have been quite concerned with a systematic approach to the interview.

pendent functions: (1) to develop a language system that will allow the client to communicate with the interviewer, and (2) mapping the child's behavior. The first function is illustrated by Goldiamond (1969). According to Goldiamond, the client's conception of human behavior may be radically different from that of the interviewer making it difficult if not impossible for useful information to be produced. Thus, either the interviewer must be capable of translating the client's language or the client must learn the interviewer's language. While clinicians operating from other theoretical bases vary in their choice of tactics at this point, behavior therapists invariably select the latter. Since the client (e.g. parents and teachers) is required to serve as therapist and perhaps observer, it follows that he must be somewhat conversant with reinforcement theory and the analysis of behavior from this point of view. The task of teaching this new language to the client is often facilitated through pre-interview "homework" provided by some recently available texts (e.g. Patterson and Guillon, 1968).

The second function of the ecological interview involves mapping the child's behavior as it is reported to occur in various environmental settings. The mapping, of course, is intended to specify what is to be observed and where it is to be observed. The authors have found the pre-interview checklists (Tables I, II, and III) to be useful sources of information in reaching these goals.

The following portions of this paper are designed to describe the ecological interview in detail, particularly its mapping function. One should keep in mind that the mapping can and should also be an educational experience for the client; he should learn something about the clinician's language system and his method of behavioral analysis.

The Client

The client in child behavior therapy is that person who, in the clinician's judgment, is capable of changing natural social contingencies for the child's behavior. Tharp and Wetzel (1969) use the term "mediator" to describe this function. Most often the child's parents and his teachers fit this definition, although recent work has suggested that members of the child's peer group (Wahler, 1970) and the child himself (Lovitt and Curtiss, 1969), may also meet the criterion.

A second criterion for client selection derives from the presenting complaint. If the child is reported to produce problems only at home, then the parents are the clients of choice; but, if his problems extend to the school classroom, his teachers must be included as well. Since evidence for generalization across natural environmental settings is sparse, one should presently assume that the child's behavior is situation specific.

The Child's Behavior

A child's behavior, deviant or otherwise, is meaningless unless its environmental setting is considered as the context for therapeutic intervention. Clients frequently have difficulty in describing the child's observable behavior and in specifying the particular subsetting in which the behavior was produced. For example, parents and teachers are inclined to be mentalistic in their descriptions of child behavior. Like most people, their units of description are abstractions of what the child did: hitting little brother is reported as "jealousy"; out of seat behavior in the classroom is reported as "inattention." Further, the typical clinical interviewer is apt to foster this style of reporting by accepting the abstraction or by translating it into another abstraction. Examine this sample taken from a clinical psychologist's interview report: "This child experiences frequent periods of depression, often to the point that he entertains thoughts of self-destruction. He is constantly angry because of his mother's attempts to keep him dependent on her. Yet, because of his anxiety concerning the expression of affect, he cannot direct his hostility outward. Consequently, he internalizes his aggression; he berates his abilities in many areas; he sees himself as inadequate and his self-esteem is extremely low."

An "abstraction count" of this sample yields a total of nine broadly judgmental terms that may be of value to many clinicians—but not to the behavior therapist. No doubt each term refers to a number of specific verbal and nonverbal child behaviors, spread over several environmental settings. Unless these behaviors are specified in terms of concrete actions, operations by the behavior therapist are impossible.

One must always keep in mind that the client will be expected to serve as the child's therapist. These non-professionals vary tremendously in translating psychological jargon into observable behaviors. Thus, to insure that all concerned are observing and treating the same child behaviors, these behaviors must be enumerated through labels that allow little variance in translation. If abstractions such as aggression and dependency are used, they must clearly appear as summary terms, designating lists of observable verbal and non-verbal child behaviors. Thus, the interviewer's account of the child's behavior must provide a wide sampling of what the child is reported to do and say—not inferences concerning these events.

Naturally, the interviewer will tend to focus his behavioral enumeration on the child's problem behaviors—as defined by the client or the interviewer, or both. However, there is also good reason to notice other parts of the child's behavioral repertoire. Any child, regardless of his degree of behavioral deviance, displays some behaviors that would be considered "normal," "positive" or otherwise desirable. Some of these behaviors may be incompatible with the child's problem behaviors and their more frequent occurrence could change client and clinician judgment about the child's degree of behavioral deviance. These behaviors warrant further attention by the interviewer.

For most deviant behaviors a child produces, one could easily imagine another more desirable behavior that would physically compete with it—compete in the sense that the two could not occur simultaneously. For example, an oppositional child cannot be oppositional and cooperative at the same time; a withdrawn child cannot avoid and approach others simultaneously. Since these kinds of competing behaviors are immediately defined when their deviant counterparts are defined, they need not be a subject of further inquiry. However, there are situations in which desirable competing behaviors are not so obviously present, and thus interviewer inquiry will be necessary. That is, some desirable behaviors may be functionally, but not physically, incompatible with the child's deviant behavior. Consider the "school phobic child" in a classroom setting. We have often received information from teachers similar to this teacher's report: "I can tell when he's going to start crying. If he starts to stare out the window I know he's thinking of home and then he's going to get frightened." This statement implies the presence of behaviors that may be functionally incompatible with crying. The logical question to this teacher would be directed at detecting those

CHILD HOME BEHAVIOR CHECKLIST

The following checklist allows you to describe your child's problems in various home situations. The situations are listed in the column at left and common problem behaviors are listed in the row at the top. Examine *each* situation in the column and decide if one or more of the problem behaviors in the row fits your child. Check those that fit the best—if any.

	Always has to be told	Doesn't pay attention	Forgets	Dawdles	Refuses	Argues	Complains	Demands	Fights	Selfish	Destroys toys or property	Steals	Lies	Cries	Whines	Hangs on or stays close to adult	Acts silly	Mopes around	Stays alone	Has to keep things in order	Sexual play
Morning:																					
Awakening																					
Dressing																					
Breakfast																					
Bathroom																					
Leave for School																					
Play in house																					
Chores																					
Television																					
Afternoon:																					
Lunch																					
Bathroom																					
Play in house																					
Chores and homework																					
Television																					
When company comes																					
Evening:																					
Father comes home																					
Dinner																					
Bathroom																					
Play in house																					
Chores and homework																					
Television																					
Undressing																					
When company comes																					
Bedtime																					

TABLE II
CHILD COMMUNITY BEHAVIOR CHECKLIST

The following checklist allows you to describe your child's problems in various situations outside the house. The situations are listed in the column at left and common problem behaviors are listed in the row at the top. Examine *each situation* in the column and decide if one or more of the problem behaviors in the row fits your child. Check those that fit the best—if any.

	Always has to be told	Doesn't pay attention	Forgets	Dawdles	Refuses	Argues	Complains	Demands	Fights	Selfish	Destroys toys or property	Lies	Cries	Whines	Hangs on or stays close to adult	Acts silly	Mopes around	Stays alone	Has to keep things in order	Sexual play
In own yard																				
In neighbor's yard or home																				
In stores																				
Public park																				
Downtown in general																				
Church or Sunday School																				
Community swimming pool																				
In family car																				

TABLE III
CHILD SCHOOL BEHAVIOR CHECKLIST

The following checklist allows you to describe your student's problems in various situations. The situations are listed in the column at left and common problem behaviors are listed in the row at the top. Examine *each* situation in the column and decide if one or more of the problem behaviors in the row fit your student. Check those that fit the best—if any.

	Out of seat	Talks to others	Always has to be told	Doesn't pay attention	Forgets	Dawdles	Refuses	Argues	Complains	Demands	Fights	Selfish	Destroys toys or property	Steals	Lies	Cries	Hangs on or stays close to adult	Stays alone	Whines	Acts silly	Mopes around	Has to keep thing in order	Sexual play
Morning:																							
Teacher explains lesson																							
Teacher discusses with group																							
Silent work time																							
Cooperative work with other students																							
Oral reading or class presentation																							
Line up for lunch or recess																							
Hall																							
Playground																							
Lunch																							
Afternoon:																							
Teacher explains lesson																							
Teacher discusses with group																							
Silent work time																							
Cooperative work with other students																							
Oral reading or class presentation																							
Line up for recess or dismissal																							
Hall																							
Playground																							

child behaviors that are rarely correlated with crying. Perhaps reading or cooperative work with other children would fit this definition. If so, these desirable behaviors should be listed as target behaviors for more systematic observation.

In summary, the interviewer's enumeration of child behaviors should include both deviant and desirable behaviors. Whatever behaviors the interviewer selects as later observational targets, they must be countable—countable by parents, teachers, and possibly the child himself.

Environmental Settings and Subsettings

It has been traditional to think of the deviant child's problem behavior as emanating from a single grossly defined environmental setting—namely, his "home life." It is commonly argued that parental interactions with the child "broadly defined" are responsible for developing and maintaining the child's deviance. Such an assumption is erroneous for two reasons. First, there is good evidence that other people (teachers and peers), while they may not be primary developmental factors in the child's deviance, do *maintain* or support the child's problem behavior in settings outside the home (Cormier, 1969; Thomas, Becker and Armstrong, 1968; Buehler, Patterson and Furniss, 1966). In fact, their support in school settings may be quite independent of parental support in home settings (Wahler, 1969a). Secondly, "home life" is to broad an environmental setting to be of much use in behavior therapy. True, inappropriate parental reactions to the child's behavior are usually a source of support for the child's deviance at home. But, few parents provide such reactions on a continual basis. It is common for parents to report that their deviant child is "fine" at certain times of the day and "terrible" at other times. The clinician needs to know those subsettings that set the occasion for deviant behavior, if for no other reason than practical use of observer time.

As stated earlier, detection of environmental settings is usefully accomplished at the same time as one constructs a list of the child's behaviors. To these goals, the enclosed pre-interview checklists for parents and teachers (Tables I, II and III) are very helpful. Essentially, the interviewer needs to specify environmental settings and subsettings for each of the child's deviant and desirable behaviors. To ignore the stimulus settings for these behaviors is to place unfounded trust in the phenomenon of generalization. Until evidence is accumulated to show that changes in child behavior transfer across settings, one should assume that each setting must be dealt with separately.

The multiple settings of deviant child behavior are of some advantage in the training of clients as observers and therapists. Although training of parents and teachers must be directed to specific subsettings, it might be unwise to instruct a mother to count child behaviors when she is in the process of fixing dinner, even though her child's deviant behaviors occur mainly at that time; it might also be a poor move to instruct a teacher to count deviant child behaviors during the arithmetic lesson. Client training ought to be geared to the success of the client's learning efforts. Therefore, why not start training in those settings that will insure such success?

Part of the interviewer's inquiry concerning environmental subsettings should be aimed at evaluating the client's opportunity to learn observational skills. In other words, to what degree does a client have free time to observe the child and his interactions with the client? Such an evaluation should permit the interviewer to select a subsetting in which to begin the training; that is, parental observations might begin during the child's bedtime and the teacher might develop her counting skills during the silent reading period. As the clients become skillful in these settings, they should be capable of similar operations in other subsettings where less client time is available for these purposes.

Social Consequences of the Child's Behavior

Ideal interview information would include a picture of how parents, teachers and peers support the child's deviant behavior and how they fail to develop his desirable, competing behaviors. Theoretically, one would expect the clients to be more attentive to the child's problem behavior than they are to his desirable behavior; or if not, the attention following desirable behavior should be aversive to the child. Limited research support for this assumption exists (Buehler, Patterson and Furniss, 1966; Patterson, Ray and Shaw, 1969).

However, the interviewer should not be optimistic in expecting this kind of information from a client. Partly, this may be due to the fact that the client is usually the primary attention dispenser in question, and self-observation is not an easy skill to acquire. In addition, other dispensers in the setting (e.g. peers and siblings) may complicate the support issue. Thus in all likelihood, direct observation may be required to understand how the child's deviant behavior obtains social reinforcement.

Despite these problems, useful information concerning social consequences can be obtained from the client. While this information might not jibe with later observational data, it can be of use in the later planning of therapeutic contingencies for the child.

Following the principles of reinforcement theory, the clinician has two options in programming therapeutic consequences for the child's deviant behavior. He may choose to instruct all social agents to ignore the behavior (extinction) or he may decide to utilize an aversive contingency (usually time-out from social attention; see Wahler, 1969b). A rule of thumb in picking tactics has to do with the social environment's ability to tolerate the child's deviant behavior. For ethical reasons, ignoring should probably always be the tactic of choice. However, this assumes that the child's deviant behavior does not produce harmful consequences to the environment, and it also assumed that the client is capable of ignoring the child. For example, suppose that a mother reports that her child's demanding behavior angers her to the point that she throws things at him. Although later observations by her or by others may reveal that she does other things as well, this information should be considered in selecting therapeutic tactics. To tell his mother to ignore her child's demanding behavior would probably be disastrous—she probably could not do it. Thus, either time-out or utilizing other social agents within the home setting would be required.

Examples like the above can easily be generated. The point is that the interviewer's assessment of a client's reactions (consequences) to the child's deviant behavior should allow him to make a judgment concerning the probable success or failure of various tactics in the later training of therapists for the child.

A Case Illustration

The following case study is presented to illustrate the previously discussed procedures of the ecological interview. This case is ideal in the sense that it clearly presents the ecological complexities of an apparently simple problem.

Willie V (age 10) was referred for psychological treatment because of his refusal to attend school. According to the school principal's referral statements, Willie often cried in class and his parents had to "drag" him to school to ensure his attendance. All concerned were mystified by the sudden onset of this problem, since Willie had been a model student up to this point (grade four). Willie's complaints to his teacher were extremely vague. He referred to excessive noise in the classroom, inability to think, and fears that unspecified other children would hurt him.

The clients for the interview were Willie, his teacher, and his parents. Prior to their interviews, the parents and the teacher completed appropriate pre-interview checklists (Tables I, II and III).

Willie's parents reported their concern about a variety of his behaviors, including his refusal to attend school in the morning. Table IV describes the interview outcome, based on the parents' responses to the pre-interview checklist. According to the parents, Willie's problem behavior reliably occurs in ten different home settings; the problem behaviors appear to be best described as non-compliance to parental instructions, demands that his mother obey him, various complaints, and "checking on mother." Notice that all of these behaviors are "countable" in the sense that Willie's parents could now be instructed to record their occurrence in any of the listed settings.

Parental social consequences for these behaviors, while they would be difficult to count, appear to provide a logical source of reinforcement for some of Willie's problem behaviors. Since one immediate goal of treatment would be to eliminate *all* parental attention following Willie's undesirable behaviors, the interviewer could simply instruct the parents to record instances of social attention provided as consequences for Willie's behaviors. (Many behavior therapists have been able to conduct effective behavior therapy programs at home and in the classroom through modifying one general, and quite countable, class of parent or teacher behavior. This class, referred to commonly as *social attention*, is a summary term for any verbal or physical action following those child behaviors one wishes to change.)

The interviewer's discussion with the parents also revealed that Willie's mother provided most social contingencies for his home behavior. Thus, she would be required to carry the major direct role of therapeutic action. Further discussion revealed that the "inside play"

TABLE IV
SUMMARY OF HOME SETTINGS FOR WILLIE'S BEHAVIOR
INCLUDING SOCIAL CONSEQUENCES*

Home Setting	Problem behavior	Social consequences	Desirable competing behavior
Awakening (school days only)	Complains about stomach or head pains	Mother gives medication and tells him he's OK	Defined by problem behavior
Dressing	Very slow	Mother prompts and sometimes helps	Defined by problem behavior
Breakfast (school days only)	Refuses to eat	Mother prompts	Defined by problem behavior
Leave for school	Refuses to go	Mother and father argue with him and sometimes spank him	Defined by problem behavior
Chores	Refuses to work or does jobs "halfway"	Mother argues or reasons with him	Defined by problem behavior
Outside play	Frequently returns to house to "ask if Mother is there"	None obvious	Defined by problem behavior
Inside play	Asks or demands Mother's help	Mother helps	Cooperative play with siblings
When Mother attends to siblings	Asks or demands Mother's help	Mother argues with him or helps	Cooperative play with siblings
When Mother plans shopping trip or visit to friends	Asks or demands to go with her	Mother complies	Defined by problem behavior
Bedtime	Complains of fears of dark and "crooks" breaking into house	Mother reasons with him and leaves room light on	Talk with siblings

*Data based on Mother's report.

and "outside play" settings would be good beginning points for the mother's observational training. According to her, she would either be too busy, too angry, or too nervous to begin the systematic observation of Willie in the other settings listed in Table IV.

At the conclusion of this interview, Willie's parents were clearly informed of the interviewer's suspicions concerning the maintenance of Willie's problem behaviors and the infrequent occurrence of his probable competing behaviors. Reinforcement theory had been discussed with them (following their reading of Patterson and Guillon, 1968) and the following observational duties had been given to Willie's mother—to be completed before the next meeting: record in longhand any requests or demands to mother during inside play and any returns to mother during outside play. Finally, record mother and father reactions to these behaviors.

During the interview, Willie's parents were told that his teacher was to be interviewed that day and a school program would soon be initiated similar to the home program. The parents were told to be certain he arrived at school the next day.

Willie was interviewed following the discussion with his parents. He was told of his parents' report concerning his behavior at school and at home, particularly his fears of school, bedtime, and what appeared to be his mother's safety. While he readily admitted his fears, he did not agree that he was demanding or oppositional at home. In addition, he pointed out that his peers seemed to dislike him and "picked on him" frequently. The latter problem and worries about his mother's health* were his explanations for his recent dislike of school.

Table V summarizes interview information from Willie. Willie pointed to five settings as the source of his difficulties. Worries concerning his mother and his peers plus his avoidance and complaints in peer presence appear to constitute his major problems. Except for Willie's observation that other children "picked on him" his version of social consequences for these problems was not helpful.

After obtaining the above information, Willie was given a brief explanation of reinforcement theory, with particular emphasis on the concepts of reinforcement and extinction. He was then told that a first step in changing any behavior involves learning how to record it. A further discussion of settings and Willie's behavior led to his agreeing to record his behavior and its social contingencies in four of the five settings (he explained that his recording would be too obvious to the other children during the free play period at school.) Complaining, avoidance of other children, and worries about mother, crooks and other children were to be checked in his school notebook or in a small notebook kept in his pocket or at his bedside. In addition, Willie was asked to record social attention from his peers, teacher, and parents whenever it occurred following this behavior.

Finally, Willie was told to begin his observational duties the next day and that his teacher and parents would be keeping records as well.

In an interview with Willie's teacher she immediately reported her

*Willie's mother had no serious health problems.

TABLE V
SUMMARY OF HOME AND SCHOOL SETTINGS FOR WILLIE'S
BEHAVIOR, INCLUDING SOCIAL CONSEQUENCES†

Home and school settings	Problem behavior	Social consequences	Desirable competing behavior
Outside play at home	Worries about Mother	None obvious to him	Talk with siblings or peers
Silent work time at school	Worries about Mother and likelihood that peers will "pick on him" later. Cries	None obvious to him	Writing or drawing
Lunch at school	Avoids peers. Complains to teacher about peer behavior	Peers "pick on him"	Talk to peers
On playground at school	Avoids peers. Complains to teacher about peer behavior	Peers "pick on him"	Talk or play with peers
Bedtime	Worries about crooks breaking into house	None obvious to him	Talk to siblings

†Data based on Willie's report.

impression that Willie was "very insecure" and that his problems undoubtedly were caused by his "overprotective" mother. After some persuasion, his teacher eventually directed her attention to Willie's school behavior, and particularly that noted by her on the pre-interview checklist. An explanation of reinforcement theory appeared to be somewhat helpful in redirecting the discussion.

Table VI summarizes the results of the discussion with Willie's teacher. She said that she could obtain observational records during the morning silent work period and during the lunch period. She agreed to check the occurrence of complaints and crying and their possible competing behaviors as well. Although she argued that school events had little to do with Willie's problems, she agreed to record her reactions and those of the peers whenever they occurred following this behavior. Because Willie's crying in the classroom was rather disruptive for all concerned, the interviewer agreed to begin the school behavior program after the teacher had obtained two days of "countable" data.

On the basis of the above interview data, it proved possible to obtain some very useful observational data. All of the data were supplied by the clients' daily tallies. For validation purposes, another observer (college undergraduate) made one home and school observation. However, since this observer's frequency data were similar to those obtained by Willie's mother and teacher, his information contributed little to the behavior therapy program.

The training of Willie's parents, his teacher and Willie himself, is too complex to describe here. Essentially, the teacher and mother were trained to reinforce differentially, behaviors competing with Willie's problem behavior and Willie was encouraged to produce some of these competing behaviors when he observed himself "worrying." All clients continued to record the designated behaviors on a daily basis, and eventually were capable of covering the behaviors in all home and school settings. [Frequency counts of the behaviors and subjective reports from all concerned indicated marked improvement in Willie.]

Selection of Observers

Interview information alone is usually insufficient to construct a successful treatment program. Its primary purpose is to instruct observers what to observe and where to observe it. For the sceptical, the dangers of operating on the basis of interview information alone are vividly illustrated by Patterson, Ray and Shaw (1969). The reader should examine Patterson and Guillon, 1968; and Bijou, Peterson and Ault, 1968; for information on the training of observers.

TABLE VI

SUMMARY OF SCHOOL SETTINGS FOR WILLIE'S PROBLEM BEHAVIOR, INCLUDING SOCIAL CONSEQUENCES*

School setting	Problem behavior	Social consequences	Desirable competing behavior
Arrival	Complains about many things	Teacher and Mother argue with him	Defined by problem behavior
Morning silent work time	Cries and complains	Teacher reasons with him	Writing
Lunch	Complains about other children "picking on him"	Peers laugh at him and teacher reasons with him	Talk to peers
Playground	Complains about other children "picking on him"	Peers laugh at him and teacher reasons with him	Talks or plays with peers

*Data based on teacher's report.

Most of the reported child behavior therapy studies have utilized observers not indigenous to the child's natural environment. This tactic was employed to insure observer objectivity as required for research purposes. However, for clinical purposes it is desirable to utilize the client, and when possible the child himself. This is not to say that outside observers should not be used for objectivity; in fact, every clinician concerned with this approach to child therapy should obtain this experience.

The advantages of using parents, teachers, peers, and the child himself as observers should be clear. They will be required to implement "contingency contracts": a shift in the reinforcement ground rules for the child's deviant and desirable behaviors. If a child is asked to change his behavior, he must first be aware of how he is currently behaving.

The pre-interview checklists (Tables I, II and III) may function as a setting operation to facilitate communication between the therapist, the client and the child. In addition, checklists can assist in mapping the kind of social attention (positive, negative, neutral or none at all) the child is receiving in a particular subsetting as a consequence of deviant as well as desirable behavior.

References

Bandura, A.: *Principles of Behavior Modification.* Holt, Rinehart and Winston, New York, 1969.

Bijou, S. W. and Baer, D. M.: *Child Development.* Vol. I, A systematic and empirical theory. Appleton-Century-Crofts, New York, 1961.

Bijou, S. W., Peterson, R. F. and Ault, M. H.: A method to integrate descriptive and experimental field studies at the level of data and empirical concepts. *J Appl Behav Anal 1,* 175-191, 1968.

Buehler, R. E., Patterson, G. R. and Furniss, J. M.: The reinforcement of behavior in institutional settings. *Behav Res & Therapy 4,* 157-176, 1966.

Cormier, W. H.: Effects of teacher random and contingent social reinforcement on the classroom behavior of adolescents. Unpublished doctoral dissertation, The University of Tennessee, 1969.

Goldiamond, I.: Justified and unjustified alarm over behavioral control. (Pos. 235-240) in *Behavior Disorders: Perspectives and Trends.* (Edited by O. H. Milton and R. G. Wahler.) J. B. Lippincott, New York, 1969.

Lovitt, T. C. and Curtis, K. A.: Academic response rate as a function of teacher and self-imposed contingencies. *J Appl Behav Anal 2,* 49-53, 1969.

Patterson, G. R. and Guillon, M. E.: *Living with Children,* Champaign, Illinois: [Research Press], 1968.

Patterson, G. R., Ray, R. F. and Shaw, B. A.: Direct Intervention in Families of Deviant Children. *ORI Research Bulletin 8*, 1969.

Tharp, R. G. and Wetzel, R. J.: *Behavior Modification in the Natural Environment.* Academic Press, New York, 1969.

Thomas, D. R., Becker, W. C. and Armstrong, M.: Production and elimination of disruptive classroom behavior by systematically varying the teachers behavior. *J Appl Behav Anal 1*, 35-45, 1968.

Wahler, R. G.: Setting generality: some specific and general effects of child behavior therapy. *J Appl Behav Anal 2*, 239-246, 1969a.

Wahler, R. G.: Oppositional children: A quest for parental reinforcement control. *J Appl Behav Anal 2*, 159-170, 1969b.

Wahler, R. G. and Erickson, M.: Child behavior therapy: A community program in Appalachia. *Behav Res & Therapy 7*, 71-78, 1969.

Wahler, R. G.: *Peers as classroom behavior modifiers.* Paper read at the American Association on Mental Deficiency, Washington, D. C., May, 1970.

Wolpe, J., Salter., A. and Reyna, L. J.: (Eds.) *The Conditioning Therapies.* Holt, Rinehart and Winston, New York, 1964.

Section II

COMMON AND LESS COMMON "PRESENTING PROBLEMS": BEHAVIORAL APPROACHES

THE READINGS OF SECTION II DEAL WITH COMMON AND LESS FREQUENT PRESENTING DIFFICULTIES ENCOUNTERED IN CHILD CLINICAL WORK. SCHOOL PHOBIA AND ENURESIS ARE FAMILIAR COMPLAINTS IN CHILD OUTPATIENT SETTINGS. NEALE'S WORK WITH ENCOPRESIS OCCURRED IN AN INPATIENT SETTING, AND HE SPECIFICALLY COMMENTS THAT THIS APPROACH IS PROBABLY APPLICABLE ONLY IN AN INPATIENT SETTING. HOWEVER, THE PRESENT AUTHORS HAVE HAD SOME SUCCESS IN MODIFYING THIS PROCEDURE FOR OUTPATIENT WORK. THE REMAINING ARTICLES REFER TO INFREQUENT, BUT OFTEN ALARMING, PRESENTING SYMPTOMS WHICH HAVE BEEN SUCCESSFULLY TREATED BY BEHAVIOR THERAPY TECHNIQUES.

Chapter 1

BEHAVIORAL MANAGEMENT OF SCHOOL PHOBIA*

T. AYLLON, D. SMITH *and* M. ROGERS

THE MOST WIDELY ACCEPTED APPROACH to neurosis is the psycho-analytic one. The phobic object is said to serve as a symbol of some danger that is extremely real to the patient and whose origins are attributed to early childhood. Concern for the underlying dynamics of school phobia has resulted in provocative speculations. For example, sometimes the cause of the child's fear of school is traced to "an unrealistic self-image" (Leventhal and Sells, 1964). More often the mother is blamed for the child's school phobia as she is said to displace her own hostility onto the school (Coolidge, Tessman, Waldfogel and Miller, 1962). It has also been suggested that the hostile impulses of sado-masochistic school personnel toward school phobics leads them to re-enact in the school setting the sado-masochistic relationship alleged to exist between mothers and their children (Jarvis, 1964). Unfortunately, such hypotheses have not led to standardized techniques for its treatment.

An alternative approach to school phobia is that of Wolpe's systematic desensitization technique. The pioneering work of Wolpe constitutes the first effective translation of the conditioning tech-

*From the *Journal of Behavior Therapy and Experimental Psychiatry*, 1970, 1, 125-138. Reprinted by permission of the author and Pergamon Press, Ltd.

★Additional experiments and related research are found in *The Token Economy: a motivational system for therapy and rehabilitation*, by T. Ayllon and N. H. Azrin, published by Appleton-Century-Crofts, New York, 1968.

niques of Pavlov and Hull to therapeutic procedures. Indeed, Wolpe's systematic desensitization technique marks a departure from methods used up to 1958 which was when his book *Psychotherapy by Reciprocal Inhibition* appeared in print.

The effectiveness of this approach, unlike the psychoanalytic one, has received empirical validation (Garvey and Hgrenis, 1966; Lazarus, Davidson and Polezka, 1965; Patterson, Littleman and Hensey, 1964). The impact of Wolpe's work has been such that even when modifications of his work have been explored, such as Patterson's (1965) use of M. & M.'s to reinforce responses to the hierarchy of stimuli presented to the phobic child or Lazarus and Abramovitz's (1962) use of so-called 'emotive imagery,' the conceptual rationale and procedural details remain those advanced by Wolpe (1958).

A complementary approach to school phobia may now be available through the use of operant techniques. In dealing with 'emotional' or behavioral problems this approach tries to determine through observation and experimentation the particular environmental event likely be responsible for the behavior. The rationale for an operant approach to school phobia, however, requires that the condition or diagnosis of school phobia be behaviorally redefined. Indeed irrespective of the interpretation to be attached to school phobia the major feature of this condition is immediately accessible to observation: the child's attendance at school. School phobia, therefore, can be redefined behaviorally as an observable event of low frequency or probability of occurrence. Two major methodological advantages are obtained by such a redefinition. First, frequencies and rates of behavior constitute the data of a large body of experimental research. Techniques to increase or decrease rates of behavior initially developed in the laboratory (Skinner, 1938; Ferster and Skinner, 1957) have been successfully extended to the treatment of pathological behaviors in clinical settings (Ayllon and Michael, 1959; Isaacs, Thomas and Goldiamond, 1960; Ayllon and Haughton, 1964; Wolf, Risley and Mees, 1964; Ayllon and Azrin, 1965; Ayllon and Azrin, 1968b).

The second advantage of redefining school phobia as a low probability behavior is that it immediately suggests what the relevant target for treatment is, namely reinstatement of school attendance. Our strategy then was to apply such behavioral procedures to the analysis and modification of school phobia.

It should be recognized that while a legitimate target of treatment may be self-understanding, growth, and insight, these are important only insofar as they are presumed to facilitate the behavioral change from not going to school to normal school attendance. The observable datum, school attendance, then is a legitimate if not the only relevant treatment objective for school phobia. Another objective of the behavioral intervention reported here was to bypass treatment in a clinical situation or in a therapist's office since success in such situations would still have to generalize into the school situation for the success to be relevant to the problem. Therefore, our attempt was to treat the phobia in the environment where it survived. In this manner if our strategy succeeded there would be no school phobia and the problem of generalization would simply not arise.

Background

The child

The subject of this study was Valerie, an eight-year-old Negro girl from a low income area. In the second grade she had exhibited episodes of gradually increasing absences from school until she stopped going to school in that grade and this continued on into the third grade.

The family

She had three siblings, a sister who was nine and two brothers ages six and 10. None of her siblings had a history of school phobia. Her father was periodically employed as a construction worker and her mother worked as a cook in a restaurant. Both had high-school level educations.

School phobia

Valerie held an above average school attendance in kindergarten and the first grade. She started skipping school only gradually in the second grade and finished that year with 41 absences. According to school records, Valerie attended no more than the first four days of school in the third grade. During her four days of attendance, her mother reported that Valerie refused to go to school. Whenever the mother attempted to take her to school, Valerie threw such violent temper-tantrums, screaming and crying, that it was nearly impossible to move her from the house.

Finally, the mother took Valerie to a number of specialists, including a school counselor, a medical specialist and a social worker. All these professionals offered extensive advice. The mother reported that the advice took several forms: 'Ignore the behavior and it will go away'; 'Give her plenty of praise and affection'; and 'Punish her severely if she refuses to go.' Unfortunately, none of this advice worked and Valerie continued to stay away from school.

Val, according to the mother's reports, had much trouble going to sleep and lay awake during much of the night. Val had no friends except for one cousin to whom she felt close. Children did not seek her nor did she seem interested in playing with children at school or in the neighborhood. According to the teacher's reports, when Val did attend school she was as quiet as a mouse in class and simply stood and watched at recess but would not join the games and activities. As the mother became convinced that Valerie had 'something wrong with her nerves' she took her to the local hospital so that she could get some 'pills for her nerves.' Valerie was evaluated by the pediatric staff and her case diagnosed as school phobia.

Diagnostic test results

Several diagnostic psychological tests were administered to Valerie while her case was being presented at the local hospital. The test results were as follows:

> Valerie demonstrated a consistent variability in her overall functioning. Her problem-solving, visual-manual skills (WISC Performance IQ = 78) are considerably below her near average verbal-expressive abilities (WISC Verbal IQ = 90). Within her verbal skills, she ranges from a defective level of functioning in comprehension of social situations and in her fund of information to an above normal level of functioning in her ability to think abstractly. Within her performance skills, she also demonstrated variability (DAP IQ = 87; Peabody IQ = 76). Valerie's variable functioning is due to an extreme inability to concentrate, since on perceptual tasks not requiring concentration she performed at a normal level (Frostig Perceptual Quotient = 98). Emotionally, Valerie's inability to concentrate is related to her extreme fears—especially her fears about men. The only way she can cope with men is to see them as dead. The inconsistency in her functioning seems to be related to the amount of concentration required by various tasks—such as classroom activities. To handle such stressful situations, she is likely to withdraw by not performing.

Social intake evaluation

A social intake evaluation was also done at the pediatric clinic.

Excerpts of this evaluation indicate that "when the mother tried to accompany Valerie to school, even as far as getting on the bus with her, as they approached the school, Valerie would become very stiff, begin shaking, screaming and hollering. When Valerie was asked about this, she stated that she was afraid to go to school, that when she went to school she thought about the time she was molested." This was a reference to an incident which took place when the child was four years old. According to Valerie's mother, a boy had "played with Valerie's 'private parts.' " Neither the extent of this incident nor any physical evidence could be obtained at the time of its occurrence. After the child had been diagnosed as suffering from school phobia, the mother was advised that the nature of Valerie's difficulties required long-term psychiatric treatment. Since the cost of such treatment was beyond the family means, the mother was left with the understanding that she should resign herself to living with the problem. Quite by accident, one of the authors of this paper was visiting the pediatric facility where Valerie's case was being discussed for the benefit of interns in pediatrics and child psychiatry. It was then that a suggestion was made by the senior author (T.A.) to attempt a behavioral treatment of Valerie's school phobia.

Methodology

Behavioral strategy

The behavioral approach to school phobia requires to break it down into three major components.

First of all there is the matter of response definition. The relevant dimension, insofar as the school, parent and child are concerned is that of school attendance. Thus, we can define school phobia as a low or near zero level of school attendance. This definition enables us to specify what the target behavior is for a treatment program. If the rate of going to school is low, our aim then is to increase it and maintain it, hopefully under the conditions that obtain in the 'natural' setting of the school environment. The next component involves the matter of CONSEQUENCES or reinforcement for staying away from school. These consequences must be examined as they affect the child and the behavior of those living with her. Finally, there is the issue of redesigning the consequences provided by the environment so as to minimize the probability of skipping school while maximizing the probability of attending school.

To identify the relevant environmental consequences responsible for the child's refusal to attend school, the child's behavior was directly observed and recorded by trained assistant-observers. The initial step was to attempt to quantify the dimensions of the relevant behaviors in the three primary environments of the child: (1) home, (2) a neighbor's home (where she was cared for) and (3) school.

The systematic observational schedule that was conducted each day on a minute-by-minute basis started at 7:00 a.m. and ended at 9:00 a.m. The sampling of observations was conducted for 10 days at home and for three days at the neighbor's house. Behavioral observations and procedures designed to reinstate school attendance were implemented by two assistant observers. One observer (M.R.) conducted the prompting-shaping procedures and participated in the observations at the neighbor's apartment. The second observer (D.S.) was responsible for giving instructions to the mother and conducted the observations at Valerie's home. Once the child returned to school as a consequence of the procedures applied, the observations were extended to include the child's behavior at school and on the way to and from school.

Valerie's behavior at home. The observations in the home revealed that Valerie was sleeping an average of one hour later than her siblings in the morning, although according to the mother she retired at the same time as they, between 9:00 and 10:00, every night. Her mother had long abandoned any hope of Valerie's going to school and simply allowed her to sleep until she awoke, or until it was time for the mother to leave for work at 9:00 a.m. The mother would usually leave for work approximately one hour following the departure of the siblings who left for school at 8:00 a.m.

Except for a few occasions when the mother made breakfast for the children they frequently fixed their own food. Valerie was given no preferential treatment, and was never asked what she would like for breakfast if she slept late. Upon arising, Valerie spoke an average of 14 sentences to the siblings, an average of 10 sentences to her mother and only two sentences to her father. The mother averaged one request each morning asking Valerie to go to school. Physical interaction such as touching, holding or other aggressive or affectionate behavior occurred seldom with her siblings and not at all with her father. On the other hand, Valerie typically followed her mother around the house, from room to room, spending approximately 80 per cent of her time within 10 feet of her mother. During these times, there was little or no conversation. When the mother left for work, she would take Valerie to a neighbor's apartment. On every observational occasion, when the mother left the neighbor's apartment to go to work, Valerie would immediately leave and follow the mother. This behavior of quietly following her mother at a 10-foot distance occurred on each of the 10 days of baseline observations. Each time this occurred, the mother would look back and see Valerie, stop and warn her several times to go back, all of which had no effect on Valerie. When the mother began walking once more, Valerie continued to follow at a 10-foot distance, with no verbal response of any type. Also, it was noted that on three occasions that the mother resorted to punishing Valerie with a switching for following, Val would cry quietly but would make no effort to return home until the mother took her back to the neighbor's apartment. Once the mother left again for work, Valerie would continue to follow at about twice the distance, or 20 feet, behind the mother. This daily scene was usually concluded with the mother literally running to get out of sight of Valerie so that Valerie would not follow her into traffic.

Valerie's behavior at the neighbor's apartment. Valerie was observed at the neighbor's apartment for three days during which the observer had no interaction with Val but remained nearby recording whatever behavior occurred. During this time Val watched the observer at times but made no effort to interact in any way.

At the neighbor's apartment, Val was free to do whatever she pleased for the remainder of the day. Val showed little interest in television or radio, preferring to be outdoors unless it was raining. If she had to stay inside she pored over a mail order toy catalogue. Very rarely did the neighbor spend time interacting with Val. The few times she did it was after Val's mother had left for work and Val was still crying.

Outdoors, Val found many ways to entertain herself. The observer watched while she played with a jump rope, exploded caps and found a dozen different ways to play with play-dough. If she ran out of things to play with, Val amused herself by hopping on one foot, jumping, running and turning in circles. In addition, Val had some money and at some time during the day made a trip to the corner store where she bought candy, gum or soft drinks.

Val was the only school age child at the neighbor's house and children from toddlers to kindergarten age sought her attention. She was somewhat aloof, but occasionally joined their play. In short, her day was one which would be considered ideal by many grade children—she could be outdoors and play as she chose all day long. No demands of any type were made on Val by anyone and she had the status of being the eldest among the children.

Valerie's behavior in school. Two visits were made to the school to get acquainted with the principal and teachers and to gather information from them about Val's past school performance, work attitude and social adjustment. Copies were obtained of the official records of Val's attendance for kindergarten, first grade, second grade, and the current year (third grade). The records showed Val's attendance to have been above average during kindergarten and first grade but that absences had increased each quarter during the second grade; first quarter, one; second quarter, seven; third quarter, 13, and fourth quarter, 20, for a total of 41 absences for the year. Excuses had been illness, oversleeping or missing the bus. Scholastic achievement had been normal or average until absences became numerous. Val, it was reported, had never cried or asked to go home. While described as shy, quiet and rather apathetic, Val had never given the impression that she was unhappy or afraid.

The behavioral assessment

The evaluation of Valerie's behavior at home, at the neighbor's apartment and finally at school suggested that Valerie's school phobia was currently maintained by the pleasant and undemanding characteristics of the neighbor's apartment where Val spent her day after everyone had left home in the morning.

Rather than speculating on the 'real' causes or etiology of the phobia itself our initial strategy was to determine the feasibility of having Val return to school by some prompting-shaping procedure (see Ayllon and Azrin, 1968a, for rationale and empirical basis for this procedure). Once this was done it would then by possible to provide for some pleasant experience associated with being in school in order to maintain her school attendance. To design the prompting-shaping procedure it was necessary first to assess Valerie's existing behaviors that had a component relation to the target behavior. Indeed, if attending school were to be meaningful, Valerie had to show sufficient interest to go to school voluntarily and consistently. In addition, she had to be prepared to work with school materials and perform academic work. To determine the presence or absence of these component behaviors, first one assistant (M.R.) took a coloring book, crayons, a set of arithmetic flash cards and other academically related items to the neighbor's apartment. While at the neighbor's apartment, she prompted Val to make the appropriate academically related responses to the stimuli. Val responded appropriately to the academic material and contrary to expectations, she did not panic, 'freeze', or become at all upset when exposed to academically related material. The next objective was to assess the difficulties associated with leaving the neighbor's apartment. Therefore, the next probe was for the observer to invite Val for a car ride after both had worked on academically related activities. Val offered no resistance and went with the observer for a car ride and later had a hamburger on the way home.

This behavioral assessment assured us (1) that a prompting-shaping procedure could start by taking Val directly to school rather than in gradually increasing steps; (2) that she would do academic work once in the classroom. The next step was to develop the desired response chain eventuating in Valerie's attendance at school. It must be remembered that Val stayed alone with her mother after her siblings left for school at about 8.00 a.m. She remained with her mother until she left for work at 9.00 a.m. If staying with her mother alone was the reinforcing consequence that maintained her refusal to go to school, we reasoned, withdrawal of this consequence might lead Valerie back to school. Before we could try such a procedure, however, it was necessary to determine the probability of Valerie remaining in the classroom once she returned to school. That was in effect the objective of the first procedure. Additional procedures were subsequently implemented to achieve the target behavior.
Specific procedures and results

Table VII shows all procedural stages as well as their behavioral effects. The target behavior of voluntary and consistent (100 per cent) school attendance was achieved in less than two months. Four distinct procedures were designed and implemented only after observing and recording their specific effects on Valerie's voluntary school attendance.

Procedure 1. Prompting-shaping of school attendance. Our plan was to manage to have Valerie visit the school at a time when school

TABLE VII

PROCEDURAL AND BEHAVIORAL PROGRESSION DURING THE TREATMENT OF SCHOOL PHOBIA

Temporal sequence	*Procedure*	*Valerie's behavior*
Baseline observations Day 1–10	Observations taken at home and at the neighbor's apartment where Val spent her day.	Valerie stayed at home when siblings left for school. Mother took Val to neighbor's apartment as she left for work.
Behavioral assessment Day 11–13	Assistant showed school materials to Val and prompted academic work.	Val reacted well to books; she colored pictures and copied numbers and letters.
Behavioral assessment Day 13	Assistant invited Val for a car ride after completing academic work at neighbor's apartment.	Val readily accepted car ride and on way back to neighbor's apartment she also accepted hamburger offered her.
Procedure 1 Day 14–20	Taken by assistant to school. Assistant stayed with her in classroom. Attendance made progressively earlier while assistant's stay in classroom progressively lessens.	Val attended school with assistant. Performed school work. Left school with siblings at closing time.
Day 21	Assistant did not take Val to school.	Val and siblings attended school on their own.
Procedure 1 Day 22	Val taken by assistant to school.	Val attended school with assistant. Performed school work. Left with siblings at school closing time.
Return to baseline observations Day 23–27	Observations taken at home.	Val stayed at home when siblings left for school. Mother took Val to neighbor's apartment as she left for work.
Procedure 2 Day 28–29	Mother left for work when children left for school.	Val stayed at home when children left for school. Mother took her to neighbor's apartment as she left for work.
Procedure 3 Day 40–49	Taken by mother to school. Home-based motivational system.	Val stayed at home when siblings left for school. Followed mother quietly when taken to school.

Procedure 4 Day 50–59	On Day 50, mother left for school *before* children left home. Home-based motivational system.	Siblings met mother at school door. Val stayed at home.
	After 15 minutes of waiting in school, mother returned home and took Val to school.	Val meekly followed her mother.
	On Day 51, mother left for school *before* children left home.	Val and siblings met mother at school door.
	On Day 52, mother left for school before children left home.	Siblings met mother at school door. Valerie stayed at home.
	After 15 minutes of waiting in school, mother returned home and physically hit and dragged Valerie to school.	Valerie cried and pleaded with her mother not to hit her. Cried all the way to school.
	On Day 53–59, mother left for school before children left home.	Val and siblings met mother at school door.
Fading Procedure Day 60–69	Mother discontinued going to school before children. Mother maintained home-based motivational system.	Val and siblings attended school on their own.
Fading Procedure Day 70	Mother discontinued home-based motivational system.	Val and siblings attended school on their own.

was almost over for the day. By having the child go to school for a short time only to be dismissed for the day along with the rest of the pupils we attempted to use the 'natural' contingencies of the school to maintain Valerie's presence in school. Permission was obtained from the teacher to bring Val to school for the last hour of the school day and for the assistant to remain in the classroom with her. The plan was to arrive at school progressively earlier until the child's presumed fears were extinguished at which time she would then initiate voluntary school attendance. The first day of this procedure the assistant (M.R.) told Val, about 1:30 p.m., that they would be going to school and that she would stay with Val. Val's eyes widened but she offered no resistance. They drove to school, arriving one and one-half hour before closing time and holding hands tightly, went to the third grade classroom. Val was given a desk and the assistant sat nearby until the day was over. The teacher, in a very natural manner, greeted Val and gave her some classroom material. Val immediately started doing some school work. On the way out of school the assistant found Val's siblings. To maximize the probability of Val's getting approval from her siblings, associated with the school, the assistant gave Val some candy to share with the siblings and left her to walk home with them.

The following day, the procedure was repeated except that the assistant left Val in the classroom about 10 minutes before school was out. Again, the teacher worked with Val just as naturally as if she had been attending all day long. The assistant before leaving the classroom instructed Val to meet her siblings and reassured her that they would wait for her to walk home with them. The next day the time of arrival was moved up so that Val spent two hours in school. By now Val had attended the third grade for a total of four hours. On the basis of her classroom performance the teacher came to the conclusion that Val was too far behind to catch up with her third grade classmates. Therefore, after careful consideration and discussion with the school principal decided to place her in a second grade class to insure her learning the material she had missed during her prolonged absence from school. Again, the cooperation of the new second grade teacher was obtained to allow Val to keep going to school at rather unusual hours, about two-three hours before the end of the school day.

The next day Val was taken to the second grade class for the first time. She gave no evidence of being upset with the shift from classrooms. On succeeding days Val was taken earlier each day. By the time Val was arriving in school at 9:30 a.m. THE ASSISTANT HAD GRADUALLY DECREASED HER OWN TIME IN THE CLASSROOM FROM THE INITIAL ONE AND ONE-HALF HOURS TO FIVE MINUTES. Each day the assistant left a sack containing some small prize like a children's magazine, a few pieces of candy, etc. with the teacher to be given to Val when school was over. On the eighth day of this procedure Val left home with her siblings and went to school without the assistant for the first time. The teacher praised her and the assistant went to school and told Val how happy she was that Val had come to school by herself.

On the next day Val stayed home until her mother left for work. As usual she was then taken to the neighbor's apartment. The assistant picked her up and took her to school where she spent the remaining four and one-half hours of the school day. The prompting-shaping procedure was discontinued at this time to allow for further behavioral evaluation. For the next six days she remained at home when her siblings went to school and, just as before, the mother took Val to the neighbor's apartment as she left for work.

Figure 1 shows the day-to-day behavior of Val under procedure one. The prompting-shaping procedure demonstrated that Val could go to school and stay all day without running away, causing disturbance in the classroom, or displaying any behavior that might suggest undue fear or panic. Just as significant, Val's behavior in school indicated that the 'natural' reinforcing consequences provided at school were adequate to keep her there once she engaged in the first activity of a COMPLEX BEHAVIOR CHAIN including getting up on time, washing, dressing, leaving the house and going to school. True, this procedure reinstated Valerie's school attendance but failed to maintain it. The problem then was how to provide sufficient motivation to insure her leaving for school. At this point it became neces-

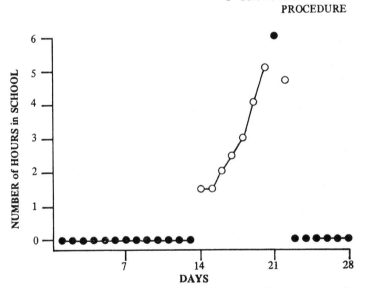

Figure 1. Valerie's school attendance both when she was escorted to school during the prompting-shaping procedure, and when she went on her own. Each dot represents the actual duration of her stay in the class room per day. The start of Procedure 1 is indicated by the gap between day 13 and day 14.

sary to examine and re-design the social consequences provided at home for Valerie's refusal to attend school.

  Procedure 2. Withdrawal of social consequences upon failure to attend school. As mentioned before, Val stayed with her mother for 1 hour daily right after her siblings had gone to school. The objective here was to eliminate such a social consequence for staying away from school. Therefore, procedure two involved instructing the mother that she was casually to inform all the children the night before that she was going to leave for work *at the same time they left for school.* When additional questions were asked, she was to reply that her working hours had been changed. Valerie gave no verbal or physical reaction to this announcement when it was given. Nothing else was changed. The children were treated the same as on previous occasions. One of the assistant-observers, who had had no interaction with Val, was in the house making standard observations the day the new procedure two was initiated and during subsequent intervention. The mother left for work along with the siblings but Val refused to go. Therefore, she was taken to the neighbor's apartment. This procedure was continued for 10 days during which Val did not attend school and was taken to the neighbor's apartment. In addition, Val increased her 'following behavior' when the mother left for work. Valerie followed at a distance of three-six feet behind the mother. When Valerie was punished by her mother she invariably dropped back to about eight-ten feet and continued following her mother. As there were no other observable effects on Valerie's behavior at the end of 10 days, this procedure was terminated. In effect, we had spent over 20 days trying various procedures and we were now back to the original behavior pattern: Val did not go to school and was taken to the neighbor's apartment. As soon as the mother started to leave for work Val followed her despite her mother's efforts to discourage her.

  Procedure 3. Prompting school attendance combined with a home-based motivational system. Despite the fact that Val appeared to have remained unchanged as ever through the various procedures, it was clear from results of procedure one that she could return to school through a prompting-shaping procedure. The problem was one of maintaining that attendance for any length of time. To find a solution, it was required that we find some source or sources of reinforcement to be used at home contingent on school attendance. Val's mother described some of the things Val liked most. Among these were having her cousin stay overnight with her, soda pop, chewing gum, and ice cream. Therefore, the strategy for designing the new procedure included the prompting-shaping procedure that previously resulted in Val's return to school and a motivational system designed to reinforce Valerie for attending school. This time, the mother rather than an assistant, was to use the prompting procedure. In addition and to facilitate implementation of the motivational system, a large chart with each child's name and the days of the week was given to the mother. She announced that a star would signify one day of going to school on a *voluntary* basis and was to be placed on the appropriate spot by each child at the end of each day. Five stars would equal perfect attendance and would result in a special treat or trip on the weekend. In addition to the above, each child who went to school on a voluntary basis would receive, each day, three pieces of a favorite candy. If anyone had to be taken to school (non-voluntary attendance), the reward was only one piece of candy. It was felt to be important to attach some reward value to the school attendance even if, in the beginning, attendance was not voluntary. The occasion of putting up stars, handing out rewards and verbal praise was to be made into a special event each evening when the mother returned home. When Valerie did not leave with the other children to go to school in the morning, the mother was to leave the house 15 minutes later taking Valerie with her to school. No excuses were to be tolerated with the exception of sickness. Since previously Valerie had used the excuse of being sick to avoid going to school, this time the mother was given a thermometer and taught to use it to decide whether or not Valerie was ill. If the thermometer reading was above 100, the mother would then be justified in allowing Val to stay home. This procedure resulted in Valerie's mother taking her to school daily for 10 consecutive days. Once, Valerie stated she was sick but since her temperature was within the normal range, her mother took her to school. Procedure three, just as procedure one, resulted in Valerie attending school but it failed to initiate Valerie's going to school on her own. In analyzing the procedure carefully, it seemed that what was happening was that the mother taking Valerie personally to school was perhaps adventitiously reinforcing and thus maintaining her refusal to go on her own. After the other children had left for school, the mother in a very matter-of-fact fashion, asked Valerie to get ready to go to school with her. On the way to school, Valerie and the mother appeared quite natural and even after 10 days of this procedure there was no particular irritation or apparent inconvenience experienced by Valerie or by her mother. It should be pointed out here that prior to the present intervention, Valerie would kick and scream and simply refused to go to school even when her mother attempted to take her by force. The results of procedure three suggested that the natural consequences for school attendance plus the motivational system employed here increased the probability of Val's going to school escorted, but it failed to prompt her going to school voluntarily. Procedure four was designed to introduce a mild aversive consequence for the mother if Val failed to go to school. In addition, the motivational system used in procedure three was maintained.

Procedure 4. The effects of aversive consequences on the mother. Procedure four involved having the mother get ready for work and leave the house 10 minutes *before* the children left for school. She was to inform all the children that she had to go to work much earlier but wanted to see that they got to school on time, so she would meet them at school each morning with a reward. This procedure was designed to have a two-fold effect: one, to prompt the behavior on Valerie's part of voluntarily leaving for school with her siblings and to provide reinforcement through the mother upon arrival at school. If Valerie failed to arrive at school with her siblings, the mother had to return home and escort Valerie to school. Since the school was about a mile away from home, Val's failure to go to school required that her mother walk back home a mile and then walk another mile to school—this time with Valerie in tow, for a total of three miles walking. By having Valerie's behavior affect her mother's directly, it was hoped that this procedure would in effect have the mother become more actively interested in conveying to Val the importance of going to school. On the first day of this procedure four, Val behaved just as she had throughout the previous ones: she remained at home after everyone, her mother and later the siblings, had left for school. The mother met the siblings at school, gave them a bit of candy and then waited for Val to come to school.

Following the previous instructions she remained at the school door for 15 minutes before going back home to find Val. Once there she very firmly proceeded to take Val by the hand and with hardly any words between them, they rushed back to school. Val did not protest and quite naturally followed her mother into school. After a few minutes Val's mother left school for work. That evening, the mother rewarded each child with praise and candy for going to school. She gave stars to the siblings and placed them on the board made for that purpose. She also gave Val a piece of candy and noted that she could not get a star since Val had not attended school on her own. The children's reaction to the stars and praise seemed one of excitement. Val, however, appeared somewhat unsure of what was happening. The second day of procedure four, Val got up along with her siblings, dressed, fixed herself some breakfast, and left for school with her siblings. When they arrived at school they met their mother who was waiting for them. The mother was obviously pleased with Val to whom she gave candy along with the siblings. At the end of the school day, the children again were praised at home and given stars by the mother on the special board that hung in the kitchen. Val appeared very interested particularly when the mother explained to her that if she collected five stars she would be able to exchange them for the opportunity to have the cousin, of whom Val was very fond, spend a night with her. The next day, Val remained at home after the mother and the siblings had left for school. Again, the mother waited for 15 minutes in school. Then she returned home. As it was raining, it was a considerable inconvenience for Val's mother to have to go back home. Once she reached home she scolded Val and pushed her out of the house and literally all the way to school. As Val tried to give some explanation the mother hit her with a switch. By the time they arrived at school, both were soaking wet. That evening, Val received some candy but no stars as she had not gone to school on her own. This was the last time Val stayed away from school. The next day she went to school along with her siblings. The mother met the children at the school door and genuinely praised them for their promptness. That evening, Val received a star along with candy and was praised by the mother in front of the siblings. Within five days Val had accumulated enough stars to exchange them for the opportunity to have her cousin stay overnight with her. She appeared in very good spirits and seemed to enjoy her cousin's visit. The next school day, Val got up with her siblings, washed, dressed, fixed herself some breakfast cereal, and left for school with them. When they arrived at school they were met by their mother, who again praised them, gave them some candy, and then the children went to their respective classrooms while the mother went off to work. Val and the children continued attending school without any difficulty, even after one aspect of the procedure was withdrawn: namely, the mother waiting for them at school. The home-based motivational system was maintained in force for 1 month and withdrawn at that time. Still, Val and the children continued attending school unaffected by the withdrawal of these formal procedures.

To gain perspective on the dimensions of the school phobia presented here it is necessary to look at Val's overall school attendance per quarter (45 days each quarter). Figure two shows that Val went from 95 per cent school attendance to 10 per cent within five quarters. This 10 per cent represented the first four days of the fifth quarter after which she quit going to school for the remainder of the quarter. The present behavioral intervention was conducted during the latter part of the sixth quarter. The net result was that Val's overall attendance in the sixth quarter increased from 10 to 30 per cent. The next quarter, the seventh, her overall attendance increased from 30 to 100 per cent. A follow-up for the next three quarters indicates that Val had maintained this perfect attendance.

Follow-up. Inquiries were made of Valerie's parents and teachers at six and nine months subsequent to Valerie's return to school. Their comments can be subsumed under school and home evaluation. Finally a psychodiagnostic evaluation was also obtained.

School evaluation. Val's academic progress is shown by her current grades. While previously she was an average C student, she now has A's and B's. Her teacher remarked that Val is well-behaved in class and helpful to the teacher. While she is pleased to volunteer for small errands and clean-up duties to assist the teacher, she has also shown sufficient social skills to be chosen as the school guide for a new girl admitted into her classroom. Val's specific duties as guide consisted of showing and explaining to the new girl the various school facilities such as the school cafeteria, the library, the gym

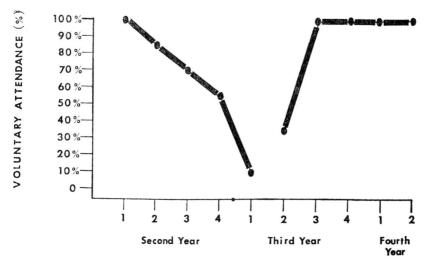

QUARTERS per SCHOOL YEAR

Figure 2. Valerie's voluntary school attendance. Each dot represents the percentage of voluntary attendance per school quarter (45 days). The behavioral intervention was initiated during the second quarter of the third year of school.

and so on. The teacher was particularly impressed with Val's performance as a guide because the new girl came from Germany and asked more detailed questions than is usually the case for a standard transfer student. Her newly developed social skills appeared to have impressed the Brownie Scouts to extend a cordial invitation for Valerie to join their group. Valerie was thrilled with the prospect and after requesting permission from her mother she joined the Brownies. Every Tuesday afternoon after class she attends the group's meeting which is held in the school. After the meeting she walks home with her girl friends.

A few months after Val resumed normal school attendance an incident took place that suggests the strength of her newly-acquired fondness for school. She was waiting for the school bus when another child snatched her money changer from her, took her bus money and ran away. Instead of crying and returning home, Val ran all the way to school since she did not want to be late.

Home evaluation. Val no longer complains of feeling sick, tired in the morning nor does she suffer from insomnia. She goes to bed about 8:30 p.m. daily with her siblings and gets up at 7:00 a.m. Valerie now fusses and hurries her siblings to finish dressing in the morning in time to go to school. She brings her math and spelling work home to show her mother. The mother very naturally praises her child as she does her other children. Whereas previously Valerie had been rather apathetic in school, she now takes pride in her work there and likes to discuss things she is learning.

Eight months after Val resumed school attendance the mother initiated divorce proceedings against her husband. This situation introduced a definite strain into the home family relations. Still, Val appeared sufficiently motivated to continue attending school without any disruption in her academic or social progress.

Neither the mother nor the school teachers have noticed any other maladaptive behavior or possible 'symptom substitution' since the child resumed normal school attendance. On the contrary, the mother as well as Valerie's teachers were very impressed with the astounding change in her behavior and the promise it now offers for her future both academically and socially.

Psychodiagnostic evaluation. Because Valerie's school phobia was initially presented and diagnosed in the psychiatric unit of a pediatric department at a large urban hospital, the formal procedures for case referral included a psychodiagnostic evaluation prior to and following treatment given to the child.

The conclusion now arrived at by the examiner in interesting !

> Her emotional development is characterized by deviations in the area of maturity and aggression. Her reality testing is marred by an extreme concern over sexuality and men, whom she sees as attacking, ever fighting animal-like creatures. On the basis of the recent results, without considerations to results previous to behavioral management, it would seem that the school phobia may have been treated successfully, but it has not meant anything to this girl.

Discussion

A child diagnosed as suffering from school phobia was cured within 45 days through the combined use of behavioral analysis and techniques. The term *cured* is used here purposely since the functional characteristics of school phobia are straightforward: chronic absence from school. Therefore, reinstating the child's school attendance constitutes the only relevant criterion of successful care.

The therapeutic intervention reported here is characterized by the following features:

1. Definition of the psychiatric problem is made in terms of behavioral dimensions. The observable and measurable dimension of school phobia is the child's frequency of school attendance. Hence this is the datum 'par excellence' in the treatment of school phobia.

2. Evaluation of the treatment objective is made in terms that are amenable to direct observation and measurement. Since the treatment objective was defined as reinstatement of voluntary school attendance, it was easy to evaluate the effectiveness of the behavioral intervention. The psychodiagnostic evaluation illustrates the dangers involved when evaluation of a treatment is on a non-behavioral basis: Speculation on personality factors often are given importance at the cost of minimizing the observable behavioral changes.

3. The behavioral intervention is conducted in the very environment where the individual's behavior is to be displayed. Hence, rather than working in a clinic or hospital situation, the emphasis is on utilizing behavioral techniques right in the field environment to which any clinic-based therapeutic efforts must generalize for these efforts to be successful.

4. Description of the procedures used here is also consistent with the stress on directly observable and measureable dimensions. The above provides a self-corrective method for approaching psychiatric problems in general. Each of the several procedures used here gave empirical quantitative information that enabled us to revise each procedure in the light of its effects on the child's behavior. This ongoing, step-by-step self-corrective evaluation is particularly critical for developing effective and inexpensive methods of treatment.

One other finding here was that the use of differential consequences for attending school was more effective than the use of either positive reinforcement or negative reinforcement (punishment) alone. It must be pointed out that during the baseline observations, the mother was observed hitting the child with no change in her refusal to attend school. Also during procedure two, she was observed hitting the child again without any effect on her refusal to attend school. Similarly, Valerie's refusal to attend school continued when positive reinforcement was made available for going to school escorted by her mother (procedure three). However, when school attendance was reinforced by the mother immediately at the school door, and at home with an incentive system that made use of the child's own motivation, while refusal to attend school was punished, it took but a few days to reinstate normal school attendance.

Why should punishment have worked this time? A parsimonious explanation of this finding lies in the fact that procedure four combined punishment for staying away from school with positive reinforcement for voluntary school attendance. Valerie's mother had used punishment previously but no positive reinforcement for going to school. These findings are consistent with those obtained by Holz, Azrin and Ayllon (1963) under more controlled conditions. In that study, they found that one of the most efficient methods for eliminating an undesirable response of mental patients was to schedule PUNISHMENT for the undesirable response and concurrently, reinforcement for an alternative competing response.

An important procedural innovation introduced here was arranging the child's refusal to attend school to affect the mother's own behavior. When procedure three required that she take Valerie to school she did so without ever appearing inconvenienced by it. It was only when Val's refusal to go to school resulted in her mother having to walk from the school back home and then again back to school that the aversive properties of the procedure led to the mother finding a 'natural' way of putting an end to such inconvenience. Only twice did she have to be inconvenienced. The second time her reaction was such as to convince Valerie that it would be easier to go to school with her siblings. The aversive properties of the procedure set up an escape-avoidance type of behavior in the mother that led Val to prevent such occurrences in the future by attending school.

References

Ayllon, T. and Azrin, N. H.: The measurement and reinforcement of behavior of psychotics. *J Exp Analysis Behav* 8, 357-383, 1965.

Ayllon, T. and Azrin, N. H.: Reinforcer sampling: a technique for increasing the behavior of mental patients. *J Appl Behav Anal 1*, 13-20, 1968a.

Ayllon, T. and Azrin, N. H.: *The Token Economy: A Motivational System for Therapy and Rehabilitation*. Appleton-Century-Crofts, New York, 1968b.

Ayllon, T. and Haughton, E.: Modification of the symptomatic verbal behavior of mental patients. *J Behav Res & Therapy* 2, 87-97, 1964.

Ayllon T. and Michael, J.: The psychiatric nurse as a behavioral engineer. *J Exp Analysis Behav* 2, 323-334, 1959.

Coolidge, J., Tessman, E., Waldfogel, S. and Willer, M.: Patterns of aggression in school phobia. *Psychoanal Study Child* 17, 319-333, 1962.

Ferster, C. B. and Skinner, B. F.: *Schedules of Reinforcment.* Appleton-Century-Crofts, New York, 1957.

Garvey, W. P. and Hgrenis, J. R.: Desensitization techniques in the treatment of school phobia. *Am J Orthopsychiat* 36 (1), 147-152, 1966.

Holz, W., Azrin, N. H. and Ayllon, T.: Elimination of behavior of mental patients be response-produced extinction. *J Exp Analysis Behav* 6, 407-412, 1963.

Isaacs, W., Thomas, J. and Goldiamond, I.: Application of operant conditioning to reinstate verbal behavior in psychotics. *Case Studies in Behavior* Modification. (Eds. L. P. Ullmann and L. Krasner). pp. 69-72. Holt, Rhinehart & Winston, New York, 1965.

Jarvis, V.: Countertransference in management of school phobia. *Psychoanalyt Q* 33 (3), 411-419, 1964.

Lazarus, A. and Abramovitz, A.: The use of 'emotive imagery' in the treatment of children's phobias. *J Men Sci 180* (453), 191-195, 1962.

Lazarus, A., Davidson, G. and Polefka, D.: Classical and operant factors in the treatment of a school phobia. *J Abnorm Psychol* 70 (3), 225-229, 1965.

Leventhal, T. and Sells, M.: Self-image in school phobia. *Am J Orthopsychiat* 34 (4), 685-695, 1964.

Patterson, G. R.: A learning theory approach to the treatment of the school phobic child. *Case Studies in Behavior Modification.* (Eds. L. P. Ullmann and L. Krasner), pp. 279-285. Holt, Rhinehart & Winston, New York, 1965.

Skinner, B. F.: *The Behavior of Organisms: An Experimental Analysis.* Appleton-Century-Crofts, New York, 1938.

Wolf, M., Risley, T. and Mees, H.: Application of operant procedures to the behavior problems of an autistic child. *Case Studies in Behavior Modification* (Eds. L. P. Ullmann and L. Krasner), pp. 138-145. Holt, Rhinehart & Winston, New York, 1965.

Wolpe, J.: *Psychotherapy by Reciprocal Inhibition.* Stanford University Press, Stanford, 1958.

Chapter 2

ELIMINATION BY THE PARENTS OF FIRE-SETTING BEHAVIOUR IN A SEVEN-YEAR-OLD BOY*

CORNELIUS J. HOLLAND

Case Report

R OBERT WAS A SEVEN-YEAR-OLD BOY, the oldest of three children, whose parents were referred to a psychiatric clinic by a private physician in order to receive counselling for family difficulties, the most distressing of which was Robert's habit of setting fires in the home. Since no child therapists were available at the time, Robert was placed on a waiting list but his parents, both high school graduates, were placed in a married-couples group for the discussion of marital and family difficulties. The author was the group therapist and saw the couple for approximately a year, once weekly. The child was not seen by the author.

It soon became apparent that the fire-setting problem was reaching increasingly serious proportions in terms of frequency and possibility of disaster for the family. Three months after the parents started the group, Robert was setting fires once or twice weekly. Usually the opportunities occurred on mornings of weekends whenever matches were available and the parents were still in bed or out of the house.

*From *Behavior Research and Therapy*, 1969, 7, 11, 135-137. Reprinted by permission of Maxwell International Microforms Corporation.

Matches were either carelessly left around the home or Robert would find them in the street and hide them until an opportunity arose. Punishments such as being slapped, locked in his room or touched with a smouldering object were successful for only short periods. Both parents, but the mother especially, by this time felt helpless and enraged so that she and Robert exchanged very little affection, and apparently avoided each other as much as possible. The mother saw the child as an oppressive duty and her feelings of impotence and anger made it difficult for her to express anything positive toward him. Her attempts to control his behaviour were almost exclusively through aversion. The father was able to be affectionate but his feelings of helplessness in coping with the problem often erupted into anger and physical punishment. The author at this time decided to attempt a more active intervention and saw the parents five times alone following the group session.

The problem was conceptualized as follows:

1. Some reinforcer obviously was maintaining the behaviour. The reinforcer was never determined although many possibilities came to mind, some through the psychological and social history reports and were available for speculation.

2. The behaviour occurred only under DISCRIMINATIVE conditions of presence of matches and absence of parents.

3. One goal was to make fire setting behaviour a DISCRIMINATIVE situation for effective punishment, thus suppressing the behaviour.

4. A second goal was to strengthen the OPERANT of bringing matches into the presence of the parents when the parents were available. This of course would prevent fire setting.

5. A third goal was to strengthen non-striking behaviour when matches were available but the parents were not present to dispense reinforcers. This goal was designed to control Robert's fire setting behaviour in the neighbourhood, or in the home when the parents were away.

Procedure

Since the mother saw little hope in changing Robert and was not willing to participate initially, the following program was carried out by the father.

1. Robert had just been given a new baseball glove which he valued highly. The father told Robert that IF HE SET ANY MORE FIRES HE

WOULD LOSE THE GLOVE IRREVOCABLY. The father said he would either give it away or destroy it in Robert's presence. It was hoped that this rather drastic threat, to Robert, would induce a strong suppression of the behaviour long enough for adaptive behaviour to be instituted. This hope was realized. The tactic was also used to help make fire-setting a discriminative situation for a significant loss.

2. At the same time the father told Robert that if matches or match covers were found around the house they were to be brought to the father immediately. That same evening the father conspicuously placed on a table an empty packet. It was assumed this was of little value to Robert so that compliance with the father's commands would be readily emitted. When Robert brought the empty packet he was immediately given 5 cents and told he could now go to the store and spend it if he wished, which he did. These instructions were given to enhance the reinforcing properties of any money Robert was to receive during the program. During the same evening and for the next few evenings the father placed around the house packets containing matches which Robert promptly brought to him. Robert was put on a CONTINUOUS REINFORCEMENT SCHEDULE for about eight trials with varying magnitudes of reinforcers, from 1 to 10 cents. He was also told during this phase of the program that he was not to expect money every time. Very shortly the desired behaviour was occurring at a high frequency so that matches or covers found outside during the day were saved and brought to the father when he returned from work. By this time the mother became interested in the program and began to reinforce Robert when he brought matches to her, although she said she found it somewhat difficult to reward the child for behaviour incompatible with what "he should not have been doing in the first place."

3. The possibility remained that Robert would find matches outside the home when either parents were not available for dispensing reinforcers. A procedure to strengthen non-striking behaviour (or anything but striking) was started after the match-bringing behaviour was believed to be strongly established. The procedure used was an approach-approach conflict. One evening about a week after the start of the program the father told Robert he could strike a full packet of matches if he wished under the father's supervision. The father also placed twenty pennies beside the pack and told Robert

that for every match unstruck he would receive one penny. Conversely one penny was removed for every match used. The first trial resulted in Robert striking ten matches and receiving ten pennies. The second trial the following evening earned Robert seventeen pennies, and the third trial, twenty pennies. Thereafter Robert systematically refrained from striking matches. The father then told Robert he was not going to know what he would receive if he did not strike a match and varied the reward for the next few trials from no money to 10 cents.

4. Throughout this program the father was instructed (it is likely he would have done so nevertheless) to give SOCIAL REINFORCERS with the monetary rewards, so that desired behaviour was brought under control of a more relevant reinforcer.

Results

The first three weeks of the program were spent in developing the procedures while the remaining two were spent in making minor modifications and discussing progress. The program was begun by the father at the end of the second week, and by the fifth week the habit was eliminated. The parents remained in the group until the author left the city 8 months later. During this period the behaviour did not recur, neither in the home nor from all evidence in the neighbourhood. It was observed during the remaining months that without further guidance the father applied a variable ratio schedule for the money reinforcer.

Secondary results developed which were unexpected but gratifying. The mother was surprised with the changes she was observing and participated to some extent in the procedures described above. In addition, she began to apply some of the principles on her own to some problems involving Robert's disobedience. Although a program was not developed for this problem the mother proved to be effective in applying the principles with desired results. Also by this time the procedures were a topic for group discussion and created much interest, and support for the mother. With her increased sense of adequacy in dealing with problem behaviour, she began to relax her aversive control and was able to express affection for Robert, something which rarely occurred prior to this time.

Discussion

The growing evidence of the possibility of replicating the results obtained in this case history is too impressive to dismiss lightly (see Russo, 1964; Wahler, Winkel, Peterson and Morrison, 1965). Shortly after the above case for example, the author had an opportunity to work with another group of parents (four couples) all of which came to the clinic for problems involving their children, such as "pathological" lying, disobedience, hyperactivity, aggression against siblings. Following the success with Robert and other cases, he defined the latter group as one employing directive parental counselling, applied operant principles systematically to analyses of the problems, taught the parents procedures for remediation, and achieved similar success. At times it was embarrassing to discuss with the rest of the staff changes in a child brought about by the parents. After much preliminary preparation by social workers, the psychological workup, the psychiatric evaluation, the ensuing staffings, the speculations and interpretations, and the often immense resulting gap between diagnosis and treatment, the problem was amenable to control within a relatively short period of time, within weeks or a few months. Although much research is needed in this area, such as a study of those personality variables of the parents which best predict success with this method, it promises to contribute at least to the amelioration of the manpower shortage in an important treatment area.

References

Russo, S.: Adaptations in behavioural therapy with children. *Behav Res & Therapy 2*, 43-47, 1964.

Wahler, R. G., Winkel, G. H., Peterson, R. F. and Morrison, D. C.: Mothers as behaviour therapists for their own children. *Behav Res & Therapy 3*, 113-124, 1965.

Chapter 3

AN INSTRUMENTAL CONDITIONING METHOD FOR THE TREATMENT OF ENURESIS*

H. D. KIMMEL *and* ELLEN KIMMEL

THIS PAPER DESCRIBES AN APPLICATION of instrumental conditioning procedures to the treatment of nocturnal enuresis in young children. The method, while hardly adequately tested, has been used in three cases with considerable success. Because of this promising initial record, and because the method has a rather different approach to the treatment of a serious and not infrequent behavior problem, it seems worthwhile to outline it and its logic so that those in a position to do so may subject it to more thorough testing.

It is well known that conditioning methods have been used with some success in the treatment of enuresis (Mowrer and Mowrer, 1938). Commercially manufactured devices are currently available and in wide use. Their usage differs from the proposed method in two fundamental respects. First, they employ CLASSICAL PAVLOVIAN CONDITIONING to achieve their effects: A deliberate arrangement is made in which interoceptive bladder distending stimuli are followed closely in time by a buzzer or bell sound which elicits waking (a sensing de-

*From the *Journal of Behavior Therapy and Experimental Psychiatry*, 1970, 1, pp. 121-123. Reprinted by permission of the authors and Pergamon Press, Ltd.

vice is placed under the bedsheet to trigger when the patient urinates and close an electrical circuit controlling the bell or buzzer which awakens him). The device is reset for additional trials. In this type of conditioning, the BLADDER STIMULATION which precedes the UN-CONDITIONED STIMULUS (buzzer) gradually becomes capable of producing a CONDITIONED VERSION of the ELICITED RESPONSE (waking). Thus, the interoceptive stimuli of bladder distension begin to become effective in awakening the patient. At first, this gradual process manifests itself in slightly earlier awakening after partial bedwetting. Eventually, the patient awakens before any actual urination occurs. The patient can then get out of bed and go to the toilet.

The second point of difference between the earlier conditioning method and the new one lies in the fact that the result of the earlier method is really not an optimal state but only the lesser of two evils. The patient has been conditioned to awaken from sleep and go to the toilet whenever bladder distension stimuli are sufficiently intense. But the optimal condition would be one in which cues of bladder distension would lead neither to bedwetting nor to the necessity of awakening to go to the toilet. This, of course, is what most normal adults manage to accomplish. The proposed instrumental conditioning method is aimed specifically at training the patient to sleep through the entire night with or without bladder distension, at the same time terminating bedwetting.

Procedure

The new method involves shaping the *desired* behavior by following it or near approximations to it closely in time with reinforcement (defined empirically in terms of effectiveness) until its occurrence has been brought under control. In the case of enuresis this becomes a matter of gradually increasing the period of time during which BLADDER DISTENSION CUES sufficiently strong to evoke urination are present but urination is voluntarily withheld. This is done, naturally, during the daytime when bladder control is typically present. The child is instructed to inform the parent each time it is necessary to empty the bladder. A record is kept for at least two days of this baseline. During this period and during training an unrestricted supply of water and other liquids is made available. It is also decided at this time what to use as reinforcement (e.g. cookies, candy, soda-pop, etc., depending upon experience with the particular child).*

On the first training day, the parent waits for the child's first report of the need to urinate. The child is asked to "hold it in" for, say, five minutes. If the child does not yet know how to tell time, the parent can instruct him/her to "hold it in" until the "big hand on the clock gets to here." The child is promised a reward (reinforcement) if this can be done. In no case should the first instance be made too demanding upon the child's retention ability. When the time has expired the reward is given and the child permitted to empty the bladder.

As it becomes clear that the time demand has become easy for the child, it is gradually increased, always in small steps to avoid failure or refusal to cooperate. In a matter of only a few days, the time can be increased to as much as 30 minutes. This may require an increase in the amount of reward as well. By this time, in the three cases referred to above, a change in rate of daytime urination was observed. Children who are troubled by nocturnal enuresis frequently are observed to urinate more often than normal during the day. This, of course, is to be expected, since such children are apparently given to emptying the bladder in response to very weak distension cues. As this tendency begins to be overcome by the training, its first manifestation is likely to be a reduction in frequency of daytime urinations.

Two of the three cases in which this method has been used involved females approximately four years of age who presented no other pathological symptoms. Both stopped bedwetting within seven days of the beginning of training and maintained control thereafter. The third case involved a 10-year-old female who was an outpatient of the psychiatric ward of a university hospital. Her major problems were of a psychotic nature and the enuresis was considered to be only a side issue. Two weeks after the beginning of the type of training described above she stopped bedwetting and also maintained

---

*Traditionally, parents have been advised in these cases to withhold liquids, especially late in the afternoon and evening to provide a reinforcing interpersonal response to any successful instances of bladder control (i.e. using the toilet) even during the day. The new method differs in that the parent avoids giving approval merely for urinating in the toilet, withholding it for those occsions when urination has been *delayed* for the desired time. The method also differs in that liquids are provided *ad libitum* (even encouraged) rather than restricted.

control thereafter. Her other problems continued without notice-able change and she was still being treated 1 year later.[†]

Discussion

A number of points may be made regarding these successful first cases. First, and perhaps most noteworthy, is the fact that complete success was achieved quickly. Although neither of the two younger children could be described an enuretics of long standing, they had both been bedwetting consistently for almost two years beyond the age at which their siblings had achieved nocturnal control. In only 1 week this was eliminated. In the case of the older psychotic child, the method was effective in spite of serious behavior problems which persisted after the enuresis ended. The ease with which the method may be employed in the home is also important. To the extent that the involvement of the parent in the successful treatment is likely to influence parent-child relations positively, it seems likely that an additional advantage may exist over the more 'mechanical' classical conditioning method. Not to be overlooked is the financial saving.

It goes without saying that extensive trials with the new method, under more controlled conditions than have so far been used, are necessary. While it cannot be considered to be more than promising at present, it is reported in the hope that readers may be interested in trying it. Variations in procedure, such as introducing *amounts* of reinforcement positively correlated to trial-by-trial *duration* of delay of urination, should result in improvements as well as clarification of the mechanism of operation.

Reference

Mowrer, O. H. and Mowrer, W. M.: Enuresis: A method for its study and treatment. *Amer J Orthopsychiat 8*, 436-469, 1938.

†In all 3 cases, follow-up indicated no more than a single recurrence of bedwetting during a period of over 1 year after the end of treatment.

Chapter 4

THE SUCCESSFUL APPLICATION OF AVERSION THERAPYTO AN ADOLESCENT EXHIBITIONIST*

M. J. MacCULLOCH*, C. WILLIAMS *and* C. J. BIRTLES

THE TERM EXHIBITIONIST derives from an article by Lasegue (1877) and has been defined by Kraft-Ebing (1912) as " . . . men who ostentatiously expose their genitals to persons of the opposite sex, whom in some instances they even pursue, without, however, becoming aggressive." This definition is still accepted in its essentials. Kraft-Ebing described two major categories of exhibitionist: patients in whom genital exhibition may be a symptom of a mental deterioration syndrome (organic psychosyndrome) and those in whom it is the outcome of an impulsive-compulsive drive.

Reports of successfully treated cases are relatively rare. In 1947 Sperling described a single case seen on five days per week for two and one-half years. The 600 sessions of analytically oriented psychotherapy resulted in the eventual marriage of the patient.

The use of conditioning techniques for the treatment of exhibitionism has been more recently described. Bond and Hutchinson (1960) successfully treated a single exhibitionist by reciprocal inhibition. A further single case (Kushner and Sandler, 1966) demonstrated the

*From the *Journal of Behavior Therapy and Experimental Psychiatry*, 1971, 2, pp. 61-66. Reprinted by permission of the author and Pergamon Press, Ltd.

successful use of a partial reinforcement schedule with imaginal stimuli. Recovery was maintained at a follow-up period of 12 months. Evans (1968) treated 10 exhibitionists by a paradigm stated to be based on the anticipatory avoidance technique of Feldman and Mac-Culloch (1965). Their subjects were asked to phantasise aspects of their sexual deviation in response to material projected on a screen. After a random delay period of three-six seconds shock was administered, and terminated by the instrumental escape response of advancing the slide projector. Five of their 10 subjects, who reported normal heterosexual masturbatory phantasy prior to treatment, reached the success criteria after a median of four weeks. The remaining subjects, who had exhibitionistic masturbatory phantasies prior to treatment, required a median of 24 weeks' treatment to achieve the same degree of improvement. Evans highlights the importance of masturbatory learning trials in the genesis and maintenance of sexual exhibiting behaviour.

The present paper reports the application of anticipatory avoidance aversion therapy to a single adolescent who showed persistent exhibiting behaviour, using apparatus which represents a technical advance over previously published techniques.

Case Summary

K was referred at 12 years of age by his family doctor because of complaints from female neighbours in February 1969. He was a reticent, neat, tidy, physically well developed young man, who only divulged his inner thoughts as his confidence was gained over several exploratory sessions.

He was an adopted child whose developmental and emotional milestones appeared normal on retrospective questioning of the parents. He had suffered no separations, emotional or sexual traumata; neither did he have any physical illness or educational difficulties. At an interview, K said "I love women's bodies," and that female bras, pants, suspenders, petticoats and stockings sexually excited him. It seemed that he was highly preoccupied with women's bodies and underwear.

One month before we saw him a female neighbour had complained to the patient's mother that he had entered her house and searched for her teenage daughter's underclothes. K described the incident: "I went into the house through a door I knew would be open, looked at the daughter's clothes and went to the mother's room. I took off my clothes and went to dress in them [the mother's clothes]."

Just before we saw him, the patient had exhibited his genitals to two women of 25 years or more when he had been left alone at home for several hours. These acts had followed a characteristic sequence. When he was alone in the house, and particularly when bored, he experienced a compulsive thought to expose his erect penis to older women, i.e. women of more than 25 years, who, by preference, should have large breasts and buttocks and well-shaped legs. He experienced an inner sense of resistance to these thoughts which he regarded as "wrong." However, they were followed by a train of compulsive thoughts to undress and exhibit himself. He positioned himself naked behind the drape of the lounge curtains, and waited for a suitably attractive older female to walk past the house. As she drew level he stepped into view (at times actually out of the home front door) and achieved orgasm when the victim appeared startled. If orgasm did not occur, he masturbated to a phantasy of himself exhibiting to the female. He also masturbated twice daily to a phantasy of himself "handling" older women. His mother's underclothes were also masturbatory items.

Although he was interested in girls of his own age, he was shy and socially unskilled with them. It was decided, as a preliminary measure, to undertake psychotherapy aimed at reducing tension about approaching girls of approximately his own age in social situations. This enabled him to talk more freely about sex, but two months later he again exhibited himself to a woman of 25.

Five months after our first meeting he reported a three-month absence of further exhibitionist acts and exhibitionist masturbatory phantasy, and said that female peers were coming to occupy more of his thoughts.

Two months later a letter was received from the Chief Superintendent of Police at K's home area, stating that the patient had exhibited himself to the wife of a policeman. There seemed the strong possibility that this case might be brought to the notice of the Director of Public Prosecutions. A rapid means of suppressing further socially unacceptable (maladaptive) behaviour was therefore sought to ward off a court appearance.

Treatment

The possibility of aversion therapy was put to the mother and the patient, who agreed to it after a full explanation of the technique and its implications. First, an analysis was made of the stimulus response sequences involved in the behaviour, to render them compatible with the most effective form of aversion therapy at our disposal (Feldman and MacCulloch, 1964; MacCulloch and Feldman, 1968). It seemed probable that the INITIAL STIMULUS to provoke sexual arousal and its consequent chain of exhibitionistic behaviour was "seeing" or phantasising well-developed mature females. There was ample evidence that the patient masturbated to female lingerie, and to "pin-ups" of older women. There seemed to be a disproportion in his sexual interest between girls of his own age, and women over 25.

It was proposed to reduce the age of the patient's heterosexual approach objects: in short, to make women of over 25 years the CS_1 (stimulus to be associated with SHOCK ONSET) and girls of his own age the CS_2 (stimulus to be associated with shock avoidance), and to apply the modified form of faradic ANTICIPATORY AVOIDANCE AVERSION THERAPY as described by Feldman *et al.* (1969).*

Measurement of sexual attitude

The Sexual Orientation Method (Feldman *et al.*, 1966) is a technique of assessing changes in sexual orientation during aversion therapy in homosexual subjects. In the present case, the object-choice of the patient was women over 25 years, and the aim of the treatment was to lower the age of preference to girls of his own age. The method was therefore modified by substituting "women of 25 years plus" for "men," and "girls of my own age" for "women." Apart from these changes the adjective pairs and the scoring remained the same as the standard form of the method.

This modified questionnaire was completed by the patient just before the first session of anticipatory avoidance aversion therapy, and repeated prior to sessions three, four, five, eight and 13; and at six and 14 weeks post-treatment.

*The successful treatment of a similar case (of age-inappropriate heterosexual object choice) in a man in his early 20s is reported elsewhere (Feldman, MacCulloch and MacCulloch, 1968). In that case, the subject was capable of sexual arousal only by women of 35 plus years.

Apparatus

Further refinements of the technical developments successively described in Feldman and MacCulloch (1964); Feldman and MacCulloch (1965) and Feldman *et al.* (1969), were as follows:

(a) *Treatment.* A single Kodak Carousel 'S' projector was modified so that it could be operated by both the therapist and the patient. Three slides were used, a blank, the CS₁ and CS₂. Figure 3 shows the operating circuit.

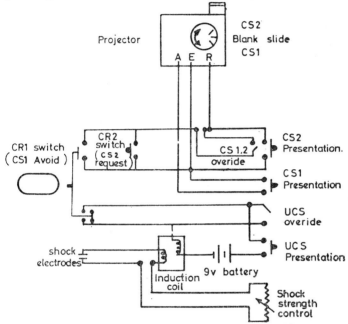

Figure 3. Operating circuit of avoidance conditioning equipment.

The projector was set to display the conditional stimuli on to a white desk top; in the between-trial intervals the projector was still running but using a blank slide. Presentation of the CS₁ and CS₂ was achieved by advancing or retarding the projector magazine.

(b) *Data logging.* The projector operating switches were monitored by a series of switches in mechanical parallel, whose output was recorded on eight-channel punched tape. The details of the encoder are reported elsewhere. (MacCulloch, Birtles and Bond, 1970; Birtles, 1970).*

*Details of the aversion/data logger "hybrid" apparatus, together with the computer program (MACRO 9) are available from the authors.

Method

A series of slides (CS_1) of fully developed women of 20-plus years was prepared. The slides were rank-ordered by the patient using the method of paired comparisons (Woodworth and Schlosberg, 1962); and eight were used in treatment. A hierarchy of slides of a second group (CS_2) of sexually immature females of approximately the patient's age, was constructed in the same way; and six were used in treatment.

The technique is described in detail by Feldman and MacCulloch (1965) together with preliminary results on the first 19 patients. Essentially, the method relation to HS/S represents the application to the treatment situation of laboratory derived escape-avoidance learning.

The slides of older females and young females were arranged in ascending and descending orders of attractiveness. The former signalled shock onset and hence anxiety, which was avoided if the patient removed the slide from the screen within eight seconds; the onset of the latter was associated with shock avoidance, and consequent anxiety relief. The technique thus combined aversion to older females and desensitization to young ones within the same treatment system.

Once the patient was avoiding consistently he was placed on a treatment programme comprising three types of trial: reinforced (R) in which his avoidance response succeeds immediately; delayed (D) in which, by special arrangement of the circuitry, the patient's attempts to switch off fail for a period of time within the eight-second period which elapses between the onset of the older female slide and recurrence of shock. He does eventually succeed before eight seconds have elapsed. The length of time for which he is delayed may be either four and one-half, six or seven and one-half seconds, after the onset of the slide, varied randomly; (NR), the patient's attempts to switch off are not allowed to succeed and he has to sit out the eight seconds and receive a brief shock of aversive strength. The shock and the slide terminate simultaneously. The programme consists of one third of each type of trial, varied randomly.

When the patient reported that (1) his previous attraction to the current older female slide had been replaced by indifference or even actual dislike, and (2) he attempted to switch off within one to two seconds of its appearance, we proceeded to the next older female slide and repeated the process.

As mentioned above, we also attempted to associate relief from anxiety with the introduction of the young female slide. However, such a slide was not introduced at every trial, to preserve what we consider to be the important principle of reducing generalization decrement—that is, reducing the disparity between the treatment situation and the real-life situation, in which of course, attempts to approach the desired females are not always likely to meet with success. We allowed the patient to request the return of the young female slide after it had been removed. (The young female slide was always removed by the therapist and not by the patient.) The patient was provided with a switch, which he could use in order to bring the young female slide back to the screen. However, his request was met in an entirely random manner, sometimes being granted and sometimes not, so that he could not predict the consequences of his attempting to switch off the older female slide, nor of his "asking" for the return of the young slide. The whole situation was designed to lead to the acquisition of two responses: avoidance of older females and approach to young females.

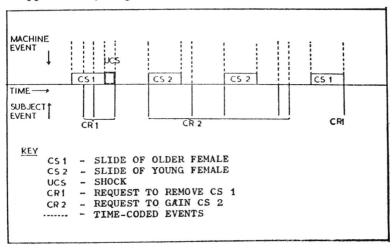

Figure 4. Sequence of treatment operations.

Figure two summarizes the treatment sequence.

The patient was given 18 20-minute sessions of anticipatory avoidance aversion therapy, using eight CS_1 and six CS_2 slides.

Results

Clinical. The prime aim of this therapy was to prevent *all* further exhibitory behaviour in order to avoid legal proceedings against the patient; he was therefore interviewed before each aversion therapy session. After three sessions he reported a gradual increase in the ease with which he could prevent such exhibitory phantasy, and the phantasy of older women during masturbation. At the completion of treatment he was able to control the start of the cognitive chain which had previously led to the exhibitory behaviour, although 25 per cent of his masturbatory phantasy was still concerned with older women. At six weeks' follow-up he reported his masturbatory phantasy exclusively concerned girls of his own age and the compulsive ideas about exhibiting himself were absent. The situation remains unchanged at the latest follow-up at five months. His heterosexual skills are improved, he has a 13-year-old "girl-friend" who visits his home, and he reports a lessening of anxiety in heterosexual relationships.

Psychometric: Sexual Orientation Measure. The scoring system for the Sexual Orientation Measure is so designed as to give scores between six and 48 on the two stimulus classes—in this case "women of 25 plus years" and "girls of my own age," where high scores indicate the direction of sexual orientation of the patient. From Figure 3 it will be seen that on first presentation K attained a maximum score on both scales indicating a high positive attitude to both girls of his own age and women over 25 years.

This high scoring on both scales was maintained through the first two treatment sessions, but by the fifth session his score on the women over 25 years concept began to drop, reaching the minimum score by the eighth session, where it has remained up to the latest follow-up.

The fall in score in relation to women of 25 plus years paralleled the increase in the patient's ability to control his compulsive thought.

We would like to suggest that aversion therapy of this type is a potent component of the behaviour therapist's repertoire provided that it is judiciously used. The main usefulness of aversion therapy appears to be in situations where MALADAPTIVE APPROACH BEHAVIOUR cannot be relieved.

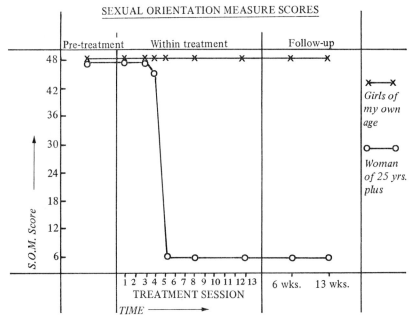

Figure 5. Sexual orientation measure scores.

References

Birtles, C. J.: A data logging system for behavioural studies. M.Sc. Thesis, University of Birmingham, 1970.

Bond, I. K. and Hutchinson, H. C.: Application of reciprocal inhibition therapy to exhibitionism. *Can Med Assn J 83*, 23-25, 1960.

Evans, D. R.: Masturbatory fantasy and sexual deviation. *Behav Res & Therapy 6*, 17-19, 1968.

Feldman, M. P. and MacCulloch, M. J.: A systematic approach to the treatment of homosexuality by conditioned aversion. Preliminary report, *Am J Psychiat 121*, 167-172, 1964.

Feldman, M. P. and MacCulloch, M. J.: The application of anticipatory avoidance learning to the treatment of homosexuality. I. Theory, technique and preliminary results. *Behav Res & Therapy 2*, 165-183, 1965.

Feldman, M. P., MacCulloch, M. J., Mellor, V. and Pinschof, J. M.: The application of anticipatory avoidance learning to the treatment of homosexuality, III. The sexual orientation method. *Behav Res & Therapy 4*, 289-299, 1966.

Feldman, M. P., MacCulloch, M. J., MacCullough, M. L.: The aversion therapy treatment of a heterogeneous group of five cases of sexual deviation. *Acta psychiat neurol Scand 44*, 113-123, 1968.

Feldman, M. P., MacCulloch, M. J., Orford, J. F. and Mellor, V.: The application of anticipatory avoidance learning to the treatment of homosexuality. Developments in treatment technique and response recording. *Acta Psychiat Neurol Scand 45*, 109-117, 1969.

Feldman, M. P. and MacCulloch, M. J.: *Homosexual Behavior: Therapy and Assessment*. Pergamon Press, Oxford, 1970.

Kraft-Ebing, R. Von: *Psychopathia Sexualis*. 12th Ed. Rebman, New York, 1912.

Kushner, M. and Sandler, J.: Aversion therapy and the concept of punishment. *Behav Res & Therapy 4*, 179-186, 1966.

Lasegue, E. C.: 'Les exhibitionistes.' troisieme serie, L'union medicale, France, 1877.

MacCulloch, M. J. and Feldman, M. P.: Aversion therapy management of 43 homosexuals. *Brit Med J 2*, 594-597, 1967.

MacCulloch, M. J. and Feldman, M. P.: Personality and the treatment of homosexuality. *Acta Psychiat Neurol Scand 43*, 300-317, 1967.

MacCulloch, M. J., Birtles, C. J. and Bond, S.: A free space-time traversal data-logging system for two human subjects. *Med & Biol Engng 7*, 593-599, 1969.

Sperling, M.: The analysis of an exhibitionist. *Int J Psychoanal 28*, 32-45, 1947.

Woodworth, R. S. and Schlosberg, H.: *Experimntal Psychology*. Holt, Rinehart and Winston, New York, 1962.

Chapter 5

BEHAVIOUR THERAPY AND ENCOPRESIS IN CHILDREN*

D. H. NEALE

THIS PAPER RECORDS EXPERIENCE in treating four boys with enco-presis. The selection of cases was fortuitous in that a group of about twenty-five children who were in-patients in the unit to which the author was assigned for a six-month period, these four were the only encopretic children. It is hoped to illustrate an approach to the problem which is therapeutically useful, which is open to theoretical development in a way in which analytic formulations are not, and, at the same time avoids the false dichotomy between psychogenic and organic diseases.

The method involves utilization of physiological and neuro-ana-tomical knowledge of bowel function, as well as learning theory. This paper abstracts a particular aspect of the children's treatment but they were of course receiving all the benefits of a children's psychiatric unit. What is reported here leans heavily on learning theory. In par-ticular the method of operant conditioning, which has a long history of study in laboratory conditions (Skinner, 1959; Ferster, 1958) is used to bring about the desired response. The concept of desensitiza-tion to phobic situations as described by Wolpe (1958) was a guide to making possible the decay of the conditioned phobic response to defaecation although in these particular children it was not necessary to use relaxation techniques. The work of Mowrer and Mowrer

*From *Behavior Research and Therapy*, 1963, 1, pp. 139-149. Reprinted by permis-sion of Maxwell International Microforms Corporation.

(1938) and others on conditioning treatment of enuresis is of great importance inasmuch as it has encouraged other applications of learning theory to clinical problems. It is not however directly applicable to the forms of encopresis described here. The two conditions of incontinence of urine and incontinence of faeces are physiologically and behaviourally different. The former requires encouragement of a conditioned inhibition of bladder emptying and the development of the ability to store urine, while the latter requires encouragement of the act of defaecation and restoration of the psysiologically normal state of emptiness of the rectum.

Using the division of neurotic behaviour into the conditioned avoidance drive (C.A.D.) and the instrumental responses by which C.A.D. is reduced (H. Gwynne-Jones, 1960) it may be seen that in this study treatment was directed at the instrumental response and in three cases this was sufficient. In the fourth case it was insufficient and cure was not achieved; probably an attack on the C.A.D. itself was required.

Encopresis is considered in terms of stimulus and response and the formation of an S-R connexion by appropriate reinforcement.

The Stimulus

In health the rectum is empty WHEN A FAECAL MASS IS MOVED INTO THE RECTUM A SENSATION OF FULLNESS is experienced which normally calls forth the response of proceeding to a lavatory and defaecating there. If defaecation does not occur then the sensation of fullness passes off. The subject then becomes unaware of his full rectum. If the rectum is distended the anus may also become dilated without the subject being aware of it and overflow incontinence can occur (Gaston, 1948). If there is impairment of the sensory path of the reflex then S-R training will be impaired or prevented. This is clearly demonstrated in cases of anatomical interruption by Goligher and Hughes (1951). It seems reasonable to suppose a similar effect where the interruption is functional. All the subjects of this study reported absence of the sensation of rectal fullness.

The Response

This consists of an expulsive act emptying the rectum and descending colon and requiring only a few moments for completion in healthy subjects. This act is itself a series of co-ordinated reflexes which can be disorganised by a failure of any one member of the series. In all four subjects discussed, this act was severely disorganised at the commencement of training. The syndrome of dyschezia (Keele & Neil, 1961) was fully developed with a constantly filled rectum from which small quantities of faeces would be expelled at short intervals without ever producing complete evacuation.

The S-R Link

Anthony (1957) has drawn attention to the subtleties of the mother child relationship in the training situation which he terms "the potting couple." Factors which appear relevant will be detailed in each case study. Prominent in these cases is inhibition of R by fear. Pinkerton (1958) in his study of psychogenic megacolon gives details of this process. Once constipation with resulting impairment of S and encopresis has developed, the child draws down upon himself extreme parental wrath which adds to the fear and further inhibits R. This is particularly the case in that the usual parental injunction is to "control yourself" and "hold it in" in order to avoid soiling.

Method of Treatment

The aim of treatment was to encourage a normal R by INSTRUMENTAL CONDITIONING while creating circumstances in which the conditioned anxiety response could decay. This latter was encouraged by the method of RECIPROCAL INHIBITION. The children were taken to the lavatory after each main meal and at bedtime (four times daily). This was done in a kindly manner by a nurse known to the child. The child was permitted to shut the lavatory door if he wished and in one case (W.S.) provided with a sweet to suck and a comic book to read, both measures designed to inhibit the anxiety reaction associated in this child with sitting on the lavatory. The procedure was fully explained to the child and every effort made to ensure that it was not unpleasant nor received by him as punitive.

In two cases (R.C. and W.S.) Isogel (Allen & Handbury) (which is dried mucilage of tropical seeds) was given to provide additional bulk for the colon to work on and to render the stools soft and not painful to pass. The child found that success in passing faeces in the lavatory was rewarded. The most powerful reinforcement was probably the approval of the nurse and the knowledge on the part of the child that he was making progress towards losing a hated symptom.

In addition he received a reward consisting of either sweets, chocolate bars, peanuts, stars in a book or pennies, these varying with the interests of the child and being changed as the child grew bored with them.

Once the child had become accustomed to using the lavatory and was free from soiling, the four times daily routine was abandoned. The child was now instructed to go whenever he felt the sensation of rectal fullness (which had returned by this stage). After reporting a successful result, he received his reward. This constituted a period of overlearning. An attempt was made to provide partial reinforcement but this ran into procedural difficulties and was abandoned as an inessential refinement of the method.

A record was kept of acts of defaecation. A score of two points was assigned to a normal bowel action. In the early stages it frequently happened that two or three pellets of faeces each the size of a pea, would be produced. A score of one was assigned to such a bowel action. If pants were soiled this was similarly scored one or two and clean pants were provided. Enquiry as to the state of pants was made tactfully and no form of rebuke was administered. All these children had previously had excessive punishment for soiling and it was considered that the fear engendered had actively interfered with learning the desired response. The records are displayed graphically as a pair of curves, one representing decay of the undesired response (involuntary and uncontrolled defaecation) and the other the growth of the desired response (defaecation in the lavatory). During treatment there was no other change in the boys' life in the ward and milieu therapy, occupational therapy and play therapy continued as before.

Case 1. R. C., age seven and one-half years I.Q. 80 (W.I.S.C.)

Reported to have been continent of urine and faeces by day and night at one year. Age three began attending day nursery where the lavatory was inconveniently situated. Faecal incontinence occurred about twice weekly. This was treated by smacking and forced sitting on the pot for long periods after the act of incontinence. This was followed, as would be predicted from learning theory, by refusal to defaecate in the pot and by the age of five he would not enter a toilet unless accompanied and if he did so he would not defaecate there. He was constantly defaecating in his trousers by day or pyjamas by night and nowhere else. His father died when he was four. On commencing primary school (age five) he showed so much aggressive behaviour that the head teacher feared for the safety of other children. We have no data by which to determine if his hostility to other children was in part determined by their dislike and scorn of his dirty conditions.

He began attending the psychiatric children's out-patient clinic weekly, aged five and one-half but neither encopresis nor behaviour improved. He became an in-patient at six years and three months. For the first two months a record was kept, solely for diagnostic purposes, which showed that he was incontinent two or three times daily and by night often passing large, formed stools involuntarily. He reported that he never felt the urge to defaecate and was unaware of the occurrence of defaecation. This record was scored in a similar manner to the present study and serves in some degree as a control. It is not quite satisfactory as a control because it is not known to what extent the child may have been rewarded by nurses' approval of bowel actions in the lavatory. The graphic record does not show unequivocally that learning did or did not take place, but if learning took place at all it did not do so at the rate achieved in the planned treatment.

At seven years and three months, after a year in hospital, his general demeanour had improved but the encopresis was worse. He never defaecated in the lavatory at all and on examination multiple faecal masses were palpable in the lower abdomen. Rectal examination was not performed but the abdominal examination indicated extreme constipation. The training procedure was instituted and within a few days he began using the lavatory and after five weeks was having only occasional accidents (Figure 6).

After three months he was considered cured by the nurses responsible for him in so far as he was never noticeably soiled. However, close inspection of his underpants showed that two or three times a week they were stained to a slight extent, as if he had been careless in wiping himself. This situation has persisted unchanged on his transfer to a boarding school for educationally subnormal children. It seems that bowel physiology has not yet returned completely to normal, but all the social disabilities previously associated with this boy's state have gone. There has been no relapse in his behaviour at

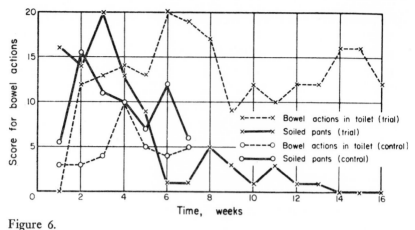

Figure 6.

the boarding school.

Comment

Normal bowel control broke down under unfavourable environmental stress and the damage was compounded by punishment. The boy's situation at the commencement of treatment was constipation with loss of rectal sensation and reflex emptying of the bowel occurring without the boy being aware of it. It seems unnecessary to relate encopresis to loss of his father one year after commencement or to postulate that encopresis and the aggressive behaviour occurring from five to six were both manifestations of the same aggressive instinct.

Case 2. J. E., age 10 W.I.S.C. I.Q. Full Scale 117; Verbal 124 Performance 108

Clean and dry from age two. Encopretic but not enuretic from age four. There had been pot phobia aged one year but this subsided. Aged four, he had an attack of diarrhoea after eating fruit and soiled himself. Father was outraged and smacked him severely; mother sympathized and a major parental quarrel ensued. He was then encopretic until father, a violent man frequently drunk, left home, eighteen months later. For six months he was clean but then father returned and had a violent quarrel with mother, striking her in front of the child. Encopresis returned and persisted. Mother threatened him, bribed him and beat him with a strap, all these measures being associated with instructions to hold in his faeces. He attended as an out-patient weekly for a year for play therapy, while his mother was the subject of social casework, but without improvement. He was admitted to the ward and after a month there was no change. At the end of this month when the training programme was commenced, faecal masses were palpable per abdomen and on rectal examination a mass of faeces was present just inside the sphincter. He never used the lavatory to defaecate and would pass bulky faeces into his trousers on average once daily. He could report brief periods, up to a week of cleanliness but in these periods he did not defaecate at all. This behaviour indicates that the only approach to continence the boy knew was to inhibit defaecation. He reported that he could not voluntarily expel faeces and that when involuntary expulsion occurred he had no conscious awareness of it.

For the training programme no purgatives were used and sweets were given as a reward. It was intended to use the first week as a control period without sweets, but as the graph shows, use of the lavatory began at once so that the sweets played only a minor part in this. It was two months before a full continence was obtained and after four months the descending colon was palpable and faeces were found on rectal examination so that the colon and rectum were not functioning with complete normality. He remained in hospital a further three months because of a legal wrangle between his parents over his custody, neither being able to provide a satisfactory home. He was discharged to a boarding school where he remains a happy and well integrated member of the community, fully continent six months after cessation of treatment (Figure 7).

Comment

The aetiology of encopresis in this case could well be formulated in terms of the Oedipus complex, and much evidence not quoted here, emerged which was consistent with such a formulation. However from the point of view of treatment it seems more profitable to see this in terms of a conditioned inhibition of defaecation by a prepotent anxiety response established by an intolerant and punitive father and maintained by a bewildered and desperate mother. The rapidity with which this boy used the lavatory in hospital when the training regime began may be explained in several ways. The anxiety response may have been conditioned to the lavatory in his own home, and so would not necessarily and completely generalize to a different lava-

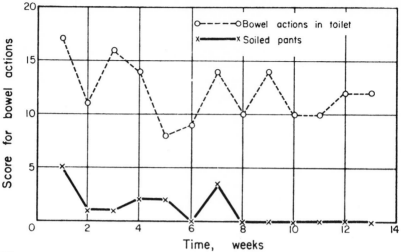

Figure 7.

tory. In addition the month in hospital prior to commencing training may have been essential in lowering his overall anxiety by providing a tolerant non-punitive atmosphere. Finally this intelligent 10-year-old may have benefited from the full explanations of what was being done, given on several occasions in a friendly and supportive manner.

Case 3. G. M., age 9 • 10/12 years. W.I.S.C. I.Q. Verbal factor 112 *Performance factor 69*

Constipation had been a great problem to mother as a girl and she was very frightened of it developing in her son. It did. He was clean and dry by two and one-half but had colic and constipation requiring enemata from three to four, again at seven and again at eight and one-half. Defaecation appeared painful and in retrospect he said he was frightened to defaecate because of the pain. In arguments with his mother one of the threats the boy made was, "If I don't get my way, I won't go to the bloody lavatory."

He was first brought to a Child Guidance Clinic at the age of six because of aggressive behaviour, phobias and sex play, but defaulted after a few visits. He was again referred at age eight for the same troubles to which scholastic retardation was now added. He received weekly play therapy but after four months, encopresis commenced. Its onset was not associated with improvement or change in any other respect, and its occurrence at this point rather than say a year earlier or later seems fortuitous. He continued weekly attendance with his mother for six months but was then admitted largely because his mother was worn out by the encopresis. Six months after admission his general behaviour was somewhat improved but the encopresis persisted. There was a continuous flow of liquid faeces and he wore napkins and plastic pants. He did not use the lavatory for defaecation at all. On examination faecal masses were palpable per abdomen. He was too nervous to permit rectal examination but on gently retracting the buttocks the anal sphincter could be seen open to half an inch diameter with bulging faeces behind it. The response to treatment was rapid and complete in that he became fully continent of faeces day and night. After three months of training the colon was still palpable per abdomen but not loaded as before. The anal sphincter was firmly closed as in normal children. The slow improvement in other aspects of his behaviour continued unchecked and he was discharged home three months after completion of bowel training, a year after first admission. After three months back in his own home there has been no relapse in bowel habit or in general behaviour. (Figure 8).

Comment

Parent and child both had bowel problems. Transmission may have been genetic but very probably it was mother's over-anxiety about the boy's use of the pot which led to mishandling of the training situ-

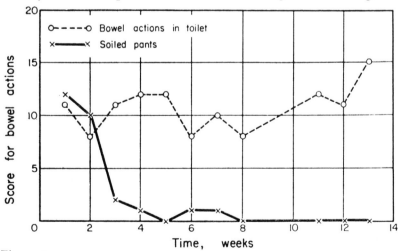

Figure 8.

ation. Judicious use of bland laxatives in the early years might have avoided encopresis but later the boy was refusing to enter the lavatory as one way of exerting his will against his mother with whom he was continuously in conflict. Constipation with overflow incontinence was the result of refusal to defaecate in the lavatory. Removal to hospital created a new situation, cutting short the conflict with his mother and providing alternative authority figures more skilled in avoiding conflict. In this setting his encopresis did not spontaneously cease but rapidly improved when the training programme commenced. At the time of his return home the total situation has been considerably improved so that parental anxiety has subsided below the point at which the whole vicious circle would start again.

Case 4. W. S., Age 10 9/12. *W.I.S.C. I.Q.* 108

As a baby he required weekly milk of magnesia for constipation but there were no battles over the pot and he was clean and dry by age two years. Encopresis began at age seven and one-half with daily incontinence of formed stools and a great deal of play with the stools, which were deposited, sometimes wrapped in paper, in various parts of the house, and smeared on walls and furniture. He would spend long periods in the lavatory without successful defaecation. He freely inserted his fingers in his rectum to obtain faeces for smearing and as a means of assisting defaecation. He was a quiet, overly good boy with a compulsion to swear, but he dealt with this by limiting himself to the initial letters F. ., S . ., S . ., C . ..

He began attending as an out-patient in May 1960 and received psychotherapy on 50 occasions. Simultaneously his mother saw P. S.W. The encopresis, smearing and swearing continued but in addition there was open rebellion and disobedience to his parents.

He was admitted as an in-patient and six months later his condition was unchanged. Examination showed hard coils of faeces-packed colon in the abdomen and hard faeces in the rectum. After an initial purge using Dulcolax suppositories, the training programme was instituted. There was no sustained improvement. Subsequently a course of rectal washouts followed by neostigmine has produced no benefit. Great difficulty exists in getting this boy to talk about his condition but he has said that at night he keeps his fingers in his rectum for long periods because he likes the sensation (Figure 9).

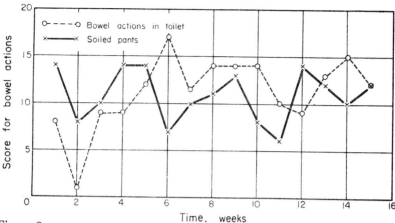

Figure 9.

Comment

This case represents a failure by a psychotherapeutic approach and by the orthodox medical approach of purgation. The method of operant training failed. However, theoretically the S-R analysis could have been pushed further although for practical reasons this was not possible for the present author. It appears that in this case, some stimulus connected with a distended rectum was a source of considerable gratification which was not outweighed by the reward we were able to offer for emptying the rectum. We never knew what the significant stimulus was, nor precisely what gratification resulted. Had we known it might have been possible to link the stimulus to an unpleasant response or to offer an alternative, socially acceptable gratification. Alternatively on a wider plane this boy appeared to delight in faeces, and an aversion reaction to faeces, real or imaginary, in a variety of contexts might have been built up.

Discussion

The four in-patients here are a small series to report, but their importance lies in part in that they were considered sufficiently disturbed on grounds other than encopresis to merit admission to a children's psychiatric in-patient unit. Probably none could have been treated in their own homes, but on the other hand admissions to the therapeutic environment of the hospital and individual psychotherapy had not of itself cured the encopresis.

In interpreting the shape of the graphs here presented, note must be made of technical imperfections in the method of scoring. In the graph of "bowel actions" occurring other than in the lavatory, what is really scored is the number of occasions on which pants or pyjamas were seen to be soiled. This has a maximum score of 10 points per day because only four inspections were made of day wear and one inspection of nightwear. Case three, with a constant trickle of faeces, scored higher than Case two who passed large, formed motions although they were both invariably encopretic at the start of training. As Case three improved, the sphincter regained its competence and the trickle stopped. This is reflected by an abrupt early fall in the curve. However after the first few weeks no boy was incontinent of a full-sized formed stool, but only of small quantities. In Case one the faecal soiling was so slight that there was doubt as to whether he had been incontinent or merely careless in wiping himself after bowel action. However a score of one was made each time soiled pants were found.

In the case of bowel actions in the lavatory there is a peak early in treatment followed by a falling off. This is misleading. Early in treatment these boys passed frequent small formed stools. Later they were passing less frequent but larger stools. The latter condition more closely resembles normality, but the size of stool could not be adequately represented in the scoring method. This alteration in the size and frequency of bowel action presumably represents a recovery of tone and co-ordination of colonic activity which is not under voluntary control, consequent on correct action of the anal sphincter which is under voluntary control. In one boy cessation of medication with Isogel reduced the total faecal material to be passed. At the time of first follow up, approximately four months after onset of treatment and one-two months after clinical continence, it was noted that none of the three continent boys were normal, if the criteria of normality is taken as an empty rectum.

Bearing these considerations in mind the scores plotted could well represent on the one hand an exponential curve representing learning to perform the act in a particular situation and on the other hand decay of a learned response to perform in another situation, which response is related to several different factors, all of which are being affected by decay of learned responses.

To obtain learning curves which would be capable of accurate and rigid interpretation in terms of learning theory would require very detailed and numerous psysiological measurements on each boy to ascertain precisely what physiological responses were contributing to the final clinical score of pants soiled or "normal" bowel actions.

The attempt to investigate them however would have caused so much discomfort to the boys as to interfere with the training programme.

In the three cases in which success was achieved it was postulated that an aversion reaction to voluntary defaecation had been built up by earlier experiences. In Case one, the inconvenience and unpleasantness of the lavatory may have been the initiating factor. In Case two, violent punishment for the initial acts of incontinence and in Case three chronic constipation with the frequent experience of pain during passage of hard faecal masses may have started the process.

Aversion reactions tend to decay unless persistently reinforced (Eysenck, 1963). If a child is punished for any act of defaecation, then the experience tends to generalize to all acts of defaecation unless other factors are at work to produce a situation in which discrimination can be learned. In the present cases a situation was reached in which every act of defaecation was punished, because they always defaecated in the wrong places. In Case one, we know that he was repeatedly punished for defaecation and the smacking was immediately followed by the further punishment of a long period of enforced sitting on a pot—when his rectum must have been empty. The consequence of emptying the rectum was punishment, whereas it should have been a manifestly gratified mother or mother-substitute.

In Case two, there were violent beatings following bowel actions, without any maternal congratulations or reward for bowel action in the lavatory. It is not surprising that discrimination failed and the boy became constipated.

The normal mother, training her child expresses pleasure when he uses the pot. In Case three, the mother's anxiety about faeces may well have prevented her from feeling or expressing this pleasure. The boy was subjected to a great many unpleasant procedures affecting his rectum and recollects the passage of faeces as painful and frightening. Lavatory refusal also became a satisfying piece of behaviour because it annoyed and alarmed his mother.

In each case the conditions for reinforcing an aversion reaction were maintained prior to admission to hospital. After admission, reinforcement largely ceased. During the treatment periods scrupulous care was taken to avoid associating defaecation with pain or unpleasantness. Simultaneously during the treatment period, DISCRIMINATION TRAINING occurred by rewarding defaecation in the right place but not in the wrong place. Once this process began it tended to be self reinforcing because the children could appreciate the significance of their success.

There is a considerable degree of agreement between authors of different view-points that learning is an essential factor in development of normal faecal continence. Thus Anthony (1957) draws attention to cues given by the child to the mother and the mother to the child but goes on to reach the conclusion that the discontinuous type of encopretic, which includes all four cases mentioned here needs prolonged psychotherapy, which is at variance with the experience reported here. Pinkerton (1958) describes the same factors as were present in the cases described here, but proceeds to make a false dichotomy when he states that treatment was "first directed to convincing the parents that what they had formerly regarded as a physical disorder was in fact of emotional origin." He ascribes his success to the disinhibitions of aggressive impulses which were finding expression symbolically in defaecation, but it may well have been that the success was equally due to his having enlightened the parents about the factors in training, of which he was himself acutely aware and his play therapy was in fact a variation of the method of reciprocal inhibition of anxiety by self-assertive behaviour.

The same false dichotomy is made by Coekin and Gairdner (1960) who successfully treated children complaining of constipation and incontinence with laxatives. They postulated a constitutional colonic inertia, although this is as yet without supporting evidence, but offered no reason as to why the use of laxatives should produce normal bowel action after the administration of laxatives has ceased. It is suggested that the use of laxatives, together with the advice offered to the parents and child when prescribing the laxatives created conditions for the decay of the aversion reaction and learning of the new pattern of bowel action. The present author's experience with successful treatment of encopresis in adolescents by laxatives in a general medical clinic is consistent with this explanation. The thesis that the child, his parents and their medical advisors should tolerate this sort of unpleasant symptom (Winnicot 1953) in the interests of the child's overall mental health requires a very powerful defence when relatively simple measures, with a sound basis in theory can be applied. Finally there seems no reason why a psychiatrist should not prescribe a laxative to assist his behaviour therapy, nor a paediatrician give advice on training based on learning theory to complete the action of his pills.

Summary and Conclusions

A method of treating encopresis based on learning theory is described. It entails the following steps:

1. Accurate diagnosis of the physiological derangement by abdominal and rectal examination and inspection of stools as is normal in medical practice.

2. Correction of the physiological derangement if required by such measures as prescription of a bulk laxative such as Isogel.

3. Accurate diagnosis of the behavioural aetiology of the encopresis.

4. If the conditioned avoidance drive is not excessive (as in Cases 1, 2 and 3) then instrumental conditioning will be adequate and the regime as described may be instituted. The child is taken to the lavatory four times a day, to sit until a motion is passed or five minutes has elapsed whichever is shorter. If a motion is passed he is congratulated and given a sweet (or other appropriate reward). If his pants are soiled he is given clean ones. No punishments or rebukes of any sort are given for dirty pants and no rewards for clean ones. Once the child is clean he should still be rewarded intermittently for successful bowel actions for several months.

If the conditioned avoidance reaction is excessive as in Case 4 (and this could have been discovered before commencing the training regime) then a programme to reduce this must be devised. It may still be necessary to use the training regime at a later date.

This method has been applied to four cases of longstanding psychogenic encopresis resistant to other methods. There was rapid success in three cases and in the case which failed this is attributable to faulty application of learning theory rather than defects in the approach. Comparisons are made with paediatric and psychotherapeutic approaches and a wide area of agreement in practice with the principles of learning theory is found.

It is concluded that learning theory can usefully be applied to encopresis but methods can be further refined.

Acknowledgments—The major part of the treatment of these children was carried out by the nursing staff of the Children's Unit, Maudsley Hospital. It would not have been possible without the sustained efforts and enthusiasm and careful record keeping of the charge nurse, Mr. I. Dimmick, R.M.N., S.R.N. and his deputy Mrs. V. Verrell, R.M.N. Thanks are due also to Dr. K. Cameron, Physician in charge of the Children's Dept., Maudsley Hospital for permission to study and report on the children in his care. I also wish to thank Dr. S. Rachman of the Institute of Psychiatry for his suggestions on the psychological aspects of this study.

References

Anthony, A.: An experimental approach to the psychopathology of childhood: Encopresis. *Brit J Med Psychol 30,* 146-175, 1957.

Coekin, M. and Gairdner, D.: Faecal Incontinence in Children: The physical factor. *Brit Med J 2,* 1175-1180.

Eysenck, H. J.: Behaviour therapy, extinction and relapse in neurosis. *Brit J Psychiat 109,* 12-18, 1963.

Ferster, C. B.: Reinforcement and punishment in the control of human behaviour by social agencies. *Psychiat Res Rep 10,* 101-118, 1958.

Gaston, E. A.: The physiology of faecal continence. *Surg Genec Obstet 87,* 280-290 and 669-678, 1948.

Goligher, J. C. and Hughes, E. S. R.: Sensibility of the rectum and colon. Its role in the mechanism of anal continence. *Lancet 1,* 543-548, 1951.

Gwynne-Jones, H.: Learning and abormal behavior, in *Handbook of Abnormal Psychology* (Ed. H. J. Eysenck). Pitman, London, 1960.

Keele, C. A. and Neil, E.: Samson Wright's *Applied Physiology.* 3rd Edn. London, 1961.

Mowrer, O. H. and Mowrer, W.: Enuresis a method for its study and treatment. *Amer J Orthopsychiat 8,* 436-459, 1938.

Pinkerton, P.: Psychogenic megacolon in children: The implications of bowel negativism. *Arch Dis Childh 33,* 371-380, 1958.

Skinner, B. F.: *Cumulative Record.* Appleton-Century-Crofts, New York, 1959.

Winnicot, D. W.: Sympton tolerance in paediatrics. *Proc Roy Soc Med 46,* 675-684, 1953.

Wolpe, J.: *Psychotherapy by Reciprocal Inhibition.* Stanford University Press, Stanford, 1958.

Chapter 6

FOOD AS THE REINFORCER IN THE OUTPATIENT TREATMENT OF ANOREXIA NERVOSA*

C. B. SCRIGNAR

IN 1868 SIR WILLIAM GULL described an eating disorder, which in 1874 was named "anorexia nervosa." This enigmatic and paradoxical condition has as its central theme an apparent self-starvation. The syndrome has attracted much attention and clinical comment through the years. The description of anorexia nervosa has not changed significantly to date. The patient is usually an energetic adolescent female who is somewhat sensitive about her weight. The condition is often precipitated by a casual remark from a friend or relative that the patient is fat or chubby. Extreme dieting, volitionally induced vomiting, or both, occur at the outset, soon leading to weight loss and symptoms of starvation, including endocrine insufficiencies, amenorrhea and changes in metabolism. This self-imposed starvation can ultimately result in death.

Psychoanalytic concepts have attached another dimension to this disorder. Fenichel (1945) described anorexia nervosa patients as having a fear of oral impregnation with sadistic wishes, an ascetic reaction formation, and characterized the condition as a compulsion

*From the *Journal of Behavior Therapy and Experimental Psychiatry,* 1971, 2, pp. 31-36. Reprinted by permission of the author and Pergamon Press, Ltd.

neurosis. Others (Nemiah, 1958: Gardner, 1959; Finch, 1967) assert that an important aspect of anorexia nervosa is the patient's fear of growing up and relate this to a fear of attaining sexual maturity.

Kolb (1968) and Char (1970) have recommended that initial medical intervention should concentrate on the nutritional needs of the patient and the use of a "common sense" approach. To date, treatment recommendations have included tube feeding, collaboration of an internist and a psychiatrist, firmness rather than force regarding food intake, hospitalization, insulin, and hormones. Prefrontal lobotomy has also been prescribed (Carmody and Vibber, 1952). Most clinicians stress the importance of the adolescent-parent conflict and recommend psychotherapy. Interestingly, psychotherapy is usually recommended only after the problem of the eating disorder has been resolved.

A different therapeutic approach is suggested by Ayllon (1964). He states that there is no need to search for an underlying cause for the anorexia but merely to analyze the current eating behavior of these patients. He bases his treatment of hospitalized (mostly psychotic) patients with eating disorders and some with chronic anorexia on concepts derived from Skinnerian learning theory. He reports extremely good results with this difficult patient population. Bachrach (1965) reported on the inpatient treatment of more typical anorexia nervosa patients utilizing environmental reinforcers. Patients were told that privileges such as visitors, television, magazines, radios, etc., were contingent on the ingestion of food and weight gain. The anorexia nervosa patients were immediately verbally rewarded by the staff for eating. This program of applying verbal and post-prandial reinforcers proved to be quite successful. Halsten (1965) has reported successfully treating one case of anorexia nervosa by systematic desentization. Blinder, Freeman and Stunkard (1970) observed the motor hyperactivity of anorexia nervosa patients and verified it by the use of a pedometer. The desire of the patients to walk was then used as a positive reinforcer. Walking privileges and passes were made contingent on ingestion of food and weight gain. The authors reported good results with several patients.

This report illustrates the utilization of food reinforcement in the outpatient treatment of one case of anorexia nervosa.

A Case Report

Diane, a 14-year-old schoolgirl, was extremely intelligent, conscientious and energetic. She participated in many extra-curricular activities and was a class leader. She was five feet two inches tall and weighed 135 lb. One evening her father made a casual remark that she was "a bit big in the hips." Diane being a sensitive girl, immediately resolved to lose weight. After her next meal she went to the bathroom and induced vomiting by sticking her finger down her throat. She then began to practice this self-induced vomiting after every meal. Soon it was no longer necessary for her to induce the vomiting; she merely had to eat a meal, walk into a bathroom and she would automatically vomit. Diane secretly continued this pattern for a year and her body weight dropped more than 50 lb.

At this point, a family friend mentioned to the parents that Diane "looked quite thin and frail." The parents only then became aware of Diane's thinness and sent her to a physician. The doctor reported that Diane was amenorrheic and cachetic, and made the diagnosis of anorexia nervosa. He recommended psychotherapy and Diane was referred to a psychiatrist.

During this period of psychotherapy, the parents became quite concerned about their daughter's food ingestion into which a hyperphagic component now entered. Diane, in a constant state of hunger, would sneak food at home. She ate voraciously, knowing she would vomit but that she would receive some immediate gratification of her hunger. On some occasions she would eat so much that in the morning no food remained for the rest of the family. Diane's desperation about food was revealed when she was involved in an automobile accident. Leaving a store after buying cookies, she was seen by her father, who followed her. Diane began to speed and wrecked her automobile. Cookies were found on the seat of the car. The accident resulted in the revocation of her driver's license and increased vigilance by the parents concerning her ingestion of food. At school Diane ate her lunch and frequently obtained from her fellow students their uneaten portions of food. She immediately went to the school bathroom and vomited.

After one year of conventional psychotherapy, her eating patterns had not changed and her body weight had not altered significantly. Her psychiatrist, sensing the conflict in the interaction between Diane and her parents, recommended that she stay with her grandparents who lived several hundred miles away. Diane lived with her grandparents for approximately one year but no substantial weight gain occurred. She was then referred to me.

Diane was given a thorough physical examination, a mental status examination, and psychological testing. Interviews were held with the parents. Diane was asked to keep a journal of her eating habits over a one week span. She was told to make a list of food preferences. Following is the list she submitted:

Like very much	Like	Dislike
ice cream	fresh fruit	milk (as a beverage)
popsicles	cottage cheese	asparagus
waffles	squash	pancakes
green or jello salads	lunch meat	lima beans
all meats	bacon	potatoes—boiled and mashed
iced tea	french fries	rye bread
coffee	baked potatoes	peanut butter
seafood (tuna and shrimp)	bread	
cookies	crackers	
vegetables	french bread	
melon and berries	pies, cakes, pastries	
eggs		
hard rolls		
English muffins		
soups		
diet soda		
dill pickles		
certain cereals		

Treatment

Diane's eating disorder was conceptualized in the following way. Her immediate desire to lose weight resulted in volitionally induced vomiting following each meal. Emesis following eating became automatic after a time. It was hypothesized that frequent vomiting reduced the size and capacity of her stomach, so that eating a normal meal led to a feeling of "stuffiness." WHEN THIS INTERNAL STIMULUS WAS COMBINED WITH THE EXTERNAL CONDITIONED STIMULI OF A BATHROOM, vomiting occurred. The habit sequence thus generated was eating—feeling full or "stuffy" in the stomach—going to a bathroom—vomiting. The hyperphagia was due to the constant state of hunger following on the inability to retain food. The concern of the parents regarding Diane's ingestion of food reinforced the hyperphagia.

Treatment was initiated by placing Diane on a "diet." She was asked to purchase a letter scale, and a regime was constructed using precise weights of all foods ingested. The amounts of the foods included in the diet were below the normal quantities eaten by a person of her age, sex, height and weight. A multiple vitamin pill was included at the beginning of each day. The diet was constructed in such a fashion that it would be well rounded in proteins, carbohydrates and fats. The most preferred foods were presented at the end of each meal to act as positive reinforcers. Below is the diet designed for the patient at the onset of treatment.

Day of Week	Breakfast	Lunch	Supper

Monday	1 multi vitamin
	1 Waffle
	¼ melon
	Coffee or tea with
	  cream and sugar
		1 cup soup
		1 cookie
		Jello salad
		Ice tea or coffee
		  with sugar
			3 oz. steak
			2 oz. peas
			½ baked potato
			1 small serving dessert
			  (half of your usual
			  portion)
			beverage

Tuesday	1 multi vitamin
	4 oz. fruit juice
	1 egg any style
	1 Eng. muffin with
	  butter and jam
	1 cup beverage with
	  cream and sugar
		3 oz. tuna salad
		1 dill pickle
		1 hard roll
		Coffee, ice tea or
		  soda pop (not diet)
			1 small green salad and
			  your favorite
			  dressing
			3 oz. chicken any style
			  (deboned)
			½ cup rice with or
			  without gravy
			2 oz. vegetable
			beverage

Wednesday	1 multi vitamin
	½ cup strawberries
	  with sugar
	½ cup cereal with
	  sugar and milk
	1 cup coffee with
	  cream and sugar
		½ cup soup
		½ sandwich with 1
		  slice meat, lettuce
		  and tomato
		2 cookies
		beverage
			3 oz. roast beef
			3 oz. vegetable
			1 hard roll and butter
			1 small portion of
			  dessert
			beverage

Thursday	1 multi vitamin
	4 oz. fruit juice
	1 egg any style
	1 slice toast with
	  jam and butter
	1 cup coffee with
	  cream and sugar
		3 oz. shrimp salad
		2 crackers
		beverage: tea, coffee,
		  nondiet soda
		potato chips (10
		  medium size chips)
			3 oz. meat loaf
			Jello salad
			1 small ear corn
			beverage

Friday	1 multi vitamin	Hamburger 3 oz.	Red beans and rice
	¼ melon	1 slice bread or ½	(½ usual portion)
	½ cup cereal with	bun with dressing	1 small green salad
	milk and sugar	beverage: tea, coffee,	and favorite dressing
	1 cup coffee with	or nondiet soda	1 hard roll
	cream and sugar	1 small piece of	beverage
		fresh fruit	
Saturday	1 multi vitamin	½ cup soup	Spaghetti (½ usual
	4 oz. fruit juice	1 piece lunch meat	portion)
	1 egg any style	1 slice bread and	french bread
	1 Eng. muffin with	dressing and lettuce	1 small green salad
	butter and jam	and tomato	and favorite dressing
	1 cup coffee with	2 cookies	beverage
	cream and sugar	beverage: tea, coffee,	
		or nondiet soda	
Sunday	1 multi vitamin	1 hard-boiled egg	3 oz. ham
	4 oz. fruit juice	Small green salad with	½ cup potato salad
	1 pastry	favorite dressing	½ portion dessert
	1 cup coffee with	1 hard roll	beverage
	cream and sugar	beverage: tea, coffee,	
		or nondiet soda	

Bedtime Snack: Fourth meal.
If no vomiting has occurred during the day, you may have:
1 serving of ice cream or pudding.

If vomiting has occurred during day, snack will consist of:
1 cup soup of choice and 4 crackers with 2 oz. cheese.

Snacks: May be eaten at any time. Limit amount in order to avoid feeling "stuffy."
popsicles
celery
carrot sticks
pickles
cucumbers
soda pop

The bedtime snacks acted as delayed reinforcers. Foods in the "like very much" category were contingent on no vomiting during the day, while foods in the "like" category were offered if vomiting after one or more meals occurred.

The hyperphagic component of Diane's eating disorder was dealt with in the following manner. At any time of the day she was allowed to eat celery, pickles, popsickles, and related foods which she highly desired but which would not cause any feeling of stuffiness.

The third aspect of the treatment program concerned the parents. Consultations were held with the mother and the father to discuss the treatment regime. Concepts of negative reinforcement were explained, and they were told to ignore the eating patterns of their daughter. Interviews with the patient consisted of a weigh-in, followed by a discussion of the diet which could be changed according to the patient's report. An illustration of the alterations in the diet following the first session are given below:

Patient's comments on diet

Monday Breakfast: Adequate, breakfast with fruits or melons seem to be better than those breakfasts not containing these foods.

Monday Lunch: Hot soup undesirable during the summer, cookies at the end extremely good. Dessert at the end of either lunch or dinner leaves a satisfying sensation in the stomach.

Monday Dinner: Quite good.

Tuesday Breakfast: Breakfast too skimpy, often substituted berries for juice, two strips of bacon should be added.

Tuesday Lunch: Very good, loves tuna fish and hard rolls.

Tuesday Dinner: Very good, but quantity of rice or vegetables should be reduced. Would rather have had some room saved for dessert. Substitute a dessert for the vegetable.

Wednesday Breakfast: For breakfast usually flaky cereals are used. Increase cereals from ½ to 1 cup.

Wednesday Lunch: Soup can be omitted here.

Wednesday Dinner: Very good, particularly roll and butter and dessert.

Thursday Breakfast: Add more to this breakfast, either two strips of bacon or two links of sausage or some fruit.

Thursday Lunch: Crackers or potato chips are preferable and dessert, such as cookies, added.

Thursday Dinner: Add small amount of dessert, such as fruits, pudding or cookies.

Friday Breakfast: Breakfast good, except increase cereal from ½ to 1 full cup.

Friday Lunch: Good.

Friday Dinner: Quite good.

Saturday Breakfast: Add bacon or sausage or grits.

Saturday Lunch: Eliminate soup.

Saturday Dinner: Quite good. Add very small portion of dessert.

Sunday Breakfast: Continue pastry, juice. Then to church and about 3½ hr later family usually eats breakfast. Add breakfast brunch —small pastry, either sausage or bacon, coffee with sugar if possible.

Sunday Dinner: Okay.

Comments on snacks in general: Soda and popsicles okay. Popsicles seem to be an ideal snack, can be used to substitute and guard against over-stuffing of undesirable foods. Pickles not desirable as a snack. Both the celery and cucumbers would be better if either cheese or some dressing were added.

Bedtime Snacks: Increase ice cream serving from 1 to 2—if any vomiting occurs during the day, continue the soup-cheese-crackers schedule.

The schedule of snacks was not consistently adhered to by the patient. There were periods of conflict with the parents about the diet, and during these the patient reverted to her indiscriminate hyperphagic pattern.

Results

At the beginning of treatment, Diane weighed 84 lb. The first four sessions were devoted to organizing a treatment program. After the fifth session approximately 1 month elapsed before Diane reappeared for treatment. During this month, she was arguing with her mother about the diet. An appointment was made with her mother to explain the treatment regime. Ten therapeutic sessions followed with two more interruptions of therapy. During these lapses, I realized that disagreements in the family were occurring and that a waiting period was in order. After these lapses the patient would call for another appointment and treatment would be resumed. At the conclusion of therapy, the patient had gone up from 84 lb to 106¼ lb. At a 6-month follow up the patient weighed 112 lb. Her appearance was markedly different. She was curvaceous and quite pretty. She had resumed menstruation and was making plans to graduate from high school and go to a college away from home. Instructions were conveyed to the patient regarding a more appropriate way of dieting if she desired to lose weight at some future date.

References

Ayllon T., Haughton, E. and Osmond, H. O.: Chronic anorexia: A behavior problem. *Can Psychiat J 9*, 147-154, 1964.

Bachrach, A. J., Erwin, W. J. and Mohr, J. P.: The Control of Eating Behavior in an Anorexic by Operant Conditioning Techniques. *Case Studies in Behavior Modification* (Edited by Ullman, L. and Krasner, L.). Holt, Winston, New York, 1965.

Blinder, J., Freeman, D. M. A. and Stunkard, A. J.: Behavior therapy of anorexia nervosa: Effectiveness of activity as a reinforcer of weight gain. *Am J Psychiat 126*, 1093-1098, 1970.

Bliss, E. L. and Branch, C. H.: *Anorexia Nervosa: Its History, Psychology and Biology.* Hoeber, New York, 1960.

Char, W. F. and McDermott, J. F.: Treating anorexia nervosa. *Medical Insight 2,* 41-49, 1970.

Fenichel, O.: *The Psychoanalytic Theory of Neurosis.* W. W. Norton, New York, 1945.

Finch, S. M.: Psychological Disorders. In *Comprehensive Textbook of Psychiatry.* (Edited by Freedman, A. M. and Kaplan, H. I.). Williams and Wilkins, Baltimore, 1967.

Gardner, G. E.: Psychiatric Problems of Adolescence. In *American Handbook of Psychiatry.* Arieti, S., Editor. Vol. I. New York: Basic Books, 1959.

Hallsten, E.: Adolescent anorexia nervosa treated by desensitization. *Behav Res Therapy 3,* 87-91, 1965.

Kolb, L. C.: *Noyes' Modern Clinical Psychiatry 11,* pp. 430-431. W. B. Saunders, Philadelphia, 1968.

Nemiah, J.: Anorexia nervosa: fact and theory. *Am J Digest Dis 3,* 249-271, 1958.

Wall, J. H.: Diagnosis, treatment and results in Anorexia Nervosa. *Am J Psychiat* 997-1001, 1959.

Chapter 7

BEHAVIOR THERAPY IN OBSESSIVE-COMPULSIVE NEUROSIS: TREATMENT OF AN ADOLESCENT BOY*

IRVING B. WEINER

A LTHOUGH SEVERAL WRITERS have described the successful application of behavior therapy in obsessive-compulsive neurosis, there has been some controversy concerning whether such treatment proceeds more efficaciously from a focus on the stimuli eliciting the neurotic behavior or on the maladaptive motor habits themselves. Walton (1960) reports a patient with a hand-washing compulsion who responded well to direct deconditioning of his motor responses but subsequently suffered complete relapse, and he concludes in agreement with Eysenck (1960) that learning theory methods achieve stable cures only if the *conditioned antonomic drives* generating a patient's neurosis are eliminated. Wolpe (1958, 1964) similarly considers the deconditioning of the neurotic anxiety to be the crux of behavior therapy in obsessional neurosis.

Yates (1958), on the other hand, asserts that merely extinguishing a compulsive patient's neurotic motor habits will sufficiently reduce his learned anxiety to obviate specific attention to the stimuli that were eliciting his maladaptive behavior. Substantiating this view,

*From *Psychotherapy: Theory, Research and Practice*, 1967, 4, pp. 27-29. Reprinted by permission of the author and the Journal.

Taylor (1963) presents a case of a woman with a 31-year history of compulsive depilation of her eyebrows who was readily and permanently relieved of her hair-pulling by negative reinforcement of the compulsive habit alone. Taylor concludes that while stimulus desensitization may be mandatory in the behavioral treatment of anxiety neurosis, compulsive disorders are so focused on the various habits involved that the entire neurosis, including its affective components, can be dissolved by reducing the habit strength of the compulsive acts at zero.

Walton and Mather (1963), however, suggest that the relative success of different treatment approaches to an obsessive-compulsive neurosis may be a function of its duration. Specifically, they hypothesize that treatment of motor phenomena, while ineffective in persons with compulsions of recent origin, may contribute to recovery from longstanding compulsive acts, since the latter have frequently become relatively autonomous and independent of the anxieties that initially triggered them. This modification of Walton's earlier position would account for Taylor's reported success with motor deconditioning, inasmuch as his patient's depilation was a symptom of many years' duration.

Further support for the Yates-Taylor arguments thus rests with demonstrating effective response-oriented treatment in obsessive-compulsive patients with symptoms of recent origin. This paper concerns such a patient, a seriously incapacitated obsessive-compulsive adolescent boy whose distress prompted a direct focus on his responses and who realized rapid improvement without relapse.

Case Material

The patient was a 15-year-old boy with a one-month history of acute onset of pervasive compulsive rituals involving washing and dressing, reading, and writing, and the compulsive placement of whatever objects he happened to handle during his daily activities. Almost every moment of his waking life was governed by one or another of these rituals, and he was terrorized by thoughts that if he failed in any way to execute them, either "something terrible" would happen to his parents or "I'll be drafted into the army and sent to Viet Nam and killed."

This boy was the only child of middle class, apparently emotionally stable parents, and he had no history of serious psychological disturbance. He had been seen for psychological consultation four years earlier when his parents had been concerned about his then mediocre school performance and overdependence on them to the exclusion of peer relationships. Interview and test data at that time had suggested a shy, somewhat withdrawn boy with a compulsive personality style, but no evidence of major psychopathology had emerged. It was concluded that he might require therapy at some future time, particularly should he develop acute symptomatology, but no treatment was then felt to be necessary. The next four years had passed without significant psychological incident, and it was only the recent onset of the patient's compulsive rituals and attendant acute distress that had led his parents to arrange the current psychotherapeutic contact.

At the end of the patient's first visit, during which the above history was obtained, he was asked, in preparation for the next session, to note during the subsequent week the exact circumstances in which his compulsions emerged. In the course of doing so, however, he experienced an intensification of his rituals and anxiety, to a point where he had difficulty eating and sleeping and was unable to study. It therefore seemed imperative, if he were to be spared hospitalization, to defer further investigation of the stimulus aspects of his disturbance in favor of a direct attack on his motor symptoms. Once this decision was made, he was helped to list five compulsive behaviors that troubled him most and was told that these rituals, taken in reverse order of their severity, would be evaluated and eliminated in the ensuing sessions.

The treatment plan for alleviating his distress was TO REPLACE THE PERVASIVE MALADAPTIVE RITUALS WITH DELIMITED RITUALS THAT WOULD INTERFERE ONLY MINIMALLY WITH NORMAL ACTIVITY. This plan was implemented in each instance by first establishing some *positive* reason for his ritual and then constructing a substitute ritual that would achieve the same end more quickly and efficiently.

The method employed can be illustrated by reference to one of his less complex rituals, a compulsive checking and relocking of his school locker at least three times whenever he locked it. When first asked why he checked the lock, he answered, "Because if I don't I'm afraid I'll end up in Viet Nam." He was then told that he had given a *negative* reason, one that indicated what was *bad* about *not* checking his lock, and that he was being asked rather to identify something *good* about checking it. After a moment's thought he replied that checking the lock was a worthwhile precaution against having things stolen, particularly since some thefts had been reported in his school. This concern with guarding his possessions was praised by the therapist as an important *positive* reason for being certain his locker was locked, and he was next requested to specify exactly what action he thought would be necessary to guarantee this positive end. He decided that locking the lock and checking it once would certainly ensure the safety of his belongings.

He was then told that during the following week every time he closed his locker he was to lock the lock, check it once, and then take one step back, put his hands in his pockets and say to himself the following: "I have checked the lock; and I can now be certain it is locked and everything in the locker is safe and protected; there is absolutely no positive reason for me to check it again; I am now going to walk away from it and go to class." He was then to leave the lock as it was until he next needed access to his locker. He was further told that he might not always be able to succeed in this assignment and that, should he feel unable to resist rechecking the lock, he was to do so; however, he was not to worry about such lapses and was by all means to try again to implement the prescribed formula the next time and every subsequent time he used his locker.

Similar procedures were followed with all of the rituals on the patient's list. For each he was helped to identify some positive value in the behavior (most of the values he specified involved neatness, cleanliness, or thoroughness); he was asked to decide what steps were necessary to ensure the positive value (in each instance he expressed confidence in actions far less extensive than his current rituals); and he was provided some alternate, relatively economic ritual based on his specifications and with a series of justifying statements to repeat to himself as he executed the modified behavior. He was also repeatedly instructed that some failures were inevitable, should not concern him and did not mean that he was losing his fight against his disturbance.

The patient carried out his instructions faithfully and in the course of six weekly sessions displayed marked behavior change. In each case the rituals prescribed served either to replace or diminish his former rituals. For example, instead of washing his face for 15 minutes in the morning, he was now using his watch to terminate his face-washing precisely after three minutes, a time period he had specified as sufficient to ensure cleanliness. As he was thus able to attenuate his rituals, his feelings of being dominated by unrealistic, uncontrollable urges and his general anxiety level abated dramatically. His eating, sleeping, and school-work returned to normal, and his parents noted that he was considerably more relaxed and engaged in recreational activities which he had felt unable to pursue at the beginning of the treatment.

After eight weekly sessions the patient was seen irregularly over the next seven months. During this follow-up period he remained essentially symptom-free and even spontaneously gave up most of the substitute rituals that had been established in the therapy. When encouraged in the last session to explore anything that might be troubling him, he spoke only of normal adolescent developmental concerns about school, parents, and social relationships.

Discussion

As recently pointed out by Phillips and El-Batrawi (1964), learning theory approaches to psychotherapy have generally focused on *stimulus* rather than *response* variables, and relatively little attention has been devoted to the potential benefits of helping a patient to develop new outputs to replace his current, pathologic output.

Much benefit seemed to accrue from the technique's simultaneous utilization and circumvention of his obsessive-compulsive personality style. On the one hand, his involvement in the treatment was probably promoted by the fact that his characterological emphases on cleanliness and neatness and his preference to conduct his life in an orderly, scheduled manner were neither demeaned nor denied him; rather, the therapist endorsed *positive* aspects of these values and encouraged him to continue to perform rituals, albeit rituals far more in tune with realistic necessity than those that brought him for help.

On the other hand, the therapeutic approach circumvented certain features of his characterological style that might otherwise have impeded his progress. First, he was instructed to act, to *do* things rather than to *think* about them, which steered him away from the ruminations and dread that initially incapacitated him. Secondly, by frequently telling him that he would probably not always be able to succeed in his assigned tasks and that failure should not concern him or prevent him from trying further, the therapist provided him with a set of standards much less harsh than his own rigidly obsessive code of success and failure.

Finally significant (once the patient began to carry out his assignments and achieve even minimal success) was the rewarding sense of confidence and self-determination he was able to realize. Each wedge he drove into his symptoms occasioned increasing optimism that he could eventually triumph over his compulsions, and his heightened feeling of competence probably contributed heavily to the general reduction in his anxiety level and to his resistance to relapse.

References

Eysenck, H. J.: Learning theory and behavior therapy. In H. J. Eysenck (Ed.), *Behaviour therapy and the neuroses*. New York: Pergamon Press, pp. 4-21, 1960.

Phillips, E. L. and El-Batrawi, S.: Learning theory and psychotherapy revisited: with notes on illustrative cases. *Psychotherapy 1*, 145-150, 1964.

Taylor, J. G.: A behavioural interpretation of obsessive-compulsive neurosis. *Behav Res & Therapy 1*, 237-244, 1963.

Walton, D.: The relevance of learning theory to the treatment of an obsessive-compulsive state. In H. J. Eysenck (Ed.), *Behaviour therapy and the neuroses*. New York, Pergamon Press, pp. 170-180, 1960.

Walton, D. and Mather, M. D.: The application of learning principles to the treatment of obsessive-compulsive states in the acute and chronic phases of illness. *Behav Res & Therapy 1*, 163-174, 1963.

Wolpe, J.: *Psychotherapy by reciprocal inhibition*. Stanford, Cal., Stanford University Press, 1958.

Wolpe, J.: Behaviour therapy in complex neurotic states. *Brit J Psychiatry 110*, 28-34, 1964.

Yates, A. J.: Symptoms and symptom substitution. *Psychological Review 65*, 371-374, 1958.

Section III
BEHAVIORAL CLASSROOM MANAGEMENT

SOME READERS MIGHT QUESTION THE RELATIONSHIP BETWEEN THE CONTENTS OF SECTION III AND THE TITLE AND THEME OF THIS WORK, "CLINICAL STUDIES IN BEHAVIOR THERAPY WITH CHILDREN, ADOLESCENTS, AND THEIR FAMILIES." AFTER ALL, IT MIGHT BE ARGUED THAT CLASSROOM BEHAVIOR MANAGEMENT IS IMPORTANT BUT NOT DIRECTLY RELATED TO BEHAVIOR THERAPY. AS COMMUNITY MENTAL HEALTH-ORIENTED PROFESSIONALS, WE RETORT THAT THE CLASSROOM ACTUALLY REPRESENTS THE NATURAL SETTING FOR MUCH PRIMARY AND SECONDARY PREVENTION IN THE CHILD CLINICAL FIELD. THUS ANY BOOK RELATED TO CHILD CLINICAL PROBLEMS WOULD BE REMISS IN OMITTING A SCHOOL-FOCUSED SECTION.

SPACE LIMITATIONS AND THE AVAILABILITY OF NUMEROUS OTHER EXCELLENT WORKS RELATED TO BEHAVIOR MODIFICATION IN THE CLASSROOM LED US TO CURTAIL THE NUMBER OF READINGS IN THIS SECTION. THE ARTICLES CHOSEN REPRESENT PRACTICAL AND, HOPEFULLY, HELPFUL READINGS (STEADMAN, ET. AL. AND CANTRELL ET. AL.) OR STUDIES RELATED TO BEHAVIOR PROBLEMS AND POPULATIONS RECEIVING LESS FREQUENT ATTENTION (MCALLISTER, ET. AL. AND MILLER, ET. AL.). IT IS OUR HOPE THAT MENTAL HEALTH PROFESSIONALS, WHO ARE INCREASINGLY ENGAGING IN CLASSROOM CONSULTATION ACTIVITIES, WILL FIND THESE PARTICULAR ARTICLES TO BE USEFUL ADDITIONS TO PREVIOUSLY PUBLISHED WORKS.

Chapter 1

CONTINGENCY CONTRACTING WITH SCHOOL PROBLEMS*

ROBERT P. CANTRELL, MARY LYNN CANTRELL, CLIFTON M. HUDDLESTON *and* RALPH L. WOOLDRIDGE

THIS PAPER DISCUSSES OUR ADAPTATION of operant methodology to deal with school children's problem behaviors in the setting of a diagnostic and remediation center. The methods described are based primarily on the structuring of available reinforcement contingencies to reinforce approximations to the desired appropriate school behaviors. The data presented are preliminary but suggest that systematic research in these methods might be very fruitful. The term "contingency contract" was borrowed from L. P. Homme (1966), who used written contracts with adolescent potential dropouts to spell out the reinforcers that were to follow completion of academic tasks. The present contract involved a somewhat different procedure. The CONTINGENCY CONTRACT was a written explanation of the changes in contingencies to be used by the natural contingency managers, parents and/or teachers. It usually also contained: (1) a written schedule of desired behaviors (such as approximations to school attendance or behaviors involved in appropriate school achievement) with assigned point values, and (2) a written sched-

*From the *Journal of Applied Behavior Analysis*, 1969, 2 (3), pp. 215-220. Copyright 1969 by the Society for the Experimental Analysis of Behavior, Inc. Reprinted by permission of the Society and the author.

ule of high probability behaviors (Premack, 1965) (individually defined rewards, privileges, preferred activities) with assigned exchange values.

The efficacy of structuring reinforcement contingencies to shape or maintain adaptive behavior in children is evident in a growing volume of behavior studies (Staats, Minke, Finley, Wolf, and Brooks, 1964; Ullmann and Krasner, 1965; Homme, 1966; Nolen, Kunzelmann, and Haring, 1967; O'Leary and Becker, 1967; Bushell, Wrobel, and Michaelis, 1968; Wolf, Giles, and Hall, 1968; McKenzie, Clark, Wolf, Kothera, and Benson, 1968; Hewett, Taylor, and Artuso, 1969). The present procedure was devised to see if viable changes in child behavior could be brought about by guiding parents and teachers in procedures of contingency control where frequency counting, direct observation, and direct manipulation by professionals were not immediately possible. Problems with which these procedures have been used have ranged from persistent school runaway behavior, school nonattendance, hyper-aggressivity, and stealing, to achievement motivation in underachieving students. Subjects were public school children, first through eleventh graders, from the seven parish areas served by the Louisiana Tech Special Education Center; all lived at a distance of 10 to 85 miles from the Center. The procedures described were initially the result of the need to deal with situational difficulties of sometimes near-crisis dimensions for the families and schools involved. Since most of these problems were of situational origin, the primary intervention procedures thought necessary were those of minimal prescriptive restructuring to alleviate the immediate problem.

Formulation of a contingency contract generally approximated the following pattern. Initially, referral information indicated if a problem might be largely one of motivation rather than academic programming. In considering the use of a contract, some sign was needed that the child could actually do or had done what was expected of him (such as inconsistent grades, intelligence test results, or adequate achievement test scores). If the child was badly in need of special academic programming, motivation by means of a contract might have been detrimental, unless that programming could have been provided in that setting. Also, if special programming would have been sufficient for motivation in and of itself, there would obviously have been no need for a contract.

After referral, the first step was to interview the child's adult agents. If the school appeared incapable of following the exigencies of a contract explicitly, only the parents and home were involved. If the home was unlikely to cooperate and the school would, only the school was involved. In most cases both agencies entered in, even though personal interviews might have been only with parents. Parents who had exhausted all available external sources of remediation and who were still concerned about their child's problems appeared to be the most willing to restructure their child-management contingencies.

Parents and teachers were told that it would be better not to attempt to write a contract unless they definitely wanted such help and were willing to involve their own personal effort in its success. This was done for at least two reasons: (1) If the system were to be attempted half-heartedly, it would not be enforced consistently and whatever extinction procedures were necessary would not occur. (2) If the agents were to give up on the system at the point where the child was testing it most severely, they would probably terminate with the maladaptive behavior at a higher peak and one even more resistant to change than before.

Initial interviews with the natural contingency managers were used to provide answers to the following questions:

1. What specifically were the key problem behaviors and how often did they occur? These primary behaviors were isolated and some provisions for counting their pre-intervention frequency were made to provide "baseline" data.

2. What was the typical or occasional consequence of these problem behaviors? Careful interviewing at this point provided a fairly complete list of usual consequences and some estimate of the schedules of their usage which appeared to be maintaining the maladaptive behavior.

3. What were the events, privileges, pastimes, foods, and material possessions which already served as reinforcements for this child? These were usually obtained by asking the parents or teachers what the child liked to do if he had the opportunity, what he spent the most time doing, what he would work for,

and if any other consequence might possibly serve as a reinforcing event. Parents and teachers were usually able to provide a fairly complete list of reinforcers for their children in a roughly hierarchical arrangement of value to the child. For each reinforcer the parent was queried as to how the child at that time gained access to these reinforcers. In almost all cases, access to desired reinforcers was not being made contingent upon approximations to the desired behavior.

4. What might be used as a definite punishment or extinction consequence of an undesirable behavior if needed? This question was usually posed to the parents in the form of asking what the child would work to avoid, what seemed to be the most effective punishment if punishment were needed, and how easily might the parents or teachers be able to legislate specific punishing contingencies if they were found to be necessary. Here again, parents or teachers were usually able to identify a rough hierarchy of events which the child would work to avoid.

Once these basic questions were answered, the problem became one of how to change the contingencies in order to utilize reinforcers already available. The written contract had to be clear, complete, useful as ongoing data to judge its effectiveness, and simple enough to carry out that its demands did not make it aversive to the agents enforcing it. The child was presented with the record sheets and the new regimen by his parents or teacher. In most cases he took his weekly sheet of earned points to school where his teacher gave him points as earned and then brought it home where his parents gave him points earned at home. Points earned at school and home were spent on a daily and weekly basis. His weekly record sheet of points spent was kept at home for easy reference by the child.

Behavioral change was monitored by building into the contract methods of measuring the problem behavior before the contract went into effect, of graphing progress continually, and of measuring the problem behavior after intervention with the contract had been completed. Independent records from the schools (such as grades, attendance records, incidences of maladaptive behavior) were obtained in addition to parental report forms.

The contracts generally fell into two ways of arranging contingencies once the problem behaviors and available reinforcers had been delineated. In the first, receipt of the reinforcers was simply made contingent on adaptive behaviors that were incompatible with the problem behaviors. For example, R's parents and teachers complained that he did not complete homework or class assignments unless he did so very carelessly and that he did not work or listen to directions without constant reminders and "pushing." R's contract was formulated as follows:

Contingency Contract:

This contract defines the ways in which R can earn points by doing specific things at school and at home that would be necessary for his academic growth (*i.e.*, completing class assignments and homework). He exchanges these points for preferred activities or money (*i.e.*, going places, watching television, Coke money, *etc.*). He can earn an approximate maximum of 50 points per day or 250 points per week under this schedule.

R's teacher marks his points earned each day on his weekly record sheet of points earned (Table VIII) and sends home an average of one graded paper per day for which he gets additional points. His mother gives him points for homework done at home and keeps a record of points spent on the appropriate weekly sheet (Table VIII). When R wants to spend his points, he is allowed to and given verbal praise for having worked well enough at school to have enough points. When he does not have sufficient points for something he wants, a simple statement that he does not yet have enough points is made. It is crucial that R receive these privileges only when he has the required number of points already on his chart.

It appears that R's non-working at school results in getting more attention from adults than his working ordinarily does. Switching the tables on him should result in increased effort on his part. Efforts should be made to give R attention and approval when he is working and behaving as we would hope. Inappropriate behavior or non-working should result in little attention (punishment, reminders, scolding included) given to him. Insofar as possible, R should learn that he will be ignored when he is not working or behaving appropriately, but when he does put forth effort and behave appropriately, people are proud of him and give him attention.

In comparing six weeks' grades for the report before intervention and the report after intervention, R's grades stayed the same in three subjects, improved one letter in two subjects, and improved two letters in one subject.

In the second general method of contract arrangement, THE BE-HAVIORAL STEPS LEADING TOWARD THE DESIRED TERMINAL BEHAVIOR WERE ARRANGED IN SEQUENTIAL, PROGRAMMED FASHION. RECEIPT OF THE REINFORCERS WAS THEN MADE CONTINGENT ON THESE STEPS. In the case of S, a "school phobic" child, points were earned for approximations or steps toward full school attendance where she had previously had problems: getting out of bed (5 points); getting dressed (5 points); having breakfast (5 points); no crying before school (5 points); no illness before school (5 points); going to schoolbus (5 points); getting on schoolbus (5 points); going to class (5 points); going into classroom (5 points); staying in class (5 points per 15 min); no crying at school (5 points); no illness at school (5 points); homework started with no reminders (15 points), with one reminder (10 points); with two reminders (5 points), completed (5 additional points.) S exchanged points for: TV viewing, renting toys or books, helping mother in kitchen (25 points per 30 min); outside play time (50 points per 30 min); having friends over or going to visit friends

TABLE VIII
WEEKLY RECORD SHEET OF POINTS EARNED
Week of: _____

R earned points for:	Mon.	Tues.	Wed.	Thurs.	Fri.	Totals

Homework:
  completed (3 points)
  well done* (5 additional)						

Class assignments:
  completed (1 point each)
  well done* (2 additional)
  with no more than 2 misspelled
    words or careless
    arithmetic errors
      (1 additional)						

Listening and complying to
  directions without reminder
  (1 point each time)

Daily grades:
  A (10 points)
  B (6 points)
  C (3 points)
  D (1 point)

Homework:
  started with no warnings (5 points)
              one warning (3 points)
              two warnings (2 points)
              three warnings (1 point)
  completed by supper time (2 additional)

TOTALS

*Bonus: Baseball glove as soon as R earns 75 points total in these two "well done"
  categories

WEEKLY RECORD SHEET OF POINTS SPENT

Week of: —————————————

R exchanged his points for:	Mon.	Tues.	Wed.	Thurs.	Fri.	Sat.	Sun.	Totals
Outdoor time (5 points per ½ hour)								
Television viewing time (5 points per ½ hour)								
Kitchen time (cooking privileges) (5 points per ½ hour)								
Driving (as parents direct) (10 points per ½ hour)								
Going out privilege (10 points per event)								
Staying with friend all night or having one over for night (25 points per event)								
Money (up to limit set by parents) (5 cents per point)								

TOTALS

(100 points); going out privilege (150 points); overnight visit with friend (200 points); spending money (1 point per penny); plus an additional bonus of one article of new clothing for going to school one full week. The terminal state desired in S's case, full school attendance without resistance, was attained on the eighth school day after the contract was initiated and maintained throughout the rest of that and the next school year.

An essential part of the program was the inclusion of a built-in feedback system. Most of the contracts provided for parents or teachers to mail completed record forms to us weekly. Upon their receipt, blank forms were sent them for another week. Agents were initially given two weeks' worth of forms to allow for one week's transit in the mails. Parents and/or teachers were encouraged to write or call as problems or questions arose. The information gleaned from the obtained record forms was used to initiate telephone conference calls or visits to the agents or to clarify or change the contracts as behavior shifts occurred. This follow-up was crucial. Even if the contingency change as designed had "hit" upon the right combination of reinforcement schedules, consistent encouragement of the parents or agents of the contract was often necessary in order to maintain the behavior until new patterns of interaction had become more solidified.

In many cases, fading procedures from the contract were instituted at the child's request. A FADING procedure was seldom needed to wean the child away from the contract system. In most cases, the children themselves gave agents clues as to when to cease the program or how to ease it back to a more natural set of contingencies. In others, external situations caused a natural change back to more natural behavior management, such as the end of the school year. Parents often indicated a reluctance to terminate the contract before the end of the school year. Only a few resumed use of the contract at the beginning of the subsequent school year.

Parents and school personnel have communicated to the contract writers their enthusiasm about the procedures and results, and have often referred other cases for similar treatment. The fact that the contracts use reinforcers already present in the child's environment, rather than introducing new ones, seems to have appeal to the natural contingency managers with whom we have worked. Training the natural contingency managers inductively through the prescriptive, precise procedures of the contracts seems to result in the principles being learned more completely than when we have attempted to teach the principles of modifying behavior before dealing specifically with the problem behavior at hand.

Optimally, the use of direct observation in the home or the school to ascertain the agent's compliance with the contract, plus the use of multiple baseline procedures to validate the efficacy of the contract on other problem behaviors for the same child, would have provided more data for the validity of the procedures beyond parent and school reportings. Even here, the establishment of a functional relationship between the instigation of the contract and the changes that accrue would be subject to the problems of indeterminacy and changes in expectation (Rosenthal and Jacobson, 1968). Relying on the agent's report of behavior alone also posed difficulties in determining the actual course of the behavior as it was occurring. On the one hand, if the contract was being consistently enforced and still was not working as expected, the possibility existed that the authors of the contract had not eliminated the salient reinforcers maintaining the problem behavior or had not provided strong enough reinforcers to change it to a more adaptive form. In this case, a new combination or revision of the old combination of reinforcers in the old contract was necessary. On the other hand, it appeared to be risky to assume that the system needed changing too soon. Many of the maladaptive behaviors were thought to have been shaped by the child's being able to "wait out" or "outlast" adult contingencies. If this were the case, the problem became one of encouraging the adult agents to maintain the newly initiated contingencies in order to break the control-counter-control cycle being tested by the child. Further studies are now in progress using multiple baseline and independent observation in the home and school to clairify further the processes involved.

A primary concern of professionals often is one of maximum efficiency in meeting the behavioral crises of individual cases while continuing their professional efforts in other endeavors. If experimentally verified, the "contingency contract" method offers one possible avenue to resolve in a clinical setting the perpetual "minimax" conflict of bringing about maximal behavioral change with minimal expenditure of professional time and money. The prospects of the natural contingency managers in the child's situation, teachers and parents, actually administering the new procedures may be one means of closing the gap between the availability of professional staff and the press of public demand for their services.

In summary, the application of reinforcement theory in the form of written contingency contracts as specific directions through which the natural contingency managers can change problem behaviors appears to be a potentially useful tool for professionals dealing with children's problems. The effect of such contracting appears to be largely dependent upon: (1) the capacity of the professionals who prepare the contingencies to derive from verbal information those contingencies that appear to be maintaining the problem behavior and then to change them, and (2) the relative ability of the adults involved to maintain the contingencies spelled out by the contract.

References

Bushell, D., Jr., Wrobel, Patricia A. and Michaelis, Mary L.: Applying "group" contingencies to the classroom study behavior of preschool children, *J Appl Behav Analysis 1*, 55-62, 1968.

Hewett, F. M., Taylor, F. D. and Artuso, A. A.: The Santa Monica Project: Evaluation of an engineered classroom design with emotionally disturbed children. *Except Child 35*, 523-529, 1969.

Homme, L.: Human motivation and the environment. In N. Haring and R. Whelan (Eds.), *The learning environment: relationship to behavior modification and implications for special education*. Lawrence: University of Kansas Press, 1966.

McKenzie, H. S., Clark, Marilyn, Wolf, M. M., Kothera, R. and Benson, C.: Behavior modification of children with learning disabilities using grades as tokens and allowances as back-up reinforcers. *Except Child 34*, 745-752, 1968.

Nolen, Patricia A., Kunzelmann, H. P. and Haring, N. G.: Behavioral modification in a junior high learning disabilities classroom. *Except Child 33*, 163-168, 1967.

O'Leary, K. D. and Becker, W. C.: Behavior modification of an adjustment class: a token reinforcement program. *Except Child 33*, 637-642, 1967.

Premack, D.: Reinforcement theory. In D. Levine (Ed.), *Nebraska symposium on motivation: 1965*. Lincoln, University of Nebraska Press, pp. 123-180, 1965.

Rosenthal, R. and Jacobson, Lenore: *Pygmalion in the classroom: teacher expectation and pupils' intellectual development*. New York, Holt, Rinehart & Winston, 1968.

Staats, A. W., Minke, K. A., Finley, J. R., Wolf, M. and Brooks, L.: A reinforcer system and experimental procedures for the laboratory study of reading acquisition. *Child Devel 35*, 209-231, 1964.

Ullmann, L. P. and Krasner, L. (Eds.): *Case studies in behavior modification.* New York, Holt, Rinehart & Winston, 1965.

Wolf, M. M., Giles, D. K. and Hall, R. V.: Experiments with token reinforcement in a remedial classroom, *Behav Res Therapy 6*, 51-64, 1968.

Chapter 2

THE APPLICATION OF OPERANT CONDITIONING TECHNIQUES IN A SECONDARY SCHOOL CLASSROOM*

LORING W. McALLISTER, JAMES G. STACHOWIAK,
DONALD M. BAER *and* LINDA CONDERMAN

NUMEROUS STUDIES HAVE REPORTED the effectiveness of operant conditioning techniques in modifying the behavior of children in various situations. Harris, Wolf, and Baer (1964), in a series of studies on pre-school children, described the effectiveness of contingent teacher attention in modifying inappropriate behavior. Hall and Broden (1967), Patterson (1965), Rabb and Hewett (1967), and Zimmerman and Zimmerman (1962) have demonstrated the usefulness of teacher-supplied contingent social reinforcement in reducing problem behaviors and increasing appropriate behaviors of young children in special classrooms. Becker, Madsen, Arnold, and Thomas (1967); Hall, Lund, and Jackson (1968); and Madsen, Becker, and Thomas (1968) extended these techniques into the regular primary school classroom and demonstrated their effectiveness there. In all of the above studies, only a limited number of children were studied in each situation, usually one or two per classroom.

Thomas, Becker, and Armstrong (1968) studied the effects of

*From the *Journal of Applied Behavior Analysis,* 1969, 2 (4), pp. 277-285. Copyright 1969, 2 (4), pp. 277-285. Copyright 1969 by the Society for the Experimental Analysis of Behavior, Inc. Reprinted by permission of the Society and the author.

varying teachers' social behaviors on the classroom behaviors of an entire elementary school classroom of 28 students. By observing 10 children per session, one at a time, they demonstrated the effectiveness of approving teacher responses in maintaining appropriate classroom behaviors. Bushell, Wrobel, and Michaelis (1968) also applied group contingencies (special events contingent on earning tokens for study behaviors) to an entire class of 12 preschool children.

There has been an effort to extend the study of teacher-supplied consequences to larger groups of preschool and elementary school subjects in regular classrooms, but no systematic research investigating these procedures has yet been undertaken in the secondary school classroom. Cohen, Filipczak, and Bis (1967) reported the application of various non-social contingencies (earning points, being "correct," and taking advanced educational courses) in modifying attitudinal and academic behaviors of adolescent inmates in a penal institution. But there is no record of investigations into the effects of teacher-supplied social consequences on the classroom behavior of secondary school students in regular classrooms.

At present, the usefulness of contingent teacher social reinforcement in the management of student classroom behaviors is well documented on the preschool and primary elementary school levels, particularly when the investigation focuses on a limited number of children in the classroom. Systematic replication now requires that these procedures be extended to larger groups of students in the classroom and to students in the upper elementary and secondary grades. The present study sought to investigate the effects of teacher-supplied social consequences on the classroom behaviors of an entire class of secondary school students.

Method

Subjects

Students. The experimental group was a low-track, junior-senior English class containing 25 students (12 boys and 13 girls). At the beginning of the study the ages ranged from 16 to 19 years (mean 17.11 years); I.Q.s ranged from 77 to 114 (mean 94.43). Approximately 80% of the students were from lower-class families; the remainder were from middle-class families. The control group was also a low-track, junior-senior English class of 26 students (13 boys and 13 girls). The ages ranged from 16 to 19 years (mean 17.04 years);

I.Q.s ranged from 73 to 111 (mean 91.04). About 76% of these students were from lower-class families, 16% were from middle-class families and 4% were from upper-middle to upper-class families. The experimental class met in the mornings for a 70-minute period and the control class met in the afternoons for a 60-minute period.

Teacher. The teacher was 23 years old, female, middle class, and held a Bachelor's degree in education. She had had one year's experience in teaching secondary level students, which included a low-track English class. She taught both the experimental and control classes in the same classroom and utilized the same curriculum content for both. She stated that she had been having some difficulties in controlling classroom behavior in both classes and volunteered to cooperate in the experiment in the interest of improving her teaching-management skills. She stated that she had been able to achieve some rapport with these students during the two months that school had been in session. She described the students, generally, as performing poorly in academic work and ascribed whatever academic behaviors she was able to observe in them as being the result of her rapport with them. She stated that she was afraid that she would destroy this rapport if she attempted to exercise discipline over inappropriate classroom behaviors.

Procedures

The basic design utilized was the common pretest-posttest control group design combined with the use of a multiple baseline technique (Baer, Wolf, and Risley, 1968) in the experimental class.

TARGET BEHAVIORS. Both classes were observed for two weeks to ascertain general occurrence rates of various problem behaviors that had been described by the teacher. Inappropriate talking and turning around were selected as target behaviors because of their relatively high rate of occurrence. Inappropriate talking was defined as any audible vocal behavior engaged in by a student without the teacher's permission. Students were required to raise their hands to obtain permission to talk, either to the teacher or to other students, except when general classroom discussions were taking place, in which cases a student was not required to obtain permission to talk if his statements were addressed to the class and/or teacher and were made within the context of the discussion. Inappropriate turning was defined as any turning-around behavior engaged in by any student while seated in which he turned more than 90 degrees in either direction from the position of facing the front of the room. Two exceptions to this definition were made: turning behavior observed while in the process of transferring material to or from the book holder in the bottom of the desk was considered appropriate, as was any turning that took place when a student had directly implied permission to turn around. Examples of the latter exception would be when the class was asked to pass papers up or down the rows of desks, or when students turned to look at another student who was talking appropriately in the context of a recitation or discussion.

Observation and recording. Behavior record forms were made up for recording observed target behaviors in both classes. A portion of the form is illustrated in Fig. 10. The forms for the experimental class contained 70 sequentially numbered boxes for each behavior; the forms of the control class contained 60 sequentially numbered boxes for each behavior (covering the 70- and 60-minute class periods, respectively). The occurrence of a target behavior during any minute interval of time (*e.g.*, during the twenty-fifth minute of class time) was recorded by placing a check mark in the appropriate box for that interval (*e.g.*, box 25) beside the behavior listed. Further occurrences of that behavior during that particular interval were not recorded. Thus, each time interval represented a dichotomy with respect to each behavior: the behavior had or had not occurred during that interval of time. A daily quantified measurement of each behavior was obtained by dividing the number of intervals that were checked by the total number of intervals in the class period, yielding a percentage of intervals in which the behavior occurred at least once. Time was kept by referral to a large, easily readable wall clock whose minute hand moved 1 minute at a time.

Behaviors were recorded daily during all conditions by the teacher. Reliability of observation was checked by using from one to two additional observers (student teachers and the senior author) who visited the class twice per week. Students in this particular school were thought to be quite accustomed to observers, due to the large amount of classroom observation done there by student teachers from a nearby university. Except for the senior author and teacher, other observers were not made aware of changes in experimental conditions. Reliability was assessed by comparing the behavior record forms of the teacher and observers after each class period in which both teacher and observers recorded behavior. A percentage of agreement for each target behavior was computed, based on a ratio of the number of intervals on which all recorders agreed (*i.e.*, that the behavior had or had not occurred) to the total number of intervals in the period. Average reliability for talking behavior was 90.49% in the experimental class (range 74 to 98%) and 89.49% in the control class (range 78 to 96%). Average reliability for turning behavior was 94.27% in the experimental class (range 87 to 98%) and 90.98% in the control class (range 85 to 96%).

In addition, two aspects of the teacher's behavior were recorded during all conditions by the observers when present: (a) the number of inappropriate talking or turning instances that occasioned a verbal reprimand from the teacher, and (b) the number of direct statements of praise dispensed by the teacher for appropriate behaviors. These behaviors were recorded by simply tallying the number of instances in which they were observed on the reverse side of the observer's form. Reliability between observers was checked by computing a percentage of agreement between them on the number of instances of each type of behavior observed. Average reliability for reprimand behavior was 92.78% in the experimental class (range 84 to 100%) and 94.84% in the control class (range 82 to 100%). Average reliability for praise behavior was 98.85% in the experimental class (range 83 to 100%) and 97.65% in the control class (range 81 to 100%).

Baseline Condition. During the BASELINE CONDITION, the two target behaviors and teacher behaviors were recorded in both the experimental and control classes. The teacher was asked to behave in her usual manner in both classrooms and no restrictions were placed on any disciplinary techniques she wished to use. The Baseline Condition in the experimental class was continued for 27 class days (approximately five weeks) to obtain as clear a picture as possible of the student and teacher behaviors occurring.

Experimental Condition I. The first experimental condition began in the experimental class on the twenty-eighth day when the teacher initiated various social consequences CONTINGENT on inappropriate talking behavior aimed at lowering the amount of this behavior taking place. The procedures agreed upon with the teacher for the

Minute No.	1	2	3	4	5	6	7	8	9	10	11	12	13	14	15	16	17	18	19	20	21
Talking																					
Turning																					

Figure 10. Portion of behavior record form used to record incidence of target behavior.

application of social consequences were as follows:

(1) The teacher was to attempt to disapprove of all instances of inappropriate talking behavior whenever they occurred with a direct, verbal, sternly given reproof. Whenever possible, the teacher was to use students' names when correcting them. The teacher was instructed not to mention any other inappropriate behavior (*e.g.*, turning around) that might also be occurring at the time. Examples of reprimands given were: "John, be quiet!", "Jane, stop talking!", "Phil, shut up!", "You people, be quiet!". It was hypothesized that these consequences constituted an AVERSIVE SOCIAL CONSEQUENCE for inappropriate talking.

(2) The teacher was asked not to threaten students with or apply other consequences, such as keeping them after school, exclusion from class, send them to the Assistant Principal, *etc.* for inappropriate talking or for any other inappropriate behavior.

(3) The teacher was to praise the entire class in the form of remarks like: "Thank you for being quiet!", "Thank you for not talking!", or "I'm delighted to see you so quiet today!" according to the following contingencies: (a) During the first 2 minutes of class, praise at the end of approximately each 30-second period in which there had been no inappropriate talking. (b) During the time in which a lecture, recitation, or class discussion was taking place, praise the class at the end of approximately each 15-minute period in which no inappropriate talking had occurred. (c) When silent seatwork had been assigned, do not interrupt the period to praise, but praise the class at the end of the period if no inappropriate talking had occurred during the period. (d) At the end of each class make a summary statement concerning talking behavior, such as: "Thank you all for being so quiet today!", or "There has been entirely too much talking today, I'm disappointed in you!", or "You have done pretty well in keeping quiet today, let's see if you can do better tomorrow!".

The concentration of praising instances during the first 2 minutes of class was scheduled because the baseline data revealed inappropriate talking as particularly frequent at this time.

Although the teacher continued to record instances of turning behavior, she was instructed to ignore this behavior in the experimental class during Experimental Condition I. In effect, baseline recording of turning behavior continued during this Condition. No changes were made in the teacher's behavior in the control class.

Experimental Condition II. After Experimental Condition I had been in effect in the experimental class for 26 class days and had markedly reduced talking behavior (see Results), Experimental Condition II was put into effect on the fifty-fourth day of the study. In this condition, the contingent social consequences for talking behavior in the experimental class were continued and, in addition, the teacher initiated the same system of contingent social consequences for turning behavior, with the aim of reducing the amount of this behavior occurring. This subsequent provision of similar consequences, first for one behavior and then for another, constitutes the multiple baseline technique.

The procedures agreed upon for providing reprimands for inappropriate turning behavior were the same as those for talking behaviors, except that the teacher referred to "turning" instead of "talking" in her reproofs. She could now also mention both behaviors in her reproof if a student happened to be doing both. The procedures regarding the application of praise contingent on not turning around were also the same as before, except that the higher frequency of praising during the first 2 minutes of class was not used. Also, the teacher could now combine her positive remarks about not talking and not turning if such were appropriate to existing conditions. Finally, since inappropriate talking behavior had been reduced considerably by this time, the procedure of praising every 30 seconds during the first 2 minutes of class was dropped. As before, no changes were made in the teacher's behavior in the control class.

Results

Because data were not collected on individual students, it is not possible to specify exactly how many students were involved in either inappropriate talking or turning behavior. The observers and teacher agreed that over one-half of the students in both classes were involved in inappropriate talking behavior and that about one-third of the students in both classes were involved in inappropriate turning behavior.

Talking Behavior

Figure 11 indicates the daily percentages of intervals of inappropriate talking behavior in the experimental and control classes throughout the study. During the Baseline Condition in the experimental class and the equivalent period in the control class (Days 1 through 27), the average daily percentage of inappropriate talking intervals was 25.33% in the experimental class and 22.81% in the control class. The two classes were thus approximately equivalent with respect to the amount of inappropriate talking behavior in each before the experimental interventions were made in the experimental class. As can be seen, the introduction of the contingencies in Experimental Condition I on Day 28 immediately reduced the percentage of intervals of inappropriate talking behavior in the experimental class. From this point on, the amount of inappropriate talking behavior in the experimental class continued to decrease and finally stabilized at a level below 5%. Meanwhile, the control class continued to manifest its previous level of inappropriate talking behavior. In the period from Day 28 through Day 62, when the study was concluded, the average daily percentage of inappropriate talking intervals in the control class was 21.51%, compared with an average of 5.34% in the experimental class.

Turning Behavior

The results obtained with the second target behavior, inappropriate turning around, can be seen in Figure 12, which indicates the daily percentages of intervals of inappropriate turning behavior in both classes during the study. During the Baseline Condition in the experimental class and the equivalent period in the control class (Days 1 through 53), the level of inappropriate turning behavior was slowly increasing in both classes. The average daily percentage of inappropriate turning intervals during this time was 15.13% in the experimental class and 14.45% in the control class. As with talking behavior, the two classes were roughly equivalent in the amount of inappropriate turning behavior observed before experimental interventions were made. The introduction of Experimental Condition

II contingencies on Day 54 again immediately reduced the percentage of inappropriate turning intervals in the experimental class. This behavior continued to decrease during the remaining days of the study. In the control class, the level of inappropriate turning behavior remained essentially the same. In the period from Day 54 through Day 62, the average daily percentage of inappropriate turning intervals in the control class was 17.22% and in the experimental class was 4.11%.

Teacher Behavior

During the Baseline period on talking behavior, the average number of instances of inappropriate talking per class period that received some type of verbal reprimand from the teacher was 25.76% in the experimental class and 22.23% in the control class. The majority of these verbal responses took the form of saying, "Shhh!". On occasion, observers noted that the teacher corrected students directly, using their names. On several occasions she made general threats, stating that she would keep people after school if talking did not subside; however, she was never observed to carry out this kind of threat. During this period there were no observations of the

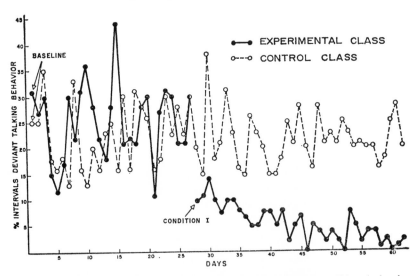

Figure 11. Daily percentages of intervals of inappropriate talking behavior in experimental and control classes during Baseline and Experimental Condition I periods.

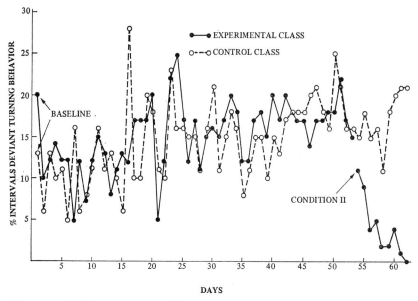

Figure 12. Daily percentages of intervals of inappropriate turning behavior in experimental and control classes during Baseline and Experimental Condition II periods.

teacher's dispensing any praise for not talking. During Experimental Condition I, the teacher disapproved of an average of 93.33% of inappropriate talking instances per class period in the experimental class. In the control class during this time, she disapproved of an average of 21.38% of inappropriate talking instances per class period. She also praised on an average of 6.07 occasions per experimental class period, contingent on not talking, during this time. With two exceptions, she was not observed directly to praise not talking in the control class.

During the Baseline period on inappropriate turning behavior, the average percentage of inappropriate turning instances per class period that received verbal reprimands from the teacher was 12.84% in the experimental class and 13.09% in the control class. Most of these were simple instructions, like, "Turn around!", and she used the student's name in most cases. During Experimental Condition II, the average percentage of inappropriate turning instances per class period that occasioned disapproving responses from the teacher was 95.50% in the experimental class and 18.50% in the control class.

In addition, she praised on an average of 5.75 occasions per experimental class period, contingent on not turning. In the control class she was not observed to provide any such praise for not turning.

Discussion

The results indicate quite clearly that the statements of praise and disapproval by the teacher had consistent effects on the two target behaviors observed in the experimental class. Both behaviors decreased. That the statements were, in fact, responsible for the observed modifications in behavior was demonstrated through the multiple baseline procedure in which the target behaviors changed maximally only when the statements were applied. The use of the control class data further substantiates this contention. The observations of teacher behavior in the study provide evidence that the program was being carried out as specified in the two classrooms.

The design of the study does not make it possible to isolate the separate effects of the teacher's statements of praise and disapproval on the students' behaviors. It is possible that one or the other of these was more potent in achieving the observed results. In addition to the possibility that statements of praise or disapproval, in themselves, might have differed in their effectiveness in modifying behavior, the different manner in which these two types of statements were delivered may have resulted in differing effects. The design, it will be remembered, called for disapproving statements to be delivered to individual students, while praise was delivered to the class as a whole. This resulted in a sudden onset of numerous disapproving statements delivered to individual students when Experimental Condition I was put into effect. The observers agreed that the students seemed "stunned" when this essentially radical shift in stimulus conditions took place. The immediate and marked decrease in inappropriate talking behavior at this point may have resulted because of this shift. The phenomenon can be compared to the sudden response rate reductions observed in animals when stimulus conditions are shifted suddenly. The decrease in inappropriate turning behavior observed when Experimental Condition II was put into effect, while immediate, was not of the same magnitude as that observed previously. Perhaps some measure of adaptation to this type of stimulus shift had taken place. Regardless of the possible reasons for the immediate effects observed when the experimental conditions were put into effect, it is also true that the direction of these effects was maintained thereafter in both experimental conditions. The combination of praise and disapproval undoubtedly was responsible for this.

Assuming that praise statements were functioning as POSITIVE REINFORCERS for a majority of the experimental class, they may have operated not only directly to reinforce behaviors incompatible with inappropriate talking and turning but also to generate peer-group pressure to reduce inappropriate behavior because such statements were contingent on the entire class' behavior. Further studies are needed to investigate the effects of peer-group contingencies on individual behavior.

Although it appears that the statements of praise and disapproval by the teacher functioned as positive reinforcers and punishers, respectively, an alternative possibility exists. These statements may have been operating primarily as instructions that the students complied with. It is conceivable that had praise statements, for example, been delivered as instructions independent of the occurrence of inappropriate behavior the same results might have been obtained. Also, it should be noted that results obtained in other studies (Lovaas, Freitag, Kinder, Rubenstein, Schaeffer, and Simmons, 1964; Thomas, Becker, and Armstrong, 1968) indicate that disapproving adult behaviors do not have a unitary effect on children's behavior. What would appear to be punishing types of statements are sometimes found to function as positive reinforcers. Informal observations indicated that this seemed to be the case in this study, at least as far as one student was concerned.

Several comments may be made regarding the practical aspects of the present approach. The study further exemplifies the usefulness of the multiple baseline technique, which makes it unnecessary to reverse variables in order to demonstrate the specific effectiveness of the experimental variables. Many teachers and school administrators will undoubtedly find this approach more acceptable in their schools. The notion of reversing variables to reinstitute what is considered to be maladaptive or inappropriate behavior is extremely repugnant to many educators who are more interested in "getting results" than in experimental verification of the results obtained.

The study differs from most previous operant research in classrooms in that the focus was on recording and modifying target behaviors without specific regard to the individual students involved. Most earlier studies have focused on observing the behavior of one student at a time. With this approach, it takes considerable time to extend observations to an entire class and usually this is not done. While observations of an entire class are not always necessary from a practical point of view (*i.e.*, only a few students are involved in inappropriate behaviors), the present approach does seem feasible when the number of students involved in one or more classes of inappropriate behavior is large. From an experimental point of view, this study was deficient in not providing more exact information as to the number of students actually involved in the target behaviors. Once this facet is determined, however, the essential approach seems quite feasible and practical.

It might be argued that a group-oriented approach will not function in the same way with all members of the group. This is potentially possible, if not probable. However, two practical aspects should be considered. In the first place, such an approach could conceivably remediate the total situation enough to allow the teacher to concentrate on those students who either have not responded or who have become worse. Secondly, perhaps a general reduction in inappropriate behavior is all the teacher desires. In this study, for example, the results obtained were, according to the teacher, more than enough to satisfy her. She did not, in other words, set a criterion of eliminating the target behaviors.

A significant practical aspect of this study was the amount of difficulty encountered by the teacher in recording behavior and delivering contingent praise and disapproval. It might be asked how she found time to teach when she was involved in these activities. Perhaps the best judge of the amount of difficulty involved with these techniques is the teacher herself. She reported that, initially, recording behaviors was difficult. The task did take considerable time and did interrupt her on-going teaching. On the other hand, the large amount of talking and other inappropriate behaviors occurring at the beginning of the study also interrupted her teaching. She felt that as the study went on she became more accustomed to recording and it became easier for her to accomplish. She pointed out that the fact that she usually positioned herself at her desk or rostrum also made recording somewhat easier because the forms were readily available. This was her usual position in the classroom; she did not change to make recording easier. Considerable time was required to deliver contingent praise and disapproval at the beginning of the experimental conditions. This also tended to interrupt teaching tasks as far as the teacher was concerned. However, she felt that this state of affairs did not last long because the target behaviors declined so immediately and rapidly. The overall judgment of the teacher was that the procedures of recording and dispensing contingent consequences did, indeed, interfere with her teaching but that the results obtained more than compensated for this. When the levels of inappropriate behavior had been lowered she felt she could carry out her teaching responsibilities much more efficiently and effectively than before. She felt strongly enough about the practicality and effectiveness of the techniques to present information and data on the study to her fellow teachers and to offer her services as a consultant to those who wanted to try similar approaches in their classrooms.

The senior author held frequent conferences with the teacher after class periods. The aim was to provide her with feedback regarding her performance in class. She was actively praised for appropriate modifications in her classroom behavior and for record-keeping behavior. Likewise, she was criticized for mistakes in her application of program contingencies.

Finally, the data of this experiment are considered significant by reason of the strong implication that teacher praise and disapproval can function to modify the behavior of high-school level students. This potentially extends the implications of earlier research accomplished on the pre-school and elementary levels.

References

Baer, D. M., Wolf, M. M. and Risley, T. R.: Some current dimensions of applied behavior analysis. *J Appl Behav Anal 1*, 91-97, 1968.

Becker, W. C., Madsen, C. H., Jr., Arnold, C. R. and Thomas, D. R.: The contingent use of teacher attention and praise in reducing classroom behavior problems. *J Spec Ed 1*, 287-307, 1967.

Bushell, D., Jr., Wrobel, P. A. and Michaelis, M. L.: Applying "group" contingencies to the classroom study behavior of preschool children. *J Appl Behav Anal 1,* 55-61, 1968.

Cohen, H. L., Filipczak, J. and Bis, J. S.: *Case I: an initial study of contingencies applicable to special education.* Silver Spring, Md.: Educational Facility Press—Institute for Behavioral Research, 1967.

Hall, R. V. and Broden, M.: Behavior changes in brain-injured children through social reinforcement. *J Exper Child Psychol 5,* 463-479, 1967.

Hall, R. V., Lund, D. and Jackson, D.: Effects of teacher attention on study behavior. *J Appl Behav Anal 1,* 1-12, 1968.

Harris, F. R., Wolf, M. M. and Baer, D. M.: Effects of adult social reinforcement on child behavior. *Young Children 20,* 8-17, 1964.

Lövaas, O. I., Freitag, G., Kinder, M. I., Rubenstein, D. B., Schaeffer, B. and Simmons, J. B.: *Experimental studies in childhood schizophrenia—establishment of social reinforcers.* Paper read at Western Psychological Assn., Portland, April, 1964.

Madsen, C. H., Becker, W. C. and Thomas, D. R.: Rules, praise and ignoring: elements of elementary classroom control. *J Appl Behav Anal 1,* 139-150, 1968.

Patterson, G. R.: An application of conditioning techniques to the control of a hyperactive child. In L. P. Ullman and L. Krasner (Eds.), *Case studies in behavior modification.* New York, Holt, Rinehart & Winston, pp. 370-375, 1966.

Rabb, E. and Hewett, F. M.: Developing appropriate classroom behaviors in a severely disturbed group of institutionalized kindergarten-primary children utilizing a behavior modification model. *Am J Orthopsychiatry 37,* 313-314, 1967.

Thomas, D. R., Becker, W. C. and Armstrong, M.: Production and elimination of disruptive classroom behavior by systematically varying teacher's behavior. *J Appl Behav Anal 1,* 35-45, 1968.

Zimmerman, E. H. and Zimmerman, J.: The alteration of behavior in a special classroom situation. *J Exper Anal Behav 5,* 59-60, 1962.

Chapter 3

DEVELOPING THE "HELPING TEACHER" ROLE: A WAY TO MOVE MENTAL HEALTH CONSULTATION ON TO THE SCHOOL CAMPUS*

JAMES M. STEDMAN *and* ALICE WALTHER

NUMEROUS INVESTIGATOR-PRACTITIONERS (Homme *et al.* 1970; O'Leary and Becker, 1967) have demonstrated that teachers can be taught to utilize behavioral principles in order to modify the academic and social actions of their students. Additionally, there have been programs designed to teach large numbers of counselors and/or school psychologists behavioral principles, in order that they might act as front line consultants to school personnel in the educational setting. The present report focuses on a slightly different problem, that of training a teacher to function as resident consultant to her peers. Additionally, this report will illustrate how behavior modification principles might be introduced to a total group of special education teachers.

The possibility of developing such a program came about with the introduction of a new special education plan for the state of Texas, known as "Plan A." Very briefly stated, this new plan stressed that all school efforts to help exceptional children should be accomplished

*Previously unpublished article, 1972.

on a "resource teacher" basis. Additionally, the plan called for the formation of the new role of "Helping Teacher" which was defined as follows: "Helping special education teachers are to be assigned to one school on a full time basis and are to assist in maintaining children in their classrooms." As is obvious from this definition, "Plan A" offered the opportunity to develop a slightly new breed of teacher, one who would essentially act as onsite consultant to her peers.

In one local setting, the Alamo Heights Independent School District, the newly designated helping teacher had three years experience in an engineered classroom setting. During those years she had received consultation from the local mental health center and had become particularly good in applying behavior modification principles within her classroom setting. Since, in an informal way, she had already aided many other teachers on campus, district officials and mental health consultants felt that perhaps that she could quickly move into the role of consultant to her peers.

Implementation began in September, 1971; and, though certain aspects of the program went well, it soon became obvious that the helping teacher was experiencing grave difficulties. Specifically, she was finding it very difficult to obtain cooperation from some of her fellow teachers, and, even when she was able to obtain entry into her colleagues' classrooms, was experiencing considerable frustration and doubt regarding her ability to work out successful behavioral and academic management plans for students. After considerable soul-searching and some thoughts on the part of the school administration that perhaps the plan should be scrapped, it finally dawned on the consultation team that our helping teacher was caught in a significant role conflict. Specifically she was finding that the role of practitioner in a self-contained, engineered classroom was quite different from the role of "Consultant on Classroom Management Problems," the new role required of her. Though she had certainly been an expert in receiving consultation and in engineering successful modification plans in her previous role as special education classroom teacher, it became obvious that application of the principles of applied learning to a variety of complex academic and behavioral problems required a consultant's "know-how." In a sense, the problem resembled one which might be created if a research technician in a large scientific study were suddenly made program director!

Once the nature of the problem was identified the solution seemed simple enough. Our helping teacher would have to absorb some of the mental health consultant's expertise. It seemed of particular importance that the helping teacher accomplish two areas of new learning, the first involving further academic understanding of applied learning principles and the second involving direct absorption of the mental health consultant's methods and procedures used in actual analysis and modification of classroom problems.

The first of these problems was easily solved, because it involved relatively formal academic training in applied learning. Thus, forty minutes of each consultation was set aside to teach applied learning principles within a case centered framework. Each week a child was discussed in light of behavior modification principles. This format proved successful, so much so, that all other "Plan A" teachers on the campus eventually participated. Often these teachers were involved with the same students, so that a general behavioral plan for a particular student could be "roughed out" during the session. Later in the year responsibility for generating behavioral plans was passed to the group, thus, giving them a chance to put their new learning into action.

The second problem, that of infusing the mental health consultant's techniques into the helping teacher, seemed more difficult. However, Social Learning Theory (Bandura and Walters 1963), which has demonstrated that a learner can rapidly acquire a complex repertoire of behavior by observational learning, offered a possible solution. Thus, it appeared that the best way to teach the consultant's accumulated knowledge, regarding approach to teachers in a consulting relationship and utilization of applied learning in the classroom setting, could be accomplished by having the consultant take the helping teacher through each specific step involved in analysis and programming for particular cases. Thus, each week the consultant and helping teacher went to classrooms and worked on actual student problems. There the mental health consultant made explicit "how he did his thing."

Once in the classroom, the mental health consultant gave a running commentary to the helping teacher, regarding such things as 1) how to gather specific data on operationally definable target behavior; 2) how to observe the classroom teacher's behavior in relationship to the child's particular target behaviors; 3) how to formulate possible behavior modification approaches to the definable target behaviors and; 4) how these programs might be sold to the classroom teacher (probably the most important step).

Much to the surprise of the helping teacher and the consultant, who had previously worked together for over three years, it became obvious that the helping teacher had never understood (got inside the mind of) the mental health consultant. Thus, both could view the same classroom situation and perceive it in very different ways. However, if the consultant made his procedures explicit in a "stream of consciousness" flow, it was found that the helping teacher very quickly absorbed this strategy of approach to classroom management problems.

At a later date, another teaching procedure proved useful. Each week the helping teacher reviewed several of the more difficult cases discussed during the previous week and developed a rough draft management plan, including specification of target behaviors, some approximation of baseline frequencies, and a plan for use for applied learning principles in managing the behavior. In the next consultative session, the consultant and helping teacher went over the material and "corrected homework."

The following are two brief case examples of what can be accomplished when mental health specialists and educators join forces in an arrangement such as has been described above.

Case Study 1

S., a five year old girl in the preschool, bilingual class, was referred to the helping teacher because of her "uncooperativeness" and "stubbornness." The consultant and helping teacher spent approximately an hour observing the girl in the classroom setting. During this time the consultant pointed out instances of deviant behavior to the helping teacher and illustrated how to record instances of these behaviors in a systematic manner. Later both questioned the classroom teacher regarding specific behaviors which were disturbing to her. At first the mental health consultant modeled appropriate questions designed to help the classroom teacher elaborate her complaints in behavioral terms. Then he listened while the helping teacher continued the process. As a result, the following positive target behaviors were identified:

1. Stay in the group for at least ten minute intervals during group activities.
2. During play periods, be friends with others—do not hit or pinch them.
3. Let others have their turn—do not always try to be first and boss others around.

In further discussion, it was decided that perhaps the PREMACK PRINCIPLE (Premack, 1965) could be utilized in establishing potential reinforcers for the girl. Specifically, this involved having S work for the privilege of doing the very things which were upsetting to the teacher, e.g. refusing to join class activities because she preferred to clean up, insisting on passing out materials, and acting in a bossy, authoritative manner with other children. The team decided that perhaps these activities could be channeled into constructive socialization, provided they occurred in a controlled way and at the proper time.

In order to implement the plan, a large "reinforcement" card was made, complete with pictures showing a typical school girl cooperating in regular classroom activities. This point card was presented to the child and she was told that she could earn points for accomplishment of the target behaviors described above. Furthermore, she was instructed that the points would be added up twice a day and, if sufficient points were earned, she would be permitted to be "class leader," to clean up the classroom, and to pass out refreshments or materials to the rest of the class.

The helping teacher, acting as consultant, supervised this program on a daily basis for one week. Under this regimen, the girl's grouping and cooperative behavior improved steadily. However, it should be noted that the plan required frequent monitoring by the helping teacher in order to deal with the usual problems encountered in implementation of behavior modification plans, e.g. REINFORCEMENT SATIATION, attention to the teacher's consistency in administering the program, etc. Thus, the helping teacher took on the role of consultant to the classroom teacher and, due to her on-campus status, could correct problems as they arose.

Case Study 2

Four regular classroom teachers, working as a team with the third and fourth grades, came to the mental health consultant and the helping teacher complaining that a minimally brain injured fourth grade boy was uncontrollable and disruptive. Once again, the consultant and helping teacher observed the child in the classroom and questioned the teachers, resulting in the following target behaviors:

1. Raise your hand to talk.
2. Stay in your seat (for intervals which increased with time).
3. Start your work.

Additionally, the classroom observation quickly revealed that teachers were reinforcing the boy's deviant behaviors by attending to him when he talked out, got out of his seat, or refused to start a task. As one step in coping with the problem the helping teacher, with the aid of the consultant, set up a role play sequence in which the four teachers got supervised practice in identifying deviant behavior, reinforcing appropriate behavior and ignoring the identified inappropriate classroom actions. Then the helping teacher constructed a reinforcement check sheet for the child, and modeled its use for the classroom teachers. Once again the helping teacher visited the classrooms for a period of time, making corrections in the program when necessary. Additionally, she set up and monitored a fading procedure in which social reinforcers were submitted for the point system. Soon the boy was no longer viewed as problematic in the classroom situation.

References

Bandura, A. and Walters, R. H.: *Social learning and personality development*. New York, Holt, Rinehart, Winston, 1963.

Homme, L., Csanyi, A. P., Gonzales, M. A. and Rechs, J.: *How to use contingency contracting in the classroom*. Champaign, Research Press, 1970.

O'Leary, D. K. and Becker, W. C.: Behavior modification of an adjustment class: A token reinforcement program. *Excep Child*, May, 1967, pp. 637-642.

Premack, D.: Reinforcement theory. In D. Levine (Ed.), *Nebraska Symposium on Motivation*. Lincoln, Neb. University of Nebraska Press, p. 132 (b), 1965.

Chapter 4

THE USE OF A TOKEN SYSTEM
IN PROJECT HEAD START*

L. KEITH MILLER *and* RICHARD SCHNEIDER

TOKEN SYSTEMS provide an effective method for generating social-ly important behaviors in a wide variety of settings (Ayllon and Azrin, 1965; Birnbrauer, Wolf, Kidder, and Tauge, 1965; Cohen, Filipczak, and Bis, 1965; Giradeau and Spradlin, 1964; Clark, Lacho-wicz, and Wolf, 1968; Staats and Butterfield, 1965; and Wolf, Giles, and Hall, 1967). The present paper describes a token system designed to develop and maintain writing skills in a group of underprivileged children in a summer Head Start program. The function of the token system in generating these skills was assessed by individual experi-ments with each of the children in the experimental token class. The overall effect of the program was evaluated by comparing the pre-test and the post-test scores of the token class with a matched control class.

Method

Subjects

Thirty students, four to five years old, who were enrolled in the regular Head Start Program of a small midwest city, served as sub-jects with the explicit agreement of their parents. Students were ran-domly assigned to an experimental token class and a control class. For reasons of health and irregular attendance four children in each class were dropped from the experiment. Of the remaining 22 chil-

*From the *Journal of Applied Behavior Analysis*, 1970, 3 (3), pp. 191-197. Copyright 1970 by the Society for the Experimental Analysis of Behavior, Inc. Reprinted by per-mission of the Society and the author.

dren, 19 were black and three were white. All children came from low-income families as defined by the Office of Economic Opportunity scale.

Staff

The staff for each class consisted of a teacher and two teacher's aides. The junior author, who had received training in behavior modification, served as the teacher in the token class. A local public school teacher taught the control class. The other staff members were welfare recipients and had no training in behavior modification.

Control Group

The control group consisted of 11 children. Their teacher was a state certified grade school teacher in the local system who had taught in the Head Start program the previous year. Although she was not instructed on how to teach her class, she was provided with the same instructional and reinforcing materials provided to the experimental group to use as she saw fit. A writing achievement test was administered to her class during the first week of the program and she was informed that it would be administered again during the final week. It was suggested that she teach the children these skills as one goal of her summer program. However, no effort was made to force her to teach these skills, whether in her own way or by using the writing program developed for the experimental class. Furthermore, no systematic observation was made of her attempts to use it. Her own reports and casual observation indicated that several attempts to use the program met with no cooperation from the children.

Experimental Group

Experimental room. The experimental space consisted of a room approximately 25 by 40 feet and an additional outside play area (Figure 13). This space was divided into six functional areas. Five of the areas were associated with reinforcement and had restricted entrances; the sixth area was associated with the opportunity to study. The areas were:

1. *Food area*: snacks of cookies and Kool Aid were served here. Lunch plates, dessert cups, and milk glasses were dispensed as children earned them before lunch. Lunch was served to the children from this area.

2. *Funroom*: this area contained a wide variety of toys that the chil-

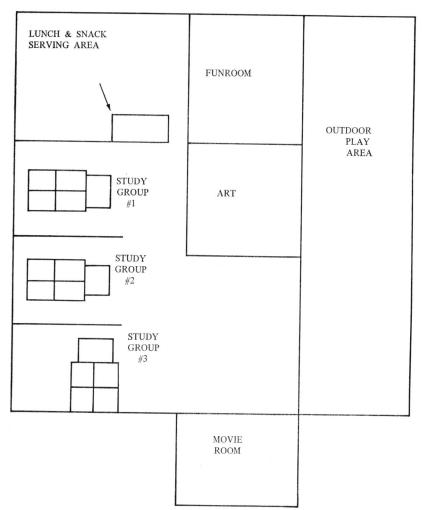

Figure 13. Floorplan of the Head Start classroom.

dren could play with. The toys included blocks, cars, dolls, dress-up clothes, a piano, blackboard, and record player.

3. *Art*: this area contained such art supplies as paints, crayons, rubber ink stamps, paste-on pictures, and paper.

4. *Outdoor play area*: this area contained outdoor toys such as a beachball, rocking horse, climbing bar, pedal car, and several water guns.

5. *Movie room*: this area contained a strip film projector and a small

TOKEN   PEGS

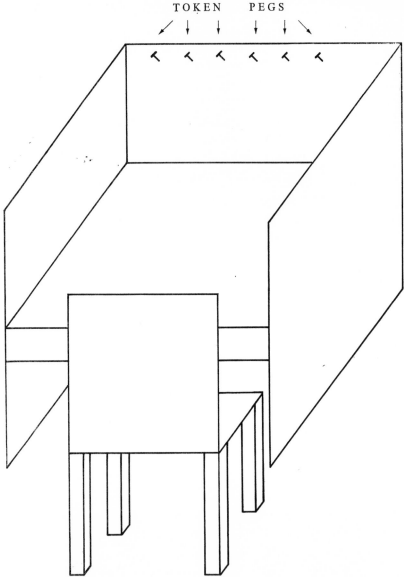

Figure 14. Individual cubicle in which each child worked during study period.

library of educational films obtained through the school system.

6. *Study area*: this area contained three groups of five children's school desks. Each desk was separated from the other four in that

same group by plywood partitions (Figure 14). Each group was separated from the other groups by folding partitions. Visual access between children required standing on their chair or table, or walking away from their desk.

Response definition. A program was prepared that was designed to teach the children the necessary skills prerequisite to learning freehand printing. These skills included: (1) how to hold a pencil, (2) how to draw a straight line at different angles, (3) how to draw curved lines at different angles, (4) how to draw freehand lines, and (5) how to draw a variety of different shapes in which lines joined and crossed at specified points. The entire program contained 15 distinct steps, several examples[2] of which are shown in Figure 15. Each step was duplicated between 24 and 48 times on a single sheet of paper. Each child in the token class worked on each step until he produced one perfect paper. He was then allowed to progress to the next step in the program. Both classes were provided with as many copies of the program as they requested.

A correct response was judged by the teacher's aides. If the child's response started at the correct point, did not cross the guidelines,

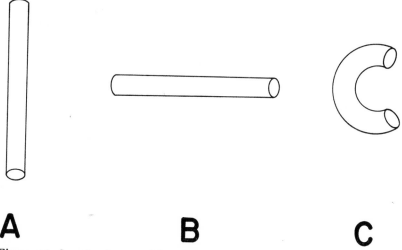

A   **B**   **C**

Figure 15. Samples from writing program.

[2]This program has been expanded and perfected by Dr. Donald Bushell. Copies of the revised program can be obtained from Dr. Bushell, Follow Through Project, Department of Human Development, University of Kansas, Lawrence, Kansas 66044.

and ended at the correct point, it was to be graded as correct. Each aide was supplied with a different colored marker so that her grading responses could be readily identified at any time. Her responses consisted of an "X" next to each incorrect response and a dot or short line next to each correct response.

Constant assessment of grading accuracy was required because of the volume of work required of the aides; they graded an average of 20 responses per minute, delivered tokens, and administered the reinforcing activities immediately after the work sessions. In addition, grading many responses at the very end of the work period was often done in a "crisis" atmosphere conducive to mistakes. It must be added that the aides were also somewhat more sympathetic toward near misses than was the teacher. In order to maintain a reasonable level of accuracy, the teacher checked each aide's grading as soon as possible and gave her further instruction until the grading was at least 95% accurate. Spot checking of accuracy was maintained for the duration of the experiment.

Procedure. The children in the token class were introduced to the token system during the first eight days. At the beginning of the first day, the aides were given explicit instructions on their duties. After this instruction period, the children were permitted to sample each of the play activities if they first repeated its name to one aide, for which they received a token, and then gave the token to another aide. During the second day, access to the snacks and activities required one token. The children were permitted to earn tokens at any time by working on the writing program; they could immediately exchange the tokens for five minutes of access to the reinforcer. During the next six days, tokens could be earned only during formal study periods, which alternated with brief play periods. Initially, the study periods were five minutes long; they were progressively increased during the six day period until there were four 30-minute study periods and four 20-minute play periods. Once this change had been introduced, the children were permitted to buy play activities only during play periods.

Table IX lists 10 reinforcers and their prices that were available to the children in exchange for tokens.

When the study periods were introduced, a response chain and a conditioned reinforcer system were developed to bridge the delay between the child's response and his access to the reinforcers. The RESPONSE CHAIN consisted of completing a fixed number of writing responses designated by the teacher and then raising his hand. When a child raised his hand, the teacher would go to that child's desk and

TABLE IX

NUMBER OF TOKENS REQUIRED FOR LUNCH MATERIALS, SNACKS, AND ACCESS TO DIFFERENT ACTIVITIES

Reinforcer	Price
Lunch Materials	
Lunch Plate	5
Second Plate	5
Dessert Cup	5
Milk Glass	5
Snacks	
Kool Aid	5
Cookie	5
Activities	
Fun Room	10
Playground	10
Art	10
Movies	10

grade each response. Tokens were given for correct responses according to a SMALL FIXED-RATIO SCHEDULE. After receiving his tokens, the child could apply them to one or more tickets, which depicted the different REINFORCERS. He bought a ticket by filling up a peg in his study booth that also held the ticket. The peg was adjusted in length so that the number of tokens that could fit onto it equalled the price of the reinforcer. This system had the advantages of (1) not requiring counting, (2) displaying a wide variety of reinforcers, and (3) not requiring any intervention or assistance by the aides.

The effectiveness of the token system in maintaining responding was experimentally evaluated after a seven-day baseline period. The evaluation used four study periods of one day. Before the first and third periods of that day, the children were given 25 tokens noncontingently and instructed to complete eight responses. After they completed those responses, the teacher graded them, praised their work, and informed them that there were no more tokens available to give out. The children were then informed that they could complete more writing responses is they wished. During the second and fourth work periods, the children were given tokens CONTINGENT upon their completion of correct responses. Each work period was 30 minutes long and was separated from the next work period by a 20-minute play period during which tokens could be spent. The design was duplicated during a second day.

In addition to this basic experiment, the effect of different work durations was also evaluated. On subsequent days, 20-minute, 30-minute, and 60-minute work sessions were scheduled with the token system in effect.

Finally, the overall effect of the token system was evaluated by an achievement test given during the first three days of the program (pre-test) and again at the end of the six week program (post-test). The test covered each target behavior of the writing program. This test was given to both the token class and the control class. The test was shown to the control class teacher before the start of classes as one target for her teaching.

Results

Figure 16 shows the day-by-day variation in response rates during the seven-day BASELINE period for a child with a high, medium, and low rate. S-5 showed considerably more variation than the other children. Most children maintained a fairly uniform daily rate during the baseline period. Two children did not, both increasing from a low rate of about two responses per minute to about seven responses per minute. In general, these data suggest a relatively stable day-to-day rate of responding during baseline.

Figure 17 shows the variation within days during the baseline period. The average number of responses in each period decreased from about 4.2 responses per minute in the first period to about 3.3 responses per minute in the fourth period. These averages are not a precise measure of the individual children, however. For example, Period 4 is the slowest work period for only three of the 11 children. These data suggest a relatively uniform rate of responding within each day, with some tendency for a decrease in rate after the first period.

Figure 18 shows the average response rate for the 10 children present during the four study periods of the experimental session. In general, the students worked at a much higher rate during the two periods when the tokens were contingent. During those periods, they

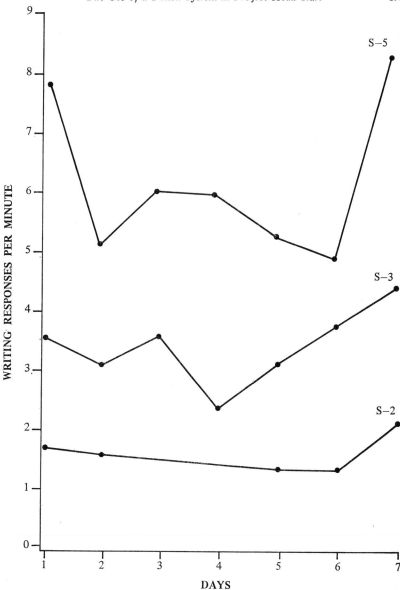

Figure 16. Writing responses per minute for a high, medium and low-rate child during first seven days of token reinforcement.

averaged about five responses per minute. During the periods when 25 tokens were given non-contingently and social attention was the only event contingent upon responding, they averaged about 0.8 and

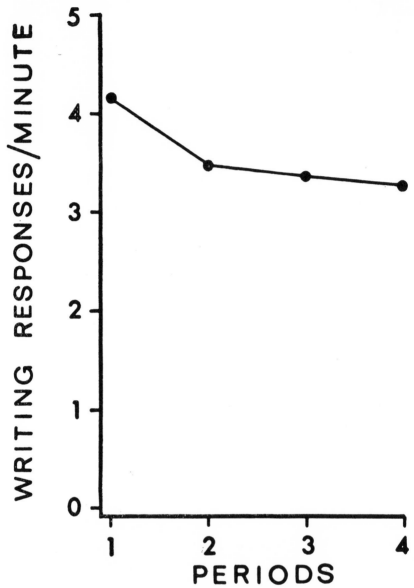

Figure 17. Mean writing responses per minute for the four daily work periods for the first seven days of token reinforcement.

0.2 responses per minute. T-tests were computed for each adjacent period. The differences between periods were significant at approximately the 0.0005 level or beyond for each comparison. Two sub-

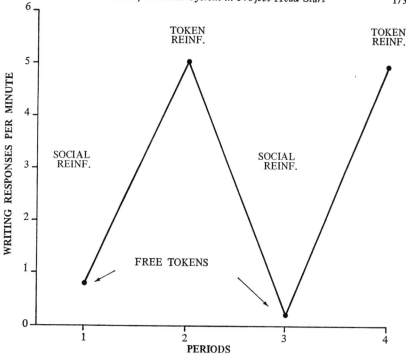

Figure 18. Mean rate of responding with and without contingent token reinforcement. Each point represents the mean rate for 10 children during a 30-min study period.

jects deviated from this statistical pattern. S-6 did not recover a high response rate during the first period. However, she showed comparable rates when tokens were delivered contingently during the other periods. S-10 worked at a high rate during the first period of non-contingent delivery of tokens but otherwise showed a pattern comparable to the other children. Six children made no responses after the eight responses they were instructed to complete. Two children maintained low rates, but still showed considerably higher rates during the periods when tokens were contingent. Virtually identical differences in rate between the reinforced and non-reinforced periods were obtained during the second experimental day. These differences between periods during the experimental days contrast sharply with the small variability between periods obtained during the baseline period. These results indicate that the tokens were effective in maintaining a high response rate among the children during the experimental days.

Figure 19 shows the effect of different study period durations on the children's rate of emitting writing responses. On the average, the children maintained a response rate of between four and five responses per minute whether the study period was 20, 30, or 60 minutes long. The rates for the individual children are similar to this average; four children showed a slight increase in rate when comparing the 20-minute and 60-minute study periods, and three showed a slight decrease in rate. The interesting thing about this experiment is that there is no evidence to suggest that the children's response rate decreased even when hour-long study sessions were used. This contrasts with the intuitive notion that four to five-year old children have a very short attention span, particularly for formal education

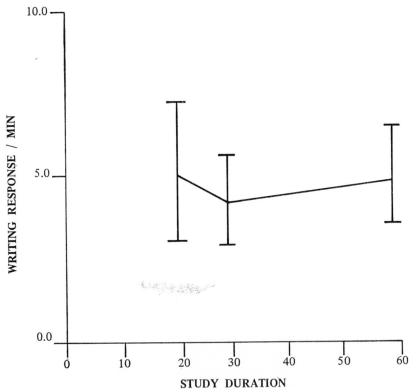

Figure 19. Mean rate of responding during study periods of different durations. Each point represents mean rate for seven children during four 20- and 30-min study periods and during one 60-min study period. Vertical bars show ranges for the seven children at each duration.

behaviors. This experiment suggests that children can work at educational activities for long periods of time with no necessary reduction in response rate—if their behaviors are adequately reinforced.

Figure 20 shows the results of the pre-test and the post-test. Both groups made about 35% correct responses on the pre-test. On the post-test, the control group showed a small gain of about 3% to a score of about 38% correct responses. The token group showed a very large gain to almost 100% correct responses on the post-test. These results indicate that the token class made very large gains on the writing achievement test while the control group made only slight gains.

Discussion and Conclusions

The differences in rates between periods with and without reinforcement contingencies suggest that the tokens were effective in maintaining writing responses. This conclusion is further strengthened by the relative lack of differences between periods during baseline when all responses were reinforced.

The data also suggest that the token system can maintain writing behavior over a period of several weeks. Counting the seven baseline days, the two experimental days, and the three days during which different durations of work periods were studied, writing behavior was maintained during the reinforced portion of 12 days. This suggests that the present reinforcing procedure has some durability.

This research indicates that token systems can be adapted to the Head Start situation. It may be that the ease with which token control was developed over these children resulted from several fortuitous features of the system. First, the development of an explicit response chain beginning with a writing response and ending with hand-raising may have effectively bridged the inevitable time delay between writing responses and token delivery. Without the hand-raising response, the aides would have had to move continually from child to child to see if they had completed their work. Not only would this have permitted unauthorized social reinforcement to occur, but it would have introduced a non-discriminated time delay between responding and token delivery. Second, the use of tickets containing a picture of the reinforcing activity may have effectively bridged the gap between token delivery and the actual access to the "back-up" reinforcing activity. It also made it possible

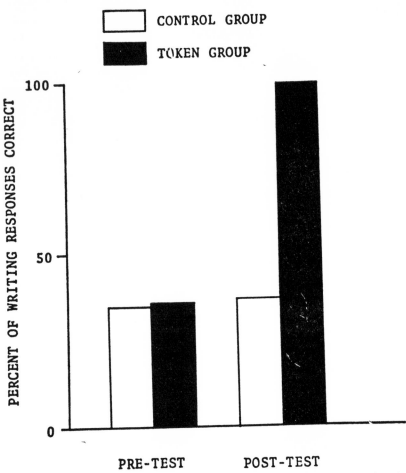

Figure 20. Comparison of pre-test and post-test achievement scores for the token group and the control group. Token group bars are averages for seven children present at both tests; control group bars are averages for 11 children present at both tests.

to display a wide variety of reinforcers to subjects with no reading ability. Third, the use of token pegs adjusted in length to count the children's tokens for them permitted the children to select their reinforcers with no intervention from the teacher or the aides. Not only might this have taught them to make responsible choices, but, by eliminating the teacher's influence, it may have heightened the probability that the tokens were exchanged for the most reinforcing events. The pegs also permitted the use of a differential pricing system without first requiring the children to learn how to count. Fourth, the fact that the children could begin to apply their tokens toward a variety of back-up reinforcers while the study period was in process may have reduced the tendency of the children to satiate on tokens. In any event, the token system reported here did rapidly develop token control in the Head Start situation. This control also produced large and measurable gains in the writing skills of these children. This success suggests that we should explore methods for applying token systems to such basic skills as vocabulary improvement, counting and adding, and reading readiness.

It should be noted that the present token system is practical as well as successful. The reinforcers used are commonly available in Head Start classrooms without additional cost. Perhaps even more important is that the token system can be administered by untrained teacher's aides. This made it practical to hire the most needy Head Start mothers: those on welfare. One of the mothers serving as a teacher's aide could not read; yet she was an excellent teacher within this system. Thus, this system was used without raising either material or personnel costs.

Informal observations suggest that the token system had several unanticipated effects. First, the token system required intense interaction between the children and the teacher's aides. Children had to learn new words in order to follow instructions successfully; the fact that the situation was relatively objective made it possible for the aides readily to observe whether instructions were understood and take corrective measures if they were not. Second, the children appeared to develop a favorable attitude toward school. Several children were kept home for a day due to a minor misunderstanding. All of them cried for several hours because they wanted to go to school. This led the parents to investigate the misunderstanding and return the children to school. Third, children gained a great deal of experience playing cooperatively with other children. One very shy child with a deformed face initially refused to play with other children. But a brief shaping period encouraged her to try playing with them. After she had tried, she rapidly overcame her shyness and became a full participant in the play periods. These and other unanticipated effects suggest that token systems may provide an environment far more suitable to developing many of the less specified behavioral changes of interest to child development specialists than one might guess. It would be of value in future token studies systematically to investigate such changes. Perhaps objective methods could be developed to increase the rate of such changes deliberately. Even if these methods could not be developed, objective data demonstrating that such changes are not incompatible with token systems would be of considerable interest.

A major failing in the present experiment was the lack of community—in particular, parent—control over the program. While a parent advisory committee was involved in all decisions from the initial hiring to the selection of teaching goals, interest and participation tended to be low. Perhaps the extension of a token system to the parents, similar to that used to maintain participation in self-help clubs (Miller and Miller, 1969), could be introduced.

References

Ayllon, T. and Azrin, N. H.: Measurement and reinforcement of behavior of psychotics. *J Exp Anal Behav 8*, 357-383, 1965.

Birnbrauer, J. S., Wolf, M. M., Kidder, J. D. and Tauge, C. E.: Classroom behavior of retarded pupils with token reinforcement. *J Exp Child Psychol 2*, 219-235, 1965.

Clark, M., Lachowicz, J. and Wolf, M.: A pilot education program for school dropouts incorporating a token reinforcement system. *Behav Res Ther 6*, 183-188, 1968.

Cohen, H. L., Filipczak, J. A. and Bis, J. S.: *CASE Project: contingencies applicable for special education.* Brief Progress Report to U.S. Department of Health, Education, and Welfare, Office of Juvenile Delinquency and Youth Development.

Giradeau, F. L. and Spradlin, J. E.: Token rewards in a cottage program. *Ment Retard 2*, 345-351, 1964.

Miller, L. K. and Miller, O. L.: Reinforcing self-help group activities of welfare recipients. *J Appl Behav Anal 3*, 57-64, 1970.

Staats, A. and Butterfield, W. H.: Treatment of non-reading in a culturally deprived juvenile delinquent: an application of reinforcement principles. *Child Dev 36*, 925-942, 1965.

Wolf, M. M., Giles, D. J. and Hall, W. V.: Experiments with token reinforcement in a remedial classroom. *Behav Res Ther 6*, 51-64, 1968.

Section IV

BEHAVIOR THERAPY WITH CHILD GROUPS

Group therapy has been utilized in child clinical work for many years, but, as Clements points out, has often represented a conceptually barren and goalless therapeutic activity. Our survey of the literature revealed few behavioral studies in this area, suggesting that perhaps this is one of the more neglected areas of application. The article by Gittelman is particularly intriguing, in light of its application to disadvantaged children.

Chapter 1

GROUP PLAY THERAPY AND TANGIBLE REINFORCERS USED TO MODIFY THE BEHAVIOR OF EIGHT-YEAR-OLD BOYS*

PAUL W. CLEMENT *and* D. COURTNEY MILNE

G ROUP AND INDIVIDUAL PLAY THERAPY TECHNIQUES are routinely used in most child guidance and psychiatric clinics. Although the therapists who use these techniques believe in their efficacy in removing unwanted, and in establishing more acceptable behavior patterns, few systematic studies have been reported on play therapy. Masling (1966) went so far as to say, "Research in child therapy is absolutely nonexistent." While the situation is no longer quite so bad, there has been a general failure to demonstrate that play therapy techniques produce predictable changes in behavior and personality (Ginott, 1961; pp. 135-158; Levitt, 1957; 1963).

The present study was designed to shed some light on the following two questions which are concerned with child psychotherapy research: (1) Within the context of group play therapy, what combination of experiences produces the largest number of changes in behavior and in emotional state and/or the greatest degree of

*From *Behavior Research and Therapy*, 1967, 5, pp. 301-312. Reprinted by permission of Maxwell International Microfilms Corporation.

change? (2) Will a treatment approach which includes the systematic reinforcement, with tangible rewards, of preselected behavior lead to more change than will a treatment approach which excludes tangible rewards?

For the present study, "group play therapy" is defined as a situation in which a specially-trained person, the therapist, establishes a relationship with a group of children who exhibit behavior patterns which are personally and/or socially unacceptable. The therapist attempts to apply a behavioral model to modify the behavior of the children so that there will be an increase in (1) productivity in school and other settings, (2) positive aspects of the self-concept, (3) social attractiveness and the ability to get along with other people, and (4) the ability to cope with the problems of life, and so that there will be a decrease in discrete, problem behavior.

We assume that "group play therapy" is *not* a single treatment approach uniformly practiced by many child therapists, but rather it is a loose concept used to categorize a very large number of poorly defined techniques used in a multitude of combinations by many practitioners. Also we assume that there are significant differences between therapists both within a given "school" of play therapy as well as across schools. The problem, therefore, is that for the present study and data "group play therapy" can only refer to the specific techniques employed. Generalization to other approaches should be done only with great care.

Regardless of the approach, behavioral terminology may be used to describe what is going on in a given type of psychotherapy. At the onset of treatment each child has a habit-family hierarchy of responses. Some of the more dominant behavior in the hierarchy is unacceptable to the child's parents, teachers, etc. More acceptable behavior is lower on the hierarchy. By selectively reinforcing more acceptable behavior and failing to reinforce unacceptable behavior, the frequency of occurrence of the desired responses should increase and that of the undesired responses should decrease.

A few attempts have been made to apply conditioning techniques to groups of adults (e.g. Lazarus, 1961), but apparently no study has been published on conditioning techniques applied to groups of children in an outpatient setting. There have been many studies, however, using operant techniques on individual children, and most of them have reported positive results (e.g. Allen *et al.*, 1964; Kerr, Meyerson and Michael, 1965).

The primary hypothesis of the present study was that children who are systematically reinforced with tangible reinforcers will change more than those who receive treatment without tangible reinforcers, and those who receive treatment without tangible reinforcers will change more than those in a control situation.

Method

Subjects

Eleven third-grade boys from the Torrance Unified School District constituted the Ss. The mean age was 8 years 10 months with a range of 8 years 2 months–9 years 3 months. The mean IQ from the California Test of Mental Maturity (CTMM), 1963 S-Form, was 100 with a range of 80-123. All of the boys were caucasian; had appropriate speech; had never received any play therapy or psychotherapy; did not exhibit psychotic or sociopathic behavior; did not present symptoms of a perceptual-motor handicap; and met Fish and Shapiro's criteria for a Type III child with a "mild" global severity rating (Fish and Shapiro, 1965). Most Type III children have a formal diagnosis within the psychoneuroses. All Ss lived with both natural parents except for two boys. One S lived with his natural mother and his step father; the other S lived with his mother only, his father having died 1 year before the study began. The mean number of years of formal education for the fathers was 13·4 years with a range of 11-16. The mothers' mean was 12·4 years with a range of 11-14.

Selection procedure

Sampling was done from 2761 third-grade children from 105 classrooms and 33 grade schools. Each principal was asked to give a letter* to each of his third-grade teachers requesting that the teacher send a form letter from the investigators to the parents of the two boys in her class who most closely fit the following description: "(1) socially withdrawn, very quiet, introverted, and friendless; (2) lacking in spontaneity; (3) maladjusted; and (4) not so withdrawn that he is unable to attend school regularly." The letter to

---

*All letters, instructions, questionnaires, etc. used in the present study which have not previously been published may be obtained in mimeographed form from the senior author.

the parents briefly described the study and asked the parents to contact the senior investigator if they would like to participate.

A group appointment was made for the mothers who applied. At the first meeting the mothers completed a social and developmental history for their boys. They also filled out a behavior problem check list, a Q-Sort (Block, 1961; pp. 154-156), and the Children's Manifest Anxiety Scale (Castaneda, McCandless and Palermo, 1956). The mothers were asked to take their boys to their family physicians or pediatricians for a complete medical examination.

About 1 week after the mothers were seen each boy received a psychological evaluation covering intellectual and personality functioning. Group administrations were used for figure drawings, the Bender-Gestalt, the Children's Manifest Anxiety Scale (CMAS), and the CTMM. Cards I, III, VI, VIII, and X of the Rorschach and a sentence completion test were administered individually.

Based on the evaluation procedure, 12 Ss were selected who met the criteria previously listed. One S had to undergo major surgery during the second week of the research program; therefore, he had to drop out, leaving a final N of 11.

Experimental design

Independent variables. There were two independent variables: (1) the type of therapy administered to the Ss and (2) time, i.e. the number of group play therapy sessions. The experimental model was for a two-factor experiment with repeated measures on the second factor with unequal groups, i.e. $n_1=4$, $n_2=4$, and $n_3=3$ (Winer, 1962, pp. 374-378). Although the primary statistical analysis was based on this factorial design, supplementary evaluations included (1) single-factor analyses of variance for the three groups taken separately, (2) trend tests, and (3) tests on all pairs of means using the Turkey (a) procedure (Winer, 1962, pp. 87-89).

There were three kinds of groups: (1) a Token Group, (2) a Verbal Group, and (3) a Control Group. The Token Group came to the hospital once a week with their mothers, spent 50 minutes in each group play session with their therapist, consisted of four boys, were treated with the procedures suggested by Ginott (1960) for doing group psychotherapy with children, and received tangible reinforcements when social-approach behavior occurred. The tangible reinforcements consisted of brass tokens which could be accumulated to purchase candy, trinkets, and small toys at the end of each therapy hour (cf. Ayllon and Azrin, 1965).

Social-approach behavior was defined as (1) walking toward another boy and/or (2) talking to another boy. Some shaping was done since tokens were initially given for single words; in the middle of therapy the S had to speak short phrases to get a token; and in the final phase of treatment only complete sentences were reinforced. A variable-ratio, variable-interval reinforcement schedule was used throughout the study. Each boy averaged about 20 tokens a session. Each token was worth approximately 1 cent in trade.

The Verbal Group received the same treatments administered to the Token Group including the verbal reinforcements usually given by a therapist, but the tangible reinforcers were excluded. This group was considered to be more similar to a typical, latency-age, boys', play therapy group found in most child guidance centers.

The Control Group met in the play therapy room without a therapist, but observers watched behind a one-way mirror. These boys were allowed to do as they wished except to endanger anyone's physical safety and to damage the play room and furnishings. The observers had to intervene actively only once.

The original 12 Ss were randomly assigned to the three groups. Each group was seen on a weekday at 9:00 a.m. for 14 consecutive weeks during the spring of 1966.

Mothers' guidance groups were held concurrently with the therapy and control sessions. The mothers were seen on the same day and at the same time as their sons. The mothers' groups were run according to the suggestions of Ginott (1960, pp. 169-189), i.e. they were guidance rather than counseling or psychotherapy groups.

Dependent variables. Table X lists (1) the dependent variables, (2) the indices to them, (3) the source person providing the data, and (4) when each index was measured. The dependent variables were taken from the definition of play therapy given in the Introduction. Valid indices to these dependent variables were sought which would provide highly objective and reliable data.

Much of the present data was obtained by directly observing through a one-way mirror the behavior of the children during the group play sessions. A time-sampling technique was used to record

TABLE X

SUMMARY OF THE DEPENDENT VARIABLES

Dependent variable (DV)	Index to DV	Persons providing data	When measured
Productivity	Grades on report card	Teachers	Quarterly during academic year
Anxiety	CMAS	Ss ———— Mothers	Pre-therapy, 7th session, and 14th session
Social adjustment	Play room observations	Research assistants	Throughout each of the 14 play sessions
General psychological adjustment	Q-sort	Mothers	Pre-therapy, 7th session, and 14th session
Problem behaviors	BPCL	Mothers	Pre-therapy, 7th session, and 14th session

the observations. The observer (O) recorded the behavior of each S by observing him every session for twelve 1-minute periods taken at 4-minute intervals. As is indicated in Table X, the time sampling provided the "social adjustment" data.

Ten classes of behavior were recorded: (1) statements to Ss, (2) statements to the therapist (T), (3) questions to Ss, (4) questions to T, (5) non-verbal vocalizations, (6) verbal and symbolic aggression, (7) physical aggression, (8) solitary play, (9) social play, and (10) proximity. Specific criteria were established for each class of behavior. The proximity measure was made as follows: Strips of tape were laid on the playroom floor so that a grid of rectangles approximately 1 yard square was formed. If the S was in the same square as another child during any part of the 60 seconds the S was being observed, the S was scored for proximity.

Only one check mark per S per class of behavior per 60 seconds was allowed, making the maximum possible score 12 per S per behavior per play session.

Because of marked session-to-session variability, the data were grouped into blocks of sessions, i.e. sessions 1–4, 5–9, and 10–14. This grouping made the data more manageable and effected easier statistical evaluation.

Attendance at all sessions was not 100 per cent; therefore, the following procedure was used for estimating raw scores for missing Ss. The mean of the Ss raw score from the session preceding and following the missed session was computed. Second, the mean raw score obtained by the Ss group on the day he missed was computed. The mean of these two means served as the Ss estimated raw score for the day he missed. Most of the boys attended all of the sessions.

During the course of the study only one O recorded the behavior of a given group. Before the study began, therefore, a check was made on inter-observer reliability. Three observers who were using the time sampling system for the first time observed a pilot group for one session. Pearson product-moment correlation coefficients yielded r's of 0·86, 0·88 and 0·93 for the three possible pairings of the three Os. A second reliability check was run on the final therapy session at the end of the present study. The r's at this time were 0·97, 0·99 and 0·99, indicating extremely high inter-observer reliability.

Personnel and equipment

The therapist for the treatment groups was the senior investigator. The leader of the three mothers' groups was the junior investigator. The three Os were volunteer research assistants. They were all young homemakers who had volunteered to work specifically on the present project and were not acquainted with any of the Ss.

The playroom measured 19 × 8½ feet. There was a one-way mirror at one end, and a sound system connected the play and observation rooms. The playroom contained a blackboard, a children's picnic table with attached benches, an easel, and a toy chest. The play materials consisted of crayons, finger paints, paper, chalk, building blocks, a doll house, two five-member doll families, four toy revolvers, a plastic war set with soldiers, tanks, jeeps, etc., a Bobo punching bag, and a small tape recorder.

Results

The results of the major statistical tests are summarized in Table XI. Columns (1), (2) and (3) present the F ratios from the two-factor analyses of variance. For the time sampling data the raw scores used in the analyses were the mean scores for each S from sessions 1—4, 5—9 and 10—14. The symbols in columns (4), (5) and (6) indicate the outcomes of the single-factor tests performed for each play group when factor A, B or AB was significant on the two-factor analysis. The symbol "O" indicates that no change occurred, "+" that the group improved on the measure, and "—" that the group got worse.

No differences between groups, no changes over sessions

Six measures of the dependent variables failed to produce any sig-

TABLE XI

SUMMARY OF THE RESULTS OF THE TWO-FACTOR AND SINGLE-FACTOR ANALYSES OF VARIANCE. XA INDICATES THE "TOKEN GROUP," XB THE "VERBAL GROUP" AND CA THE "CONTROL GROUP"

Measure	F ratios			Results of single-factor analyses of variance			Criterion for improvement
	(1) Groups	*(2)* Sessions	*(3)* Inter-action	*(4)* XA	*(5)* XB	*(6)* CA	
Achievement	0.43[a]	0.38[b]	1.75[c]	0	0	0	Increase
Citizenship	9.31*[a]	0.74[b]	0.07[c]	0	0	0	Decrease
Boys' CMAS	0.79[d]	0.15[e]	0.05[f]	0	0	0	Decrease
Mothers' CMAS	6.17[d]	0.46[e]	2.67[f]	0	0	0	Decrease
Statements to Ss	8.52†[d]	3.44[e]	7.04†[f]	+*	0	0	Increase
Statements to T	0.79[g]	6.81*[b]	3.58[b]	0	+†	0	Decrease
Questions to Ss	11.25†[d]	2.51[e]	1.26[f]	0	0	0	Increase
Questions to T	0.32[g]	0.14[b]	0.11[b]	0	0	0	Decrease
Non-verb. vocal.	2.58[d]	1.75[e]	3.28*[f]	0	0	0	Increase
Aggression (V & S)	2.33[d]	0.27[e]	0.40[f]	0	0	0	Increase
Aggression (Phys.)	2.61[d]	1.84[e]	3.78*[f]	0	0	0	Decrease
Play (Solitary)	38.94†[d]	3.47[e]	1.57[f]	0	0	0	Decrease
Play (Social)	16.99†[d]	0.23[e]	24.52†[f]	+†	—†	0	Increase
Proximity	29.02†[d]	37.23†[e]	15.75†[f]	+†	+†	0	Increase
Q-Sort	0.10[d]	0.50[e]	2.35[f]	0	0	0	Increase
BPCL	9.09†[d]	3.00[e]	0.71[f]	+*	0	0	Decrease
		Improved	(+)	4	2	0	
		No change	(0)	12	13	16	
		Worse	(—)	0	1	0	

*P < 0.05
†P < 0.01
[a]With 2 and 6 df; [b]With 2 and 12 df; [c]With 4 and 12 df; [d]With 2 and 9 df; [e]With 2 and 18 df; [f]With 4 and 18 df; [g]With 1 and 6 df.

nificant Fs for groups, sessions, or groups-sessions interaction (see Table XI. The measures were achievement (i.e. the mean grade in reading, English, spelling, arithmetic, and social studies), boys' scores on the CMAS, mothers' scores on the CMAS, questions to T, verbal and symbolic aggression, and the Q-Sort.

In Table XI and the subsequent figures the Token Group is identified as "XA," the Verbal Group as "XB," and the Control Group as "CA."

Differences between groups, no changes over sessions

In five cases the "groups" or "interaction" factor was significant, but the "sessions" factor did not reach significance. In all of these instances single-factor analyses of variance revealed no reliable changes over sessions in the three groups. Although Table XI shows a reliable difference between groups for "citizenship," this difference existed on the pre-therapy grades in citizenship ($P<0\cdot05$). For "questions to Ss" the same kind of problem existed. The groups were different on the very first play session ($P<0\cdot05$). For the time sampling data a significant F on the first play session was taken to mean that due to sampling error the groups started out different at the beginning of treatment. "Non-verbal vocalizations" and "physical aggression" produced significant interactions only. The groups were different on "solitary play" (XA<XB, $P<0\cdot01$; XA<CA, $P<0\cdot05$; and XB>CA, $P<0\cdot01$) but the "sessions" factor was not significant.

Changes over sessions

No indication was given by the preceding measures that the treatment procedures had any effect on the dependent variables. The results are more positive for the remaining measures.

Statements to Ss. Table XI indicates that only XA exhibited a reliable increase in the amount of verbal communication between the early part of treatment and the latter part. A trend test on group XA indicated a significant linear trend ($P<0\cdot01$). For the time factor, sessions 1—4 are indicated as "b_1," sessions 5—9 as "b_2," and sessions 10-14 as "b_3." Tests on all pairs of means for XA showed that $b_1<b_3$ ($P<0\cdot05$), but $b_1=b_2$ and $b_2=b_3$ (see Figure 21).

Statements to T. A reliable decrease in scores on this measure was defined as improvement. The assumption underlying the definition was that shy, withdrawn children are overly-dependent on adults at the beginning of therapy. As they become less dependent on T, they talk to him less and to the other children more. Trend analysis for XB indicated a significant linear trend ($P<0.01$). Tests on all pairs of means produced the following results: $b_1>b_2$ ($P<0.05$), $b_1>b_3$ ($P<0.01$), but $b_2=b_3$ (see Figure 22).

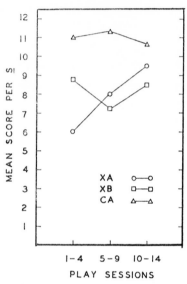

Figure 21. Frequency of "statements to Ss" averaged for the first four, middle five, and last five play sessions, XA indicates the "Token Group," XB the "Verbal Group" and CA the "Control Group."

Social play. Both XA and XB changed during the course of treatment; however, the boys in XA increased in the amount of time they spent playing with each other, whereas the Ss in XB decreased (see Figure 23). Trend tests on XA revealed a significant linear trend ($P<0.01$), but both the linear and quadratic trends were significant at the 0·01 level for XB. Tests on all pairs of means for XA demonstrated that $b_1<b_3$ ($P<0.01$), $b_2<b_3$ ($P<0.01$), and $b_1=b_2$, and for XB $b_1>b_2$ ($P<0.01$), $b_1>b_3$ ($P<0.01$), and $b_2<b_3$ ($P<0.05$).

Proximity. XA and XB exhibited reliable increases during treatment on this measure (see Figure 24 and Table XI). Trend tests indicated significant linear and quadratic trends for both XA and XB. Tests on all pairs of means showed that for XA $b_1<b_3$ ($P<0.01$),

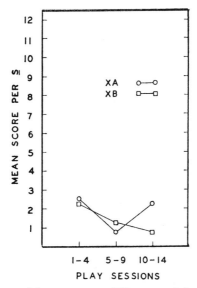

Figure 22. Frequency of "statements to T" averaged for the first four, middle five, and last five play sessions.

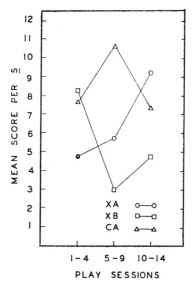

Figure 23. Frequency of "social play" averaged for the first four, middle five, and last five play sessions.

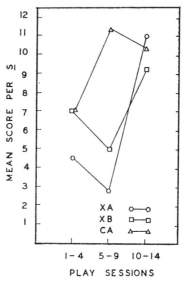

Figure 24. Frequency of "proximity" averaged for the first four, middle five, and last five play sessions.

$b_2 < b_3$ ($P<0.01$), $b_1 = b_2$, and for XB $b_1 > b_2$ ($P<0.01$), $b_1 < b_3$ ($P<0.01$), and $b_2 < b_3$ ($P<0.01$).

Behavior problem check list. The four preceding indices were based on in-therapy measures. The behavior problem check list provided the only extra-therapy data which suggested that the treatments used affected the dependent variables under study. Although the groups did not differ on the pre-therapy measures, they became reliably different during treatment (see Table XI). Tests on all pairs of means for the groups factor revealed that XA<XB ($P<0.01$), XA=CA, and XB<CA ($P<0.01$). All three groups had lower raw scores on the post-therapy measures than on the pre-therapy measures, but the over-all time effects were not significant. A trend analysis of XA's data, however, showed a significant linear trend ($P<0.05$), and tests on all pairs of means indicated that for XA $b_1 > b_3$ ($P<0.05$), $b_1 = b_2$, and $b_2 = b_3$.

Mothers' subjective evaluations

At the end of treatment the mothers of the eleven Ss were asked to write about any change which they had observed in their boys during the time they were coming to the group sessions. Ten of the mothers listed changes. One said that her boy's stealing had gotten worse. All of the other mothers listed positive changes only. Even the mother of the stealing boy indicated that her son's teacher felt he had improved at school.

The types of changes which were listed were "more assertive," "happier," "more concerned about doing well in school," "more self-assured," "now has a good attitude toward himself," "is branching out," "his tears are less frequent," "more stable," "less shy," "tells stories to his dad and relates the happenings of the day," "neighbors report him as more aggressive," "teacher says he speaks up for himself now," "not so fearful," "not so hard to get along with," "is enjoying his PE class now," "plays more with kids outside," "more competitive," "more energetic," etc.

There was no apparent difference in quality or quantity of these responses between the three groups.

Discussion

A common belief found in many child guidance centers is that emotional conflicts can lead to underachievement in school work but that psychotherapy usually leads to an increase in academic productivity (e.g., Bills, 1950a; 1950b). No such increase was noted in the Ss of the present study; however, the boys had not been referred as underachievers. Inspection of their grades suggested a fairly normal mean and distribution, indicating that on the average the boys had been working up to capacity before treatment began. The use of school grades as a dependent variable was probably inappropriate for boys with the presenting symptoms of these Ss.

Another common belief held by child therapists is that anxiety decreases as therapy progresses. The measure of anxiety used in the present research showed no reliable change during the course of the treatment. The length of treatment may have been too short to produce any consistent changes; but, the Ss' raw scores indicated that the lack of change in CMAS scores may have had the same cause as the lack of change in grades, i.e. the mean anxiety score was close to the mean for all 8- and 9-year-old boys. In order for the Ss as a group to have improved on this measure would have required them to exhibit less anxiety than typical boys their age.

After reviewing the literature on child psychotherapy research,

Levitt (1957; 1963) said, "...the inescapable conclusion is that available evaluation studies do not furnish a reasonable basis for the hypothesis that psychotherapy facilitates recovery from emotional illness in children (1963)." The present study has provided data which contradict the impression that child therapists are unable to demonstrate that formal treatment makes a difference. The primary hypothesis stated in the Introduction appears to have been supported by the present data. The Token Group improved on four variables; the Verbal Group improved on two and got worse on one; and the Control Group did not show any improvement. The present study randomly assigned Ss from the *same* population to the treatment and control groups; whereas, although Levitt claimed to use a well-matched control group for his comparisons, his control and experimental Ss were not obtained from the same population and at the same point in time.

The problem of evaluating parents' subjective reports of improvement in their children during and following therapy is pointed out in the present results. All of the mothers except one reported improvement in their boys. Their comments implied more improvement during the course of treatment than was observed on the objective data. The assumption has been made in writing this Discussion that the mothers' subjective reports were unreliable; however, their subjective reports provided the kind of data typically used in clinical settings to evaluate outcome of child treatment. The discrepancy between objective and subjective data points out the need for systematic study of the causes of the obtained differences.

Ayllon and Azrin (1965) demonstrated the effectiveness of treating adult psychotic patients with metal tokens which could be traded for desired objects. The present study showed a similar type of operant conditioning technique which is effective in treating shy, withdrawn eight-year-old boys in a group play situation. Figure 21 indicates most clearly the impact the tokens had on the Token Group's behavior. Although some child therapists may be repulsed by the idea of giving brass tokens to the children they are treating, the use of such a procedure will probably increase the therapeutic impact of the therapist on his clients.

There is so much session-to-session variability in the behavior of eight-year-old boys in a group play situation that week-to-week predictions are very precarious. Accurate prediction becomes more possible when T looks for general trends based on data averaged on groups of sessions, i.e. meaningful predictions may be made from month to month but not from week to week.

The major criticisms of this study are as follows: (1) There was only one T. (2) The senior investigator and T were the same person. Ideally T should not be aware of the major hypotheses of the research project. (3) The sample size was very small. (4) The sample represented only one type of presenting problem out of the many which confront the typical child guidance clinic. (5) The data do not lend themselves to reasonable generalization to other groups representing other kinds of problems. (6) Although an attempt was made to avoid the major criticisms of psychotherapy research (e.g. Kiesler, 1966), the present paper did not solve the most important problem of providing an adequate research paradigm which will lead to systematic theory construction and modification.

Finally there has been relatively little systematic research on psychotherapy with children. One of the reasons for this lack of research has been the apparent difficulty in obtaining an adequate sample. The present study demonstrates an effective approach for obtaining reasonably homogeneous groups of children. Adult samples could be obtained in much the same manner; however, institutions other than schools would have to be used as the source. For example, all ministers, priests, and rabbis in a community could be contacted as the school principals were in the present study and asked to make referrals having particular types of problems.

Acknowledgments—This study was supported by Grant P-389 from the Attending Staff Association, Harbor General Hospital, Torrance, California. The authors wish to thank the following for their assistance on this project: Robert S. Dollarhide and Louis Kaplan of the Torrance Unified School District as well as the many principals and teachers who cooperated; Katherine Clement, Anita Congelliere, Paula Heindel, and Lee Ann Robertson who were the observers; the staff of the Department of Psychiatry, Harbor General Hospital; and the staff and students of the Department of Psychology, Pepperdine College.

References

Allen, K. E., Hart, B. M., Buell, J. S., Harris, F. R. and Wolf, M. M.: Effects of social reinforcement on isolate behavior of a nursery school child. *Child Dev 35*, 511-518, 1964.

Ayllon, T. and Azrin, N. H.: The measurement and reinforcement of behavior of psychotics. *J Exp Anal Behav 8*, 357-383, 1965.

Bills, R. E.: Nondirective play therapy with retarded readers. *J Consult Psychol 14*, 140-149, 1950a.

Bills, R. E.: Play therapy with well-adjusted readers. *J Consult Psychol 14*, 246-249, 1950b.

Block, J.: *The Q-Sort Method in Personality Assessment and Psychiatric Research.* Springfield, Thomas, 1961.

Castaneda, A., McCandless, B. R. and Palermo, D. S.: The children's form of the Manifest Anxiety Scale. *Child Dev 27*, 315-326, 1956.

Cox, F. N.: Sociometric status and individual adjustment before and after play therapy. *J Abnorm Soc Psychol 48*, 354-356, 1953.

Fish, B. and Shapiro, T.: A typology of children's psychiatric disorders. I. Its application to a controlled evaluation of treatment. *J Am Acad Child Psychiat 4*, 32-52, 1965.

Ginott, H. G.: *Group Psychotherapy with Children: The Theory and Practice of Play-Therapy.* McGraw-Hill, New York, 1961.

Kerr, N., Meyerson, L. and Michael, J.: A procedure for shaping vocalizations in a mute child. In *Case Studies in Behavior Modification.* (Eds. Ullmann, L. P. and Krasner, L.), pp. 366-370, Holt, Rinehart & Winston, New York, 1965.

Kiesler, D. J.: Some myths of psychotherapy research and the search for a paradigm. *Psychol Bull 65*, 110-136, 1966.

Lazarus, A. A.: Group therapy of phobic disorders by systematic desensitization. *J Abnorm Soc Psychol 63*, 504-510, 1961.

Levitt, E. E.: The results of psychotherapy with children: An evaluation. *J Consult Psychol 21*, 189-196, 1957.

Levitt, E. E.: Psychotherapy with children: A further evaluation. *Behav Res & Therapy 1*, 45-51, 1963.

Masling, J.: One man's viewpoint on training. *Newsl Sectn Clin Child Psychol, Div Clin Psychol—Am Psychol Assn 5*, No. 2, 1966.

Winer, B. J.: *Statistical Principles in Experimental Design.* McGraw-Hill, New York, 1962.

Chapter 2

BEHAVIOR REHEARSAL AS A TECHNIQUE IN CHILD TREATMENT*

MARTIN GITTELMAN

Introduction

SINCE ITS INCEPTION, behavior therapy has been characterized by the development and innovation of a wide range of technical strategies. Beginning with the earliest work of Jones (1924), and Rayner and Watson (1920), new approaches based on learning theory have continued to proliferate, providing the therapist with a considerable armamentarium in the treatment of neurosis. However, as Rachman (1962) has pointed out, the focus in the investigation and treatment of behavior disorders has been on work with adults, and relatively less in the area of children's disturbances. Rachman ascribes this disparate advance to the difference in the nature of disturbances in children and adults. Whereas adults manifest behavior patterns which are unadaptive and must be broken down, children are more often seen for their inadequate or inappropriate development of desired behavior. While this is often the case, children are frequently seen who require help in breaking down behavior patterns, as well as those who need to adopt developmentally appropriate behavior.

This is particularly so with children whose primary disturbance

*From the *Journal of Child Psychology and Psychiatry,* 1965, 6, pp. 251-255. Reprinted by permission of Maxwell International Microfilms Corporation.

is manifested in the expression of inappropriate aggression and hostility towards their peers, parents, or other authority figures (most often teachers). Such children are readily provoked into rage and 'acting out' by minimal instigation. While the roots of such behavior are often traceable to parental practices (Bandura, Ross and Ross, 1963; Schaefer and Bayley, 1963; Sears, Maccoby and Levin, 1957) and can often be modified by parent counselling, more immediate intervention is frequently required, particularly with older children. As is well known with such children, efforts to point out the unadaptive nature of their responses are met with little or only temporary success. Even when the child states that he knows he has nothing to gain by expressing anger, he often feels powerless to resist striking out against real or imagined provocation. This paper is a report of an attempt to apply learning theory principles to the treatment of such children. Since children on the whole appear to have difficulty in deliberately producing the vivid visual images necessary for desensitization therapy, a method which more closely approximates the elements of the instigatory situation is required. The method, as it has developed, involves the use of role-playing or BEHAVIORAL REHEARSAL, whereby various instigatory situations are played out by the child and, in the case of group therapy, by various members of the group.

Method

While the are many variations of the technique, that which has proved to be clinically most useful requires the elicitation from the child of various situations which in the past have provoked him to aggression or defiance. These situations are then presented, through acting, in a hierarchical manner, with the mildest situation presented initially. As the child develops tolerance for these mild situations, those of a higher instigatory valence are gradually introduced. An arbitrary point score is constructed and the child's responses to instigation are rated by other group members and by the therapist.

An example of such a scoring system is: Two minus points for overt expression of aggression, e.g. striking out; one minus point for an 'emotional' response, e.g. flushing, clenching fists, tightening of the facial musculature, etc. No points are given for a neutral response. On the positive side, one point is scored for a passive reaction, as for example when the child goes 'limp' as he is lifted or pushed. Finally, two points are given for a reaction involving a verbal response which in some way serves to disarm or mollify the instigator. The point system, as noted, is an arbitrary one and can doubtless be improved. However, in practice it serves to quickly differentiate for the child which behaviors are acceptable, and which are not. Moreover, the points received by the child, and possibly more important, the approval he wins from the group for particularly ingenious responses, may be conceptualized as a form of social reinforcement.

The procedure is one which children find enjoyable—often, of course, because (for the instigator) it serves as a way of expressing aggression, albeit a socially acceptable one. That is, the instigator is helping the other child to inhibit his own aggression, and as such is functioning in a therapeutic manner. Even the child who is provoked finds his role bearable, since it will be his turn next to play the part of the instigator. Even extremely passive children, who fear aggression, gradually find behavior rehearsal is not threatening in the context of the protective therapy setting.

Other variants of the technique can be used with children who are not physically aggressive, but who, for example, are having school difficulties because of 'clowning' or who express hostility or defiance by facial or gestural cues. Of course such behavior is often based on underlying difficulties, which can be helped by insight therapy. However, one is impressed by how often a child appears to have obtained genuine insight into the basis of his behavior, and yet finds it difficult to change an established pattern. In such cases, behavior rehearsal would seem to be a valuable adjunct.

In practice, the method draws upon the techniques of psychodrama (Moreno, 1959), that described by Wolpe (1958) in establishing assertive responses, and to training given to civil rights workers in passive resistance (Belfrage, 1965). Recently, young Negro children have been prepared for entry into desegregated schools by subjecting them to sorts of abuse they might expect upon entering the school. Because such preparation is often traumatic for young children, the attrition rate prior to entry has reportedly been high, and it has been suggested that gradual introduction to a hierarchy of provocation would be less traumatic (Gittelman, 1964).

Case Illustration

To illustrate behavior rehearsal with children, a case is described.

The context of the treatment was in a group of seven boys ranging from 12-14 years of age who met for 2 hours each week as outpatients at a community mental health clinic. The group was mixed, in the sense that three of the boys presented varying degrees of 'acting out' behavior, one child was extremely constricted and fearful of aggression, and the remaining three showed a variety of problems. Most of the children were having learning difficulties as well as problems in the home.

One of the group members, Ralph, a 13-year-old whose parents were divorced and who lived with his mother, presented the greatest problems in the expression of aggression. His temper outbursts had proved so violent that he had been expelled from one school and was threatened with expulsion from his new school. The boy was extremely small in stature, giving the impression of a child some two or three years younger. It is likely that this was due to the fact that he had been a premature infant, weighing only two pounds 10 ounces (1.19 kg) at birth. Despite his prematurity and a slow rate of physical growth for the first six months, development had proceeded within normal limits and no signs suggestive of cerebral dysfunction could be inferred from his developmental course. Intelligence testing as well as clinical impression indicated that his intellectual functioning was in the high average range. While he was extremely small in size, he was physically agile and an excellent fighter, feared by many of his peers and, most likely, by some of his teachers.

Ralph's pattern of response to stress was generally as follows: The slightest stimulus would cause him to feel singled out and provoked. Another child who might brush his shoulder in passing, or a teacher's criticism of his work, would cause him to become enraged. Under these conditions, he would respond impulsively, striking out at the other child without waiting for an apology or explanation. During his first session with the group, Ralph provided an example of how easy he was to provoke. While presenting the group with his background and school difficulties, one of the group members asked him whether he was a 'good fighter.' Ralph turned quickly to the boy, his eyes narrowed in anger, and said "You want to try me?" With his teachers he could not resist answering back and was at all times prepared to strike out. In discussing these incidents in the group, he reported feeling that unless he responded aggressively others would think him weak and he would face even greater provocation. Ralph's difficulties had approached a crisis point when he threatened to kill his mother's boy friend with a knife. Following this incident, Ralph said that he understood his reaction was inappropriate and that he felt anxious and guilty, but felt powerless to inhibit his immediate uncontrolled reaction.

Treatment with Ralph proceeded along lines previously described. Behavior rehearsal was initiated after four two-hour weekly sessions. Ralph was first asked to describe, in as great detail as possible, situations which aroused unadaptive affective responses. Subsequently several of the situations were acted out with Ralph and the therapist, or another group member, alternating roles. This was done to provide a more detailed picture of Ralph's behavior, but was also incidentally found to be useful in suggesting alternative modes of behavior to him. Following this procedure, the group members alternately acted out instigating and provocative situations. Initially only the largest group members were used, since Ralph found himself unable to refrain from striking out. A hierarchy of provocative situations was then constructed and individual group members each acted out one. In practice it was not possible to follow the usual formal course of desensitization, proceeding from the least to increasingly provoking situations, since the group members differed in their ability to make 'real' the instigatory situation. However, a gradient of provocative situations was generally adhered to, and ratings made of Ralph's reactions. Illustrations of some of the instigatory situations presented to Ralph, as well as his initial response, included: (1) Being approached and 'accidentally' bumped, with an immediate apology made by the instigator (low intensity reaction). After Ralph was able to tolerate this provocation, the situation was modified by having the instigator follow the 'accidental' brushing with an attempt to provoke Ralph to fight. This was done initially by verbal provocation (e.g. implying that Ralph was cowardly for not responding). Still later, physical instigation was used such as pushing, stepping on his toes, and lifting him. (2) Another situation presented to Ralph involved the enactment of a robbery (high intensity reaction). In this situation the aggressor asked Ralph to empty his pockets, remove his tie and jacket. As the situation was enacted, Ralph was constantly rated by the group. For example, when be slowly complied with the demands to empty his pockets, he was given one negative point. In contrast, he was given two plus points when, as the instigator carefully folded Ralph's tie and placed it in his pocket, he commented that he (the instigator) was welcome to it and did he also need a wristwatch? (3) With two group members acting as classmates and one playing the role of teacher, Ralph was subjected to a number of instigatory situations. Following a pre-arranged plan, developed while Ralph waited outside the room, the boy sitting next to him asked him a question. The 'teacher,' who pretended to be writing on the blackboard, turned to Ralph and asked him to be quiet. One plus point was given him when he did not proclaim his innocence. While Ralph was initially unable to inhibit aggression in the early scenes, he was gradually able to avert rage, but still showed signs of anger, clenching his fists, flushing, etc. Still later, following his chance to provoke several of the other boys, he was noticeably able to tolerate increasingly instigative acts. After the formal aspects of the game, the group was encouraged to discuss their subjective reactions to the roles they had played.

After four group sessions in which behavior rehearsal was employed, Ralph reported a considerable improvement in his behavior out of the group. At that point he had completed eight weekly two-hour sessions over approximately a two and a half month period. He said that while he often felt angry and provoked by many situations, he now felt much more able to inhibit aggressive responses. While he continued to have difficulties in school, involving learning problems, his school guidance counselor reported much diminution of his aggressiveness, which had previously been almost a daily occurrence. Follow-up lasted four months after therapy was initiated, with consistent absence of any major 'flare-ups.' Post-treatment follow-up and direct examinations were precluded when he stopped treatment on moving to another city, after having attended some 12 group-meetings. However, contact with Ralph's mother nine months after termination revealed that he continued to show progress in his school work and had not shown a further outbreak of impulsive or aggressive behavior.

Conceptually, behavior rehearsal with children may be viewed as an attempt to intervene in, or inhabit, unadaptive responses and provide and reinforce more socially acceptable ALTERNATIVE RESPONSES.

In children who exhibit impulsive and aggressive behavior and who are motivated to change, the technique may serve a useful therapeutic role.

Summary

This paper describes a technique in the treatment of aggressive, 'acting-out' children in an out-patient group setting. The method involves the use of role-playing or behavior rehearsal, whereby various instigatory situations are played out by the child and other group members. While the technique is similar in many respects to psychodrama, an effort has been made to introduce certain learning theory concepts, particularly that of desensitization. A case illustrating the technique is presented.

References

Bandura, A., Ross, D. and Ross, S. A.: Vicarious reinforcement and imitative learning. *J Abnorm Soc Psychol 67*, 601-607, 1963.

Belfrage, S.: *Freedom summer*. Viking Press, New York, 1965.

Gittelman, M.: Report on the Work of the Medical Committee for Human Rights in Mississippi. Paper read at Albert Einstein College of Medicine in New York, November 25, 1964.

Jones, M. C.: A laboratory study of fear: the case of Peter. *Pedag Semin 31*, 308-315, 1924.

Moreno, J. L.: Ch. 68: Psychodrama. *American Handbook of Psychiatry*. Edited by Arieti, S. Basic Books, New York, 1959.

Rachman, S.: Learning theory and child psychology: therapeutic possibilities. *J Child Psychol Psychiat 3*, 149-163, 1962.

Rayner, R. and Watson, J. B.: Conditioned emotional reactions. *J Exp Psychol 3*, 1-14, 1920.

Schaefer, E. S. and Bayley, N.: Maternal behavior, child behavior, and their intercorrelations from infancy through adolescence. *Monogr Soc Res Child Dev 28*, 1-127, 1963.

Sears, R. R., Maccoby, E. E. and Levin, H.: *Patterns of child rearing*. Row, Peterson, New York, 1957.

Wolpe, J.: *Psychotherapy by reciprocal inhibition*. Stanford University Press, Stanford, California, 1958.

Chapter 3

APPLICATION OF A TOKEN SYSTEM IN A PRE-ADOLES-CENT BOYS' GROUP*

JAMES M. STEDMAN, TRAVIS L. PETERSON, *and*
JAMES CARDARELLE

Pᴿᴱ-ᴬᴰᴼᴸᴱˢᶜᴱᴺᵀˢ would seem highly amenable to operant techniques in groups. However, the fact that there is only one report, by Gittelman (1963), suggests that this application has received little attention. We attempted to utilize the principles and guidelines reported by Ayllon and Azrin (1969) to establish an operant motivational system (ᴬ ᵀᴼᴷᴱᴺ ᴱᶜᴼᴺᴼᴹʸ) in a pre-adolescent boys' group. This paper will report the procedures we used in establishing the system, our attempts to extend it to academic and social behaviors in the school, and its effectiveness in eliminating deviant behavior in two group members.

Method

General Characteristics of the Group

The group comprised eight boys, ranging in age from 10 through 12.5 years, and met on a weekly basis for approximately one hour. The group was composed of a mixture of overtly aggressive and withdrawn types. In fact, however, the prevailing mood was one of hostile interpersonal relationships and generally aggressive behavior. Even the withdrawn and anxious children were continually drawn

*From the *Journal of Behavior Therapy and Experimental Psychiatry*, 1971, 2, pp. 23-29.

into hostile interactions because of the exceptionally aggressive behavior of two of the group members. Behavior, as ascribed to the boys in the "real world," followed the patterns familiar to child guidance workers. At home they acted out the prevailing patterns seen in the group, manifesting aggression, manipulation or seclusion, depending on the modal behavioral deviation of the particular individual. In school, group members showed inconsistent to poor academic performance, with frequent D's or F's in conduct.

Both before and during our experiment with the token economy, the group was conducted according to an activity group orientation. Sessions began with a brief discussion of the plan for the day, with activities sometimes structured by the therapists and sometimes decided upon by group members. It was at these weekly activities that therapeutic interventions occurred.

Characteristics of the Experimental Subjects

In order to evaluate behavioral changes as a function of the token economy system, two boys in the group were chosen as test subjects. Subject No. 1, age 11, had been diagnosed as "Unsocialized Aggressive Reaction of Childhood." Behavioral problems at home and in school included fighting with peers, temper tantrums and the use of "bad" language. At the time of his group participation he was in a special education class placement for children with minimal brain injury, receiving academic grades of B's and C's. As part of his treatment he had been placed on stabilizing medication and, though this medication had shown effects in the school and home situation, its positive impact was not observable in our group setting. His behavior during group sessions could be characterized as hyperaggressive and unpredictable, for the least provocation often led to physical or verbal aggression or both. All other group members were obviously afraid of him, verbalized their feelings of relief on days he missed the group and generally regarded him as a powerful and uncontrollable boy. Before instituting the token economy, the therapists had seriously considered removing him from the group because of his disruptive influence.

Subject No. 2, age 12.5, carried the diagnosis of "Anxiety Reaction." His behavior both at home and in school was seen as erratic, swinging from extreme politeness and conformity to aggressive outbursts directed toward others. Moreover, teachers complained that he often made loud, disruptive noises and manifested other attention-getting behaviors. Academic grades varied unpredictably from A's to F's. This child was also receiving medication but observable effects were negligible. His group behavior was characterized by attention-getting "stunts," childish clowning and provoking aggressive reactions from others.

Prosocial Target Behaviors for the Group

Table XII presents behavioral clusters and the "token" values for specific prosocial TARGET BEHAVIORS. These clusters were established after informal but detailed observations of the behaviors which seemed to be most disruptive for the group as a whole and least adaptive for the particular members. After negative target behaviors were specified, we tried to restate each item positively; however, it became apparent that many behaviors needed dual specification in terms of the positive behavior expected and the negative counterpart to be avoided. Perhaps this process helps group members to DIFFERENTIATE positive, rewardable responses from negative, non-rewardable ones. After a process of elimination from several previous lists, the items represented in Table XII emerged.

It should be noted that the group members themselves contributed to this item evolution process and were especially active in modifying the token schedule for behaviors outside the group. Our experience suggests that changes in target behavior lists be made in cooperation with group members for both therapeutic and practical reasons.

As inspection of Table XII will indicate, the behaviors chosen were specific in keeping with the basic principles of behavior modification which call for precise determination of target behaviors (Ayllon and Azrin, 1969). However, no attempt was made to specify individualized behavioral programs for each member. Instead, the therapists established an informal consensus regarding rewardable individual conformity to the items of Table XII, thereby establishing a certain degree of individualization.

Section IV, Table XII, represents an attempt to bridge the gap between the activity group and the school room. As is obvious from inspection, reception of tokens is contingent upon academic and conduct behaviors. Though some of the items are rather arbitrary (such as Item 3—"Academic grades—same and show you are trying."), the therapists felt that a reasonably accurate subjective judgment could be made regarding a child's attempts to cope with academic work. The emphasis on conduct grades reflects the therapists' special interest in modifying social behavior.

Negative Target Behaviors for the Two Test Subjects

After informal but detailed observation, two habitual behavior patterns were chosen for each of the test subjects. For Subject 1 these were: (1) acts of physical aggression or threatening gestures and (2) acts of verbal aggression (e.g. "I'll get you," or "I am going

TABLE XII

SCHEDULE FOR EARNING TOKENS AS POSITIVE REINFORCEMENT FOR CHILDREN IN GROUP THERAPY

I. Beginning Group
1. Come to group (1 token)
2. Stay in waiting room until group starts (1 token)
3. Good behavior in the waiting room prior to the group (1 token)
4. Come to place where the adult group leaders are and stay there (1 token)
5. Take part in group decision about today's activity (1 token)

II. Cooperation in Group
1. Participate and try in group activities—sports, discussions, hikes (1 token at beginning, middle and end of group session)
2. Act like a friend—do not hit, pinch, call names or hurt others (1 token at beginning, middle and end)
3. Try to help people be friends and get along—do not stir up one against another (1 token at beginning, middle and end)
4. Stay with the group (1 token at end)

III. Cooperation in Group Discussion
1. Listen to others—don't hog the time (1 token at beginning, middle and end)
2. Talk about the problem—don't act silly, shout, hit others (1 token at beginning, middle and end)
3. Make helpful comments to the other boy about his problem (1 token at beginning, middle and end)
4. Raise hand (1 token at beginning, middle and end)

IV. Behavior Outside Group (as indicated on school report card)
1. Same conduct grades as on previous report card period
A, 5 tokens
B, 4 tokens
C, 3 tokens
2. Any improvement in conduct grades (20 tokens)
3. Academic grades—same and show you are trying (10 tokens)
4. Academic grades—improved
A, 5 tokens per grade
B, 4 tokens per grade
C, 3 tokens per grade

to murder you," or "I hate you"). For Subject 2, behaviors included: (1) verbally interrupting conversations between a therapist and another child or another therapist and (2) interrupting such conversations by physical action, such as swinging hands, dropping a chair, or otherwise producing a loud noise or distracting behavior. Before we began the token system, Subjects 1 and 2 were observed for four sessions in order to establish a base line of occurrence for each of the behaviors mentioned above (see Figure 25). One observer recorded the frequency of occurrence of these behaviors during the session. The same observational procedure was followed at the four base line sessions and at the experimental sessions after the token economy was begun.

Procedure

Initiation of the Program

Before starting the token economy, we explained the system to parents; and in view of the closeness to the supper hour, we obtained permission from the parents for a session-ending "party" with refreshments. Parents were also requested not to send money for the purchase of food from the clinic's vending machines, so that neither appetite nor desire for a snack would be dampened.

Implementation and Operation of the Token System

At the start of the experiment, printed schedule sheets, similar to Table XII, were given to each group member and discussed in detail. This ensured that members understood the nature of the program and provided an opportunity to clarify questions regarding items on Table XII. The program was fully implemented the following week.

Inspection of Table XII will reveal that the TOKENS, consisting of 1 ¼ inch steel washers, were dispensed according to two basic schedules. Some responses (such as I, Item 3) were reinforced on occurrence. Most of the other responses were reinforced after a fixed time interval, with receipt of tokens occurring at definite periods during the session (after 10, 30, and 45 minutes of the activity portion of the session). Responses reinforced after the fixed time interval required the therapists to pay particularly close attention to specific behaviors occurring during the intervals. Token dispensation was decided by therapists' consensus during each reinforcement period, and, if any deviant behavior had been noted during the interval, the group member was informed of his infraction and token reinforcement omitted. Though it is obvious that reinforcement after fixed time intervals probably led to many errors of observation, our experience suggests that the system, with the built-in correction offered by therapist caucus, produced satisfactory results.

Most tokens were dispensed according to the schedules shown in Table XII. Occasionally, however, bonus tokens were given for outstanding adaptive behaviors. For example, when one boy returned a token which a therapist had accidentally dropped, this "honest" response was promptly rewarded. Dispensing of such bonus tokens occurred after therapists publicly consulted and agreed that a particular response constituted an obvious example of desirable behavior.

Token "earnings" were tallied at the end of each activity portion of the session (after 45 minutes) and recorded on a tally sheet. Tokens were then "spent" for the following reinforcement events: (1) the right to return for the next group session; (2) the right to attend the "party" during the last ten minutes of each session; and (3) the privilege of going on occasional field trips away from the clinic. The reinforcement value of Items 2 and 3 seems obvious, but Item 1 may strike some readers as inappropriate and even risky, as a child might easily forego returning to the group. However, as Ayllon and Azrin (1969) point out, research indicates that any behavior with a high probability of occurrence is capable of functioning as a reinforcing event. Since all our boys had been group members for some time, we reasoned that group attendance was a highly probable event for them and, therefore, reinforcing. The problem involved in applying this reasoning to any new group member was recognized and will be discussed briefly in the results section.

At the end of the session each child was required to "pay" ten tokens for the right to return to the next group meeting, and five tokens for the right to attend the "party" during the current session. During a normal meeting, each child could earn 14 to 16 tokens. Though this amount did not allow much leeway, our experience suggests that there is some value in making the child "stretch his budget" in order to acquire Reinforcers 1 and 2. Accumulation of a "bank account" was possible through the child's participation in the group; however, most "bank accounts" were swelled considerably by tokens received for improved behavior in the school situation. Improvement was determined on the basis of report cards, and, invariably, each member earned a substantial number of additional tokens. These were "spent" for Reinforcer 3 (special field trips), for which the number of tokens required was established by the therapists before each occurrence.

Reinforcer 3 was made more attractive by the fact that group members determined the nature of each field trip.

Results and Discussion

For the Test Subjects

Figure 25 presents observed occurrence of unacceptable behavior for the two experimental subjects, under BASELINE and token economy conditions.

Analyses of average weekly occurrence of deviant behaviors for baseline vs. token economy conditions were highly significant (all t's, $P < 0.001$), except for Verbal Aggression exhibited by Subject 1 ($t = 1.09$, $P < 0.15$). Inspection of Figure 25 will show that unusually high occurrences of Verbal Aggression during sessions No. 11 and No. 15 account for this finding.

Though this grouped data is of interest, perhaps the weekly behavior trends charted in Figure 25 are more important. Inspection reveals a dramatic and marked decrease in all forms of deviant behavior, particularly on the part of Subject 2. Though our quantitative analysis was restricted to decreasing the deviant behaviors, we can report that competing, socially positive responses (the behaviors described in Table XII) were increasing for both test subjects, while their socially deviant behaviors were decreasing.

Results for Subject 1 indicate that he too reacted rather well to the structure provided by the token economy. The relapses, occurring during sessions No. 11 and No. 15, happened on days when the subject had failed to use his stabilizing medication; and on those days, he came to the meeting in a hyperactive condition and grew progressively worse. During session No. 11 he refused to accept tokens (the only occasion on which he or any of the other children showed disregard for the token system) and proceeded to emit physically and verbally aggressive responses at an increased rate. His behavior during session 15 was similar. The fact that verbal aggression occurred more frequently than physical aggression during both sessions might be significant, for this might indicate a tendency to use words rather than fists, a situation generally regarded as indicative of therapeutic movement in conventional treatment of aggressive children.

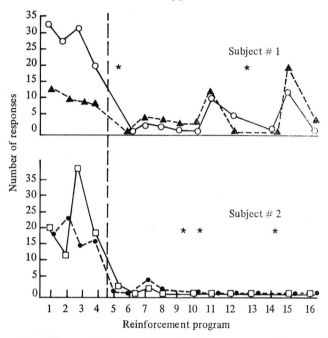

Figure 25. Occurrence of deviant behavior for two test subjects (O Physical aggression or threatening gestures; ▲ Verbal aggression; □ Verbal interruption; ● Physical interruption; * Child absent for session).

Lack of medication certainly seemed to contribute to decreased effectiveness of the token system during both these sessions, and reasons for this are not clear. However, it may be possible that Subject 1 arrived in such a "stirred up" state that the reinforcement system was simply not powerful enough to counteract fully expression of aggressive responses, although inspection of Figure 25 indicates a decreased rate of responding, at least for Physical Aggression. Previously medication alone had never proved powerful enough to counteract either form of aggression in this patient.

The group's reaction to his behavior was interesting. In the past they had become immediately embroiled in any aggressive action by Subject 1. On these occasions, however, they made supportive statements and generally attempted to draw him back in the group. Despite their efforts, Subject 1 continued to act out and was removed from the group for a "time-out" period during both sessions. It should be noted, however, that he was able successfully to rejoin the group activity on both occasions.

There are no quantitative data for other group members. Our observations suggest, however, that the token economy system served as a positive facilitator of group therapeutic process. The children accepted the rationale behind the reward system without question or protest, and there was little or no loss of interest in group attendance or group participation. Whereas initially the "game" aspect itself offered some appeal, the children quickly accepted the system as routine and sought tokens with much fervor. On only one occasion did a boy fail to earn sufficient tokens to participate in the "party" at the end of the session and at no time did any member fail to earn sufficient points to return to the group the following week. Though the design of the study obviously does not take account of previous base rates for all group members (with the exception of Subjects 1 and 2), it is certainly our impression that, following initiation of the token system, the rate of socially acceptable behavior increased greatly, while socially deviant behavior declined.

Qualitative inspection of the trends in report card grades from the beginning of the token economy to the end of the spring semester suggested that five group members had either maintained adequate academic and conduct grades, or had actually improved in both areas. Two others showed mixed patterns, with some scattered improvements. One member manifested little observable change, although his group behavior improved markedly.

Though these data are uncontrolled, they at least suggest some impact on the school behaviors of some group members. We can also report that members presented their cards during each grading period and were eager to point out areas of improvement. Furthermore, at least one teacher spontaneously indicated that two of the group members (both of whom were her students) seemed very aware of the relationship between their school room behavior and receipt of tokens. Her impressions were supported by the fact that one of her students chose to fulfill an English assignment by writing a paragraph regarding the token economy aspects of his therapy sessions.

Nevertheless, Wahler (1969) has recently reported that contingency programs do not automatically generalize from one setting to another (from home to school in his case). This finding suggests that maximal behavioral improvement will occur only when all settings operate with similar contingency systems, and it implies that to be most effective operant programs should be installed simultaneously in several settings. No doubt any attempt to modify behavior in two or more settings can best be achieved by simultaneous and systematic introduction of similar operant programs in all settings.

Finally we should comment on the difficulty involved in introducing a new member to the group. Theoretically this seems to pose a problem, as the new member presumably would not be "hooked" on the group and therefore might not experience group participation as a reinforcing event. One new member entered the group during our experiment. He and his family were thoroughly briefed regarding the structure and operation of the group; and upon entering the following week, he began to seek tokens as actively as any other member. Though this limited and uncontrolled experience with one case does not settle the issue, at least it suggests that participation in the group might be established as a reinforcing event merely by defining it as such during an intensive family session before group entry. Further research, systematically controlling all other sources of reinforcement is needed to settle this issue.

References

Ayllon, T. and Azrin, N. H.: *The Token Economy*. Appleton, Century, Croft, New York, 1968.

Gittelman, M.: Behavioral rehearsal as a technique in child treatment, *J Child Psychol Psychiat 6*, 251-255, 1965.

Wahler, R. G.: Setting generality: Some specific and general effects of child behavior therapy, *J Appl Behav Anal 2*, 239-246, 1969.

Section V

BEHAVIOR THERAPY WITH DELINQUENTS

SECTION V CONCENTRATES ON DELINQUENT MALADAPTIVE BEHAVIOR. AGAIN OUR SURVEY SUGGESTS A DEARTH OF QUALITY ARTICLES, EXCEPT FOR THOSE RELATED TO RESIDENTIAL PROGRAMS (E.G. PHILLIPS). BURCHARD, AND TYLER'S WORK REPRESENTS AN EARLY, CASE ORIENTED APPLICATION TO DELINQUENT BEHAVIORAL PROBLEMS. THE LATER WORK OF STUART MAY WELL REPRESENT A REAL BREAKTHROUGH IN DEALING WITH DELINQUENT BEHAVIOR, AS WELL AS A LARGE RANGE OF MALADAPTIVE BEHAVIORS MANIFESTED BY ADOLESCENTS. OF PARTICULAR IMPORTANCE IS THE FACT THAT STUART'S ARTICLE PRESENTS A METHODOLOGY WHICH INCORPORATES THE FAMILY INTO THE TREATMENT PROCESS.

Chapter 1

THE MODIFICATION OF DELINQUENT BEHAVIOUR THROUGH OPERANT CONDITIONING*

JOHN BURCHARD *and* VERNON TYLER, Jr.

IN RECENT YEARS there has been an impressive demonstration of the modification of maladaptive behaviour with psychotherapeutic techniques which are based upon principles of learning (Bandura, 1961; Eysenck, 1960; Rachman, 1963; Wolpe, 1958). In most instances the behaviour being modified has involved some form of neurotic disorder and the therapeutic technique has been based upon the principles of classical conditioning (i.e. desensitization, aversion-relief therapy). There has also been an increasing number of studies in which pathological behaviour has been significantly modified with techniques based on operant conditioning (Ayllon, 1963; Ayllon and Haughton, 1962; Lindsley, 1956; Rickard, Dignam and Horner, 1960; Wolf, Risley, and Mees, 1964). There have, however, been few attempts to modify the antisocial behaviour of the delinquent (Slack, 1960; Schwitzgebel, 1960; Schwitzgebel, 1963; Schwitzgebel and Kolb, 1964).

In the exploratory study to be reported here, a programme was developed to eliminate antisocial behaviour utilizing the principles of

*From *Behavior Research and Therapy*, 1965, 2, pp. 245-250. Reprinted by permission of Maxwell International Microforms Corporation.

operant conditioning. It was hypothesized that the frequent disruptive and antisocial behaviour of the subject used in this study was a function of the contingencies existing between such behaviour and the social reinforcements received from peers and staff within the institution, and it was felt that such behaviour could be eliminated through a systematic modification of those contingencies.

Case History

Donny has been institutionalized since he was nine years old, a period of four and a half years. He was committed to the Department of Institutions of the State of Washington due to his mother's inability to handle his "destructive and disruptive behaviour" which included destruction of property, cruelty to domestic animals and small children, stealing, starting fires, bed-wetting, etc. Diagnostic labels have ranged from possible childhood schizophrenia to psychopathic personality and in each psychiatric or psychological evaluation he has received, it was concluded that his general adjustment had deteriorated and that his behaviour was becoming more difficult to control.

A psychiatric report written shortly after Donny was committed to the institution set the pattern of his treatment for the next two years. The report stated that Donny would be a perfect candidate for regressive therapy; that he should be regressed to the point of taking a bottle from his therapist, that he should have as much physical contact as possible, even if only to sit on the therapist's lap for an hour and suck candy, and that if he could be brought to smearing faeces it would surely be good for him. The report continued that the only alternative would appear to be to lock Donny up for the remainder of his life and that the worst outcome of the recommended procedure would be that he would remain at an early level of development and then be suitable for a mental hospital.

After this two year period of regressive therapy, other methods of treatment were undertaken including a more behaviourally oriented approach, but they were all ineffective in controlling Donny's behaviour and were therefore abandoned. In conjunction with the various psychotherapeutic endeavours, Donny was also receiving various types and dosages of tranquilizers, none of which seemed to have a consistent or enduring effect.

During the year prior to this study, Donny's behaviour led to his confinement in an individual isolation room* on more than 40 occasions where he spent a total of 200 days. His most serious offences included: smearing paint over the walls and curtains of his room, breaking and entering, glue-sniffing, damage to property, attempted escape, and inflicting injuries on himself and others.

Approximately three months prior to the beginning of the study, it was the staff consensus that Donny could not be controlled in a cottage setting.† Therefore he was placed in an isolation room on a continuous basis and it was recommended that he be transferred to an institution where greater external controls were available.

Procedure

Analysis of Donny's behaviour with its consequences strongly suggested that his antisocial behaviour was controlled by various CONTINGENCIES that existed within the institution. Observation of the interaction between Donny and the institutional staff indicated that much of his antisocial behaviour was followed by rewards rather than punishment. The events which were acting as reinforcers and thereby increasing the probability of this behaviour seemed to be the following:

1. Increased staff attention as a consequence of his disruptive or antisocial behaviour. Whenever Donny was placed in a cottage for the first time (e.g. after transfer from isolation), he would gradually become more difficult to control. Associated with this behaviour was a temporal sequence of staff reactions which appeared to be reinforcing; efforts to ignore the behaviour as long as possible, attempts at supportive persuasion to desist, frustration, ambivalence, expression of anger, the administration of punishment (placement in isolation), and then guilt reactions with sympathy and visits to isolation.

*The isolation room was one of several rooms, 8 × 10 ft, in a security unit and contained a stationary metal bed and toilet. The isolation unit was on a separate floor from the cottage and was checked hourly by a security man.

†The cottage consisted mainly of a large dormitory and dayroom containing a ping-pong table, TV, pool table. Although the total population varied, there were usually 20 to 22 boys residing in the cottage. The cottage and the institution provide an "open" setting inasmuch as there are no physical barriers to prevent unauthorized leave. The staff assigned to the cottage consisted of a cottage supervisor and five cottage parents all of whom had at least a high school education. On all occasions there was one staff-member in the cottage, although during the day shift on weekdays, the regular staff were frequently assisted by the cottage supervisor.

Although the time Donny spent in the isolation unit far exceeded that of any other boy in the institution, it was apparent that he was also receiving far more individual attention than anyone else.

2. Snacks which were given to Donny by the staff while he was in his isolation room.

3. Peer attention, praise and sympathy as well as considerable gratification from inciting the boys in the cottage to the point where they became emotionally upset, vocal and assaultive. Also, because the isolation rooms were in close proximity to each other, Donny was able to communicate verbally with other boys in the security unit and actually obtained these same types of rewards while in isolation.

Associated with the administration of these reinforcers were other factors which could explain why there was such a high operant level of antisocial behaviour. The immediate reinforcement of staff and peer attention appeared to be considerably more potent than the delayed PUNISHMENT (isolation). In addition, the competing, socially-acceptable, "good" behaviour, which in Donny's case mainly consisted of apathetically watching TV and suppressing unacceptable behaviour, was not sufficient to evoke much reinforcement from others. In a cottage setting where one staff-member is responsible for 15 to 25 boys, considerable attention must be focused on problems which develop within the cottage and in many instances there is little time to direct attention toward the boy who is not acting out. In general, the contingencies described above indicate that the staff were actually shaping and maintaining Donny's antisocial behaviour.

During the five months of this study, Donny was taken off all medication, placed in a regular cottage setting and routine and removed from all the conventional forms of psychotherapy. The contingencies of his behavior were systematically modified to produce the following programme of concurrent punishment of antisocial behaviour and the differential reinforcement of all other behaviour.

1. In order to avoid the reinforcement of antisocial behaviour, Donny was immediately and perfunctorily PLACED INTO HIS ISOLATION ROOM upon displaying any "unacceptable" behaviour. He was to remain there for a period of three hours unless he was sent in the late evening in which case he remained there until 7.00 a.m. All staff-members who were in contact with Donny were given the following

instructions:

> Whenever Donny displays any unacceptable behaviour, he is to be immediately placed in isolation. Unacceptable behaviour is defined as any behaviour which would normally require a sanction, verbal or otherwise. If you don't feel the behaviour should warrant isolation, then the behaviour should be ignored. However, if any action is taken to modify or eliminate the behaviour, it should be isolation. The use of isolation should be on an all-or-none basis; that is he should never be threatened with the possibility of being sent to isolation. He should be sent to isolation in a "matter-of-fact" manner. He should be told in simple terms why he is being sent and any further verbal interaction with Donny should be held to a minimum. It is important that you do not become too emotionally involved with Donny. Anyone who feels guilty or for some reason does not send Donny to isolation when his behaviour warrants it is not participating in the treatment plan. As long as Donny is "fouling up," the more he is sent to isolation, the more effective the treatment programme will be.

2. In order to remove possible POSITIVE REINFORCEMENT from the punishing situation, while Donny was in isolation, a radio immediately above his room was played at moderate volume between the hours of 7.00 a.m. and 10.00 p.m. The purpose of the radio was to prevent communication between Donny and any other boys who might be in the isolation unit or any unnecessary communication with staff who might be in the area.

Aside from a metal bed without any mattress and a toilet, there were no objects within Donny's isolation room. If Donny had to remain in isolation overnight, he was given a mattress and blankets at 10.00 p.m.

All staff were instructed not to pay unnecessary attention to Donny while he was in isolation. Whenever Donny acted out while he was in isolation, his length of stay in isolation was extended by an hour.

3. For each hour that Donny remained out of isolation between the hours of 7.00 a.m. and 10.00 p.m., he was given a token (poker chip). (If Donny remained in the cottage for the entire overnight period between 10.00 p.m. and 7.00 a.m., he was given three tokens at 7.00 a.m.)

4. With his tokens, Donny was permitted to buy such things as cigarettes, soda pop, trips to town, recreational activities, attendance at movies, and so on. These privileges were only available to Donny when he was able to pay for them with the appropriate number of tokens. At irregular intervals, approximately three times a week, he was given an opportunity to spend his tokens in the institution canteen. The opportunity to purchase nonmaterial rewards (i.e. recreational activities) usually occurred on a daily basis.

After two months of this procedure, the following changes were made in his programme:

1. Donny was required to stay out of isolation for two hours rather than one hour in order to receive one token. Whenever Donny remained out of isolation for a period of 24 hours, he received a bonus of seven tokens. These changes represented an attempt to shape longer periods of acceptable behaviour by increasing the time interval between reinforcements and by increasing the reinforcement for a long interval (24 hours) of "other behaviour."

2. Trips to the canteen were made at regular, predetermined intervals, three times a week. After two months of the study, it was evident that the intermittent schedule for primary reinforcement (trips to the canteen) created anger and frustration for Donny. Therefore that scheduled was changed.

3. Time in isolation was changed from three to two hours. It was felt that two hours was sufficient "time-out" and this gave Don an opportunity to spend more time in the cottage.

Results

The results show a gradual but consistent decline in the frequency of unacceptable behaviour. Donny was placed in isolation 18 times during the first month and 12 times during the fifth month, a decline of 33 per cent. The significance of these results was enhanced by a subjective analysis which indicated that as the study progressed, the seriousness of the offences decreased. Donny's most serious offences during the first one-month period included glue-sniffing on two occasions, attempting to sniff purex which he pilfered from the storeroom, stealing fish while visiting a fish hatchery, stealing from the staff, and fighting with peers. During the last month, Donny's most serious offences were: fighting, running in the cottage, disrupting his classroom at school, insolence to cottage staff and general disruptive behaviour in the cottage. It should also be mentioned that it was the opinion of some of the staff that as the study progressed they had raised their criterion for "unacceptable" behaviour to include behaviours which were previously unpunished (e.g. running in the cottage). Several comments made by the staff during the study indicated that Donny was much easier to control and that, for the most part, his attempt verbally to manipulate staff (cajoling and begging) decreased.

Regarding the procedural changes made at the close of the second month, there was no noticeable change in the number of trips to isolation to suggest that the procedure for the succeeding three months was any more or less effective than the procedure for the preceding two months.

Discussion

In general, it is felt that many of the initial objectives of this study were accomplished. As an exploration into the use of operant techniques in modifying the antisocial behaviour of delinquents, useful information was obtained, especially with regards to methodology. Because there were many relatively untrained institutional staff members who were responsible for applying the contingencies and recording the data, it was impossible to obtain laboratory precision and therefore, it was impossible to ascertain which aspects of the procedure were responsible for the behavioural changes which occurred. Nevertheless, this study does provide evidence which strongly suggests that Donny's antisocial behaviour was shaped and maintained by the natural contingencies within the institution and that the overall modification of those contingencies was responsible for the obvious decline of that behaviour. After five months on this programme, the *grossly* unmanageable aspects of Donny's behaviour were eliminated so that he could be controlled in an open cottage setting.

One factor that contributes to the lag in applying operant techniques to the treatment of delinquents is the delinquent's ability to conceal his "pathology" (Cleckley, 1955). Most delinquents possess considerable control over their behaviour and can adapt to significant alterations in their environment. Unlike the neurotic whose anxiety attacks are consistent and stimulus-bound, or the psychotic who frequently displays grossly atypical behaviour, the delinquent may function quite adequately in certain situations for relatively long periods of time, especially if his environment possesses considerable structure and control. Therefore it is difficult to study the effects of operant techniques on any one particular type of antisocial response (e.g. stealing), because of its extremely low operant level in most situations where such techniques could be applied.

In order to avoid this problem a subject was chosen for this study who displayed a wide variety of antisocial behaviour within the institution and the dependent variable was defined in terms of an extremely broad class of behaviour (unacceptable behaviour) providing an operant level of sufficient magnitude for study. At the present time, however, the investigators are evaluating two other ways of resolving this problem. The first consists of systematically removing considerable structure and control from the institutional environment so that the delinquent is given progressively greater responsibility and freedom. It is felt that under such conditions an individual will be more apt to display the type of behaviour that led to his institutionalization. It is also apparent that this would serve to increase the similarity between the institutional and home environments thereby facilitating any generalization that might take place.

A second way in which antisocial behaviour might be made more susceptible to this type of investigation would be to create situations which simulate certain simulus characteristics of the environment which are associated with the expression of antisocial behaviour. For example, under moderately controlled conditions the experimenter could build into the institutional environment a certain amount of deprivation or frustration in order to precipitate antisocial behaviour which could then be followed by certain prearranged consequences. Because this would provide the experimenter with some control over the occurrence of antisocial behaviour there would be a corresponding increase in the control and precision associated with the administration of contingencies and the collection of data.

With regard to the effect of operant techniques on the behaviour of the delinquent, it is probable that more information could have been obtained if a more specific and readily definable behaviour had been selected. While further work will be done in this area, the objective of the present study was to develop a set of operant techniques which would modify the antisocial behaviour of a delinquent.

Acknowledgments—The authors are indebted to E. G. Lindquist, Superintendent, and Robert Koschnick, Assistant Superintendent of the Fort Worden Treatment Center, Port Townsend, Washington, for their co-operation and encouragement throughout the course of this study. Also Montrose Wolf and Todd Risley of the University of Washington deserve credit for their valuable counsel concerning certain problems which arose during the study.

We wish to express special appreciation to the cottage staff members who worked closely with Donny, Joe Peters, Val Widner, James Lindley, Byron Ruby, Larry Williamson, Jack Gallager and to Gordon Allie and his security staff, without whose co-operation this study could not have been satisfactorily conducted.

This paper was presented at the American Psychological Association, Los Angeles, California, 1964.

References

Ayllon, T.: Intensive treatment of psychotic behaviour by stimulus satiation and food reinforcement. *Behav Res Ther 1*, 53-61, 1963.

Ayllon, T. and Haughton, E.: Control of the behavior of schizophrenic patients by food. *J Exp Anal Behav 5*, 343-352, 1962.

Bandura, A.: Psychotherapy as a learning process. *Psychol Bull 58*, 144-159, 1961.

Cleckley, H.: *The Mask of Sanity* (3rd ed.), C. V. Mosby, St. Louis, 1955.

Eysenck, H. J.: *Behaviour Therapy and the Neuroses*. Pergamon Press, Oxford, 1960.

Lindsley, O. R.: Operant conditioning methods applied to research in chronic schizophrenia. *Psychiat Res Rep 5*, 118-139, 1956.

Rachman, S.: Introduction to behaviour therapy. *Behav Res Ther 1*, 3-16, 1963.

Rickard, H. C., Dignam, P. J. and Horner, R. F.: Verbal manipulation in a psychotherapeutic relationship. *J Clin Psychol 16*, 365-370, 1960.

Slack, C. W.: Experimenter-subject psychotherapy: a new method of introducing intensive office treatment for unreachable cases. *Ment Hyg 44*, 238-256, 1960.

Schwitzgebel, R.: Delinquents with tape recorders. *New Soc* Jan. 31, 1963.

Schwitzgebel, R. and Kolb, D. A.: Inducing behaviour change in adolescent delinquents. *Behav Res Ther 1*, 297-304, 1964.

Wolf, M., Risley, T. and Mees, H.: Application of operant conditioning procedures to the behaviour problems of an autistic child. *Behav Res Ther 1*, 305-312, 1964.

Wolpe, J.: *Psychotherapy by Reciprocal Inhibition*. Stanford University Press, Stanford, Calif., 1958.

Chapter 2

ACHIEVEMENT PLACE: TOKEN REINFORCEMENT PROCEDURES IN A HOME-STYLE REHABILITATION SETTING FOR "PRE-DELINQUENT" BOYS[†][*]

ELERY L. PHILLIPS

Contents

A LTERNATIVES ARE BEING SOUGHT to the placement of juvenile delinquents in large state reformatories. While reformatories are steadily increasing their standards they still have had less than adequate records of success (Block and Flynn, 1966; Berelson and Steiner, 1964).

The current trend away from the reformatory can be seen in the establishment of small home-style, residential treatment programs by individual communities. These often involve a pair of house-parents and from three to eight youths. The adjudicated youths live in these homes, attend the local schools, and continue to participate in their communities.

Achievement Place, the program described in this report, is an example of a home-style, community based, treatment facility. The treatment program at Achievement Place employed a "token economy" based on those described by Cohen, Filipczak, and Bis (1965), and Burchard (1967) for institutionalized delinquents; by Ayllon and Azrin (1965) for institutionalized psychotics; and by Wolf, Giles, and Hall (1968), Clark, Lachowicz, and Wolf (1968), and Birnbrauer, Wolf, Kidder, and Tague (1965) for classroom management.

The aim of the present research was to develop and evaluate the effects of a token economy (based on naturally available reinforcers) in a home-style, residential treatment program for "pre-delinquent" boys.

Program

Subjects

Three boys who had been declared dependent-neglected by the County Court and placed in Achievement Place served as subjects. The boys, all from low-income families, had committed minor offenses ("thefts," "fighting," and "general disruptive behavior") and had histories of "school truancy" and "academic failure."

Jack was 13 years old. His school records reported an I.Q. of 85

†I wish to thank Montrose M. Wolf for his advice and guidance throughout this research. I am also indebted to Elaine Phillips for assistance in conducting the experiments and in preparing this manuscript. This study is based on a thesis submitted to the Department of Human Development in partial fulfillment of the requirements of the Master of Arts degree. The research was partially supported by a grant (HD 03144) from the National Institute of Child Health and Human Development to the Bureau of Child Research and the Department of Human Development, Univeristy of Kansas.

and a second-grade reading level. Concern had been noted regarding a "speech problem," "poor grammar," "aggressiveness," "poor motivation," and "a general lack of cleanliness."

Don was 14 years old. School records indicated that academically he was performing two years below his grade placement, but that he had a normal I.Q. rating. Reports from school also described this youth as "possessing an inferior attitude," "rejected" by his classmates, and "aggressive."

Tom, who was 12, was described as having an I.Q. of approximately 120. His disruptive behavior in school had resulted in his being placed in the fifth grade, three years below his level of achievement as indicated by the Iowa Basic Skills Test. School records also noted that he was "dangerous to other children" and "openly hostile toward teachers."

Facilities and Routine

The purpose of Achievement Place was to provide a home situation in the community for boys who had been termed pre-delinquents by local juvenile authorities (boys who had committed only minor offenses thus far, but whom the Court felt would probably advance to more serious crimes unless steps were taken to modify their behavior). The author and his wife were the house-parents.

The daily routine was similar to that of many families. The boys arose at 7 A.M. They showered, dressed, and cleaned their bedrooms and bathrooms. After breakfast, some of the boys had kitchen clean-up duties before leaving for school. After school the boys returned home and prepared their homework, after which they could watch TV, play games, or engage in other recreational activities if these privileges had been earned via the token economy. Some boys were assigned kitchen clean-up duties after the evening meal. Bedtime was 9:30 P.M. Trips, athletic events, and jobs, both around the home and away from the home, were scheduled for weekends and school holidays.

The Target Behaviors and the
Token Reinforcement System

TARGET BEHAVIORS were selected in social, self-care, and academic areas considered to be important to the youths in their current or future environment. A further requirement was that a target behavior had to be definable in terms of observable events and measurable with a high degree of inter-observer agreement.

Token reinforcers were used which could be easily and rapidly administered and thus could bridge the delay between the target behavior and the remote BACK-UP REINFORCING EVENTS. The TOKENS took the form of points. The boys earned points for specified appropriate behavior and lost points for specified inappropriate behavior. Points were tallied on 3-by-5-inch index cards that the boys always carried with them. Thus, the points could be earned or lost immediately and points later redeemed for the back-up reinforcers.

Items and events which were naturally available in the home and which appeared to be important to the boys were the back-up reinforcers. Access to these privileges was obtained on a weekly basis. At the end of each week the boys could trade the points they had earned that week for privileges during the next week. Some of the privileges are described in Table XIII.

TABLE XIII
PRIVILEGES THAT COULD BE EARNED EACH WEEK WITH POINTS

Privileges for the Week	*Price in Points*
Allowance	1000
Bicycle	1000
TV	1000
Games	500
Tools	500
Snacks	1000
Permission to go downtown	1000
Permission to stay up past bedtime	1000
Permission to come home late after school	1000

The prices of the privileges were relatively constant from week to week, although they were occasionally adjusted as their importance appeared to vary. For example, during the winter the price of television was increased.

The economy of the system (the relationship between the total number of points that could be earned and the total cost of all the privileges) was arranged in such a manner that if a youth performed all the tasks expected of him and lost a minimum of points in fines, he could expect to obtain all the privileges without performing any extra tasks.

There was another set of privileges for "one-of-a-kind" opportunities which had no fixed price but which were instead sold to the highest bidder, auction style. One example was the "car privilege" which entitled the purchaser to his choice of seating in the car for the week. Another auctioned privilege was the opportunity for a boy to obtain authority over the other boys in the execution of some household chore. Each week these managerships were auctioned. The purchaser was made responsible for the maintenance of the basement, the yard, or the bathrooms. Each manager had authority to reward or fine the other boys under his direction for their work at the task. The manager, in turn, earned or lost points as a result of the quality of job done (as judged by the house-parents).

Most of the behaviors which earned or lost points were formalized and explicit to the extent of being advertised on the bulletin board. Rewards and fines ranged from 10 to 10,000 points. Some of the behaviors and approximate points gained are indicated in Table XIV.

A few other CONTINGENCIES were less formalized but still resulted

TABLE XIV

BEHAVIORS AND THE NUMBER OF POINTS THAT THEY EARNED OR LOST

Behaviors That Earned Points	*Points*
1) Watching news on TV or reading the newspaper	300 per day
2) Cleaning and maintaining neatness in one's room	500 per day
3) Keeping one's person neat and clean	500 per day
4) Reading books	5 to 10 per page
5) Aiding house parents in various household tasks	20 to 1000 per task
6) Doing dishes	500 to 1000 per meal
7) Being well dressed for an evening meal	100 to 500 per meal
8) Performing homework	500 per day
9) Obtaining desirable grades on school report cards	500 to 1000 per grade
10) Turning out lights when not in use	25 per light

Behaviors That Lost Points	*Points*
1) Failing grades on the report card	500 to 1000 per grade
2) Speaking aggressively	20 to 50 per response
3) Forgetting to wash hands before meals	100 to 300 per meal
4) Arguing	300 per response
5) Disobeying	100 to 1000 per response
6) Being late	10 per minute
7) Displaying poor manners	50 to 100 per response
8) Engaging in poor posture	50 to 100 per response
9) Using poor grammar	20 to 50 per response
10) Stealing, lying, or cheating	10,000 per response

in point consequences. For example, even though there was no formal rule the boys would sometimes earn or lose points as a result of their overall manners while guests were in the home.

EXPERIMENT I: AGGRESSIVE STATEMENTS

One behavior pattern that had led to the classification of these youths as deviant juveniles had been the "aggressiveness" they exhibited. The terms "aggression" and "aggressiveness" were noted in school records, psychological test reports, Court notes, and in general comments from individuals who were familiar with the youths. Inquiry into the nature of this "aggressiveness" revealed it to be inferred almost completely from comments the boys emitted such as: "I'll smash that car if it gets in my way" or "I'll kill you." The following experiment describes the house-parents' program to measure and to reduce the aggressive verbal behavior.

Procedures and Results

"Aggressive" phrases were recorded for the three boys simultaneously for 3 hours each day (one session) while the youths were engaged in woodworking activities in the basement workshop.

Response Definition

Phrases or clauses emitted by the youths were considered to be aggressive statements if they stated or threatened inappropriate destruction or damage to any object, person, or animal. For example, the statement "Be quiet" was not counted as an aggressive response, while "If you don't shut up, I'll kill you" was recorded as an aggressive statement. Over 70% of the aggressive statements were from a list of 19 phrases used repeatedly.

Conditions

Baseline. No contingencies were placed on the youths' responses.

Correction. The boys were told what an aggressive statement was and that such statements were not to be used. A corrective statement by one of the house-parents, such as "That's not the way to talk" or "Stop that kind of talk," was made contingent on the youths' responses. An arbitrary period of approximately 3 to 5 seconds was allowed to elapse after a response (or responses) before the corrective comment was made. This meant that a correction did not follow every aggressive statement; sometimes many responses were emitted before a corrective statement was made. The delay interval was employed in order to increase the chance that the boy would have completed his speech episode before correction was administered by the parent.

Fines. A FINE of 20 points was made contingent on each response. The fines, like the corrections of the previous condition, were not delivered until approximately 3 to 5 seconds had passed without a response. No announcement of this condition was made in advance.

No fines. No fines or corrections were levied on responses. This condition was introduced unannounced. There were occasional threats to reinstate the Fines condition if the rate of responding did not decrease. The threats were worded approximately as follows: "If you boys continue to use that aggressive talk, I will have no other choice but to take away points." These threats were not carried out.

Fines. This condition was identical to the first Fines condition except that fines were 50 points instead of 25. The onset of this condition was announced.

In Figure 26 it can be seen, by comparing Correction rate with the BASELINE RATE, that Correction reduced the responding of only one boy, while Fines (20 points per response) produced an immediate and dramatic decline in each youth's aggressive statements. Responses gradually returned when fines were no longer levied but were eliminated when the Fines condition was reinstated. Although the first threat (indicated by the arrows) in the No Fines condition did appear to have a large suppressive effect on the rate of behavior, the last two threats appeared to have much less, possibly due to the fact that the first threat had not been carried out.

Inter-observer agreement about the occurrence of aggressive statements was measured by the use of a second observer during 14 of the 75 sessions. Agreement averaged 92%.

EXPERIMENT II: BATHROOM CLEANING

The youths in the home were assigned a number of household chores, such as aiding in the upkeep of the yard and cleaning their rooms and bathrooms. They originally failed to complete these chores in most instances. Programs involving the point system were designed to increase the boys' contribution to the maintenance of these areas. The cleaning of the bathrooms was studied under a number of conditions.

Procedures and Results

Sixteen cleaning tasks in the bathroom involving the sinks, stools, floors, *etc.* were scored as accomplished or not accomplished. The bathrooms were scored every day between 12:00 and 12:30 P.M., except in the Baseline condition, where recording was done as soon as the boys reported that the cleaning had been completed (usually before noon). Consequences, if there were any, were levied immediately after inspection.

Response Definition

As stated above, the bathroom cleaning was divided into 16 tasks. In order to obtain a high degree of inter-observer agreement, each task had a specified set of criteria to be met in order to be considered accomplished. For example, one of the 16 tasks was described in the following manner:

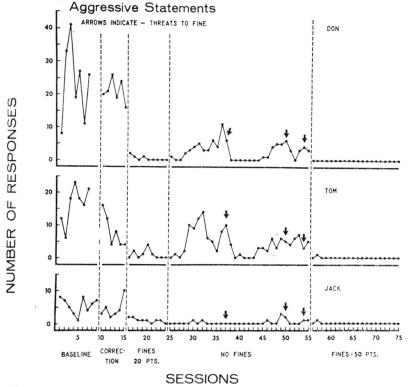

Figure 26. Number of aggressive statements per 3-hr session for each youth under each condition.

Floor and Rugs—The floor has to be clear of all objects greater than ¼ by ¼ by ¼ inch and clear of all visible water. If rugs were removed for cleaning, they should be replaced and centered under the sink within one foot of the wall.

Conditions

Baseline. The Baseline condition consisted of instructing all the boys to clean the bathrooms. No consequences were contingent on their behavior other than the instruction that they clean the bathrooms again, if fewer than four of the tasks had been accomplished.

Manager. During the Manager condition one boy was given the responsibility for cleaning the bathrooms daily. He picked the individual, or individuals, to clean the bathrooms each day and then paid or fined the workers (20 points lost or gained per task) according to the quality of their work as judged by him. Later, when the bathrooms were checked by the house-parents, the manager received or lost points (20 points per task). The manager earned points only if 75% or more of the tasks were completed. The privilege of being manager was auctioned each week.

Group. The Group condition consisted of all boys being responsible for cleaning the bathrooms and subject to the same fines. There was no manager. The boys were fined when less than 75% of the 16 tasks were completed. The amount of the fines varied from 25 to 300 points.

Manager. This condition was identical to the first Manager condition.

Group. Identical to the first Group condition except that the fines were 100 points.

Manager. Identical to the first and second Manager conditions.

The point contingencies levied by the manager under the Manager condition were more effective than the fines administered by the house-parents under the Group condition, even when the values of the fines under the Group condition were greater than those administered by the manager. The greater effectiveness of the manager condition may have been the result of the differential contingencies for each boy administered by the manager.

Table XV shows the average number of points lost per boy each day under each condition. Table XV shows clearly that the man-

Bathroom Cleaning Behavior
MANAGER SYSTEM VS. GROUP CONTINGENCY

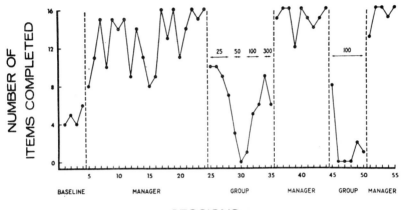

SESSIONS

Figure 27. Number of tasks accomplished per session for each condition. The numerals above the arrows indicate the possible number of points lost or gained for the sessions indicated by the horizontal arrows.

agership was not purchased because it was possible to earn a large number of points as a manager. The manager consistently lost more points than the workers he supervised.

Item by item, inter-observer agreement about the accomplishment of the bathroom cleaning tasks for 20 sessions ranged from 83% to 100% agreement and averaged 97%.

EXPERIMENT III: PUNCTUALITY

One of the boys in particular failed to respond to instructions about promptness. This led to an analysis, over a series of behaviors, of the effectiveness of point contingencies on punctuality.

Procedures and Results

Promptness was recorded for three separate behaviors:

TABLE XV

AVERAGE NUMBER OF POINTS LOST PER SESSION BY WORKERS
AND MANAGER UNDER EACH CONDITION

	Baseline	First Manager	First Group	Second Manager	Second Group	Third Manager
Worker	0	18	73	13	100	0
Manager	0	64	—	20	—	16

(1) Returning home from school.
(2) Going to bed.
(3) Returning home from errands.

Instructions were posted which stated times to be home from school and to retire to their bedrooms at night. When a boy was sent on an errand the time he was due to return was determined before he departed.

The house-parents recorded the number of minutes late or early up to 30 minutes.

Conditions

Before Fines. If the boy was late from school or an errand, he was reprimanded by one of the house-parents, "Why are you late? You know what time I told you to be here." Tardiness in going to their bedrooms resulted in a reminder every 10 minutes, "Go to bed; it's past your bedtime." No other contingencies were involved.

Fines. The youths were fined 20 points for every minute that they were late. Other than being initially informed of the change in contingencies, they were given no reminders or verbal reprimands. The fines were dispensed when the youths returned home or departed for bed. There were no programmed consequences for being early.

Punctuality for school was dealt with first. The termination of the baseline (Before Fines) involving school marked the beginning of the baseline of errands. Completion of the baseline for errands corresponded to initiation of the baseline for bedtime behavior.

The development of Tom's punctuality in all three areas can be seen in Figure 28. The other two boys had a consistent punctuality problem only at bedtime, and this disappeared at the onset of the Fines condition. The fines were very specific in their effect on the subjects' behavior. Fining tardiness from school had no apparent effect on promptness in returning from errands, and punishing lateness from errands did not seem to produce punctuality at bedtime. Interobserver agreement was greater than 95% for the 53 checks which occurred throughout the study.

EXPERIMENT IV: HOMEWORK

Failure in school is frequently associated with juvenile delinquency. The school records of the boys sent to Achievement Place all con-

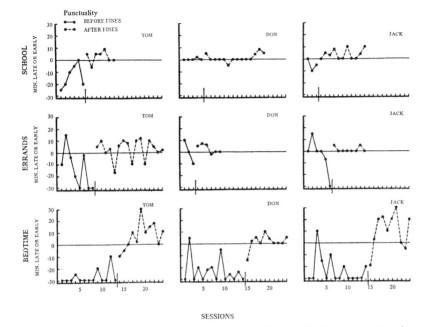

SESSIONS

Figure 28. Number of minutes early or late before and after the application of point contingencies. Each youth's punctuality was measured for school, errands, and bedtime.

tained accounts of truancy and lack of academic success throughout the boys' school years. One apparently severe deficiency in their school repertoires involved their failure to prepare routine classroom assignments and homework. This experiment compared the effect of several contingencies on preparation of homework tasks.

Procedures and Results

The study was carried out during the summer, when the youths were not in school. Daily assignments were described on 3-by-5-inch index cards which were available after 8:00 A.M. each morning. The work was scored at 5:00 P.M. of the same day. Each boy was instructed that failure to pick up an assignment card during the day would result in a fine equal to the number of points he would have received if he had completed the assignment. None of the youths ever failed to pick up his assignment card. The house-parents were available to aid in the preparation of the assignments during two periods each day, 10:00 to 11:00 A.M. and 2:00 to 3:00 P.M.

Response Definition

The assignments were pages out of self-teaching workbooks which required approximately 1 hour to complete. The workbooks used were *The Practice Workbook of Arithmetic*, Grade 5 and 6, Treasure Books, Inc., 1107 Broadway, New York, N.Y., and *The Practice Workbook of Reading*, Grades 2 and 3, also by Treasure Books, Inc.

The assignments, usually two or three pages, were divided into five approximately equal parts on the assignment cards. Each part required an accuracy of 75% to be considered complete. The boys received one-fifth of the maximum number of points, money, or time obtainable for each assignment completed, as explained below.

Conditions

Money. Under this condition each boy could earn 25 cents for each day's assignment if he had completed the assignment with less than 25% errors. The youths had the choice of receiving the money daily or at the end of the week. All three chose the latter, and the amount of money they earned was accumulated on an index card carried by each boy.

Weekly late-time. The boys had the opportunity to earn up to 1 hour of late-time per assignment. Late-time could be spent on the weekends to stay up beyond the youths' normal bedtime (9:30 p.m.). A maximum of 7 hours could be spent by a boy during a weekend and the boys could share their late-time with each other.

Daily late-time. Throughout this condition the boys could use the late-time the same day earned or save it for the weekend.

Points. The points phase allowed the youths to earn 500 points per assignment.

Money. This was the same as the first Money condition.

Points. This was the same as the first Points condition.

Figure 29 shows that the Points condition was by far the most effective in producing homework preparation. Daily Late-Time compared favorably to other conditions. Money, at the one value tested, yielded relatively poor results.

It should be noted that no effort was made to equate the points with the money and it seemed quite likely that at some higher value money would have been as effective as points. It was thought that the low rate of behavior in the first Money condition might have been due to the youths' lack of experience in using money. Thus, after the first condition, an allowance of $1.50 was given each week until the second Money condition (a period of seven weeks). During this interim the youths spent their money and appeared to understand what could be obtained with money. However, the reinstatement of the Money condition produced no better performance than the original Money condition.

Observer agreement in scoring the assignments was measured for four separate sessions, one in each of the first four conditions. The agreement on the proportion of the assignment completed was 100%.

EXPERIMENT V: "AIN'T"

Poor grammar was an obvious problem for one of the boys. The present study describes a program designed to correct a grammatical problem both with and without manipulation of the point system.

Procedure and Results

The verbal response "ain't" was recorded for one boy for 3 hours

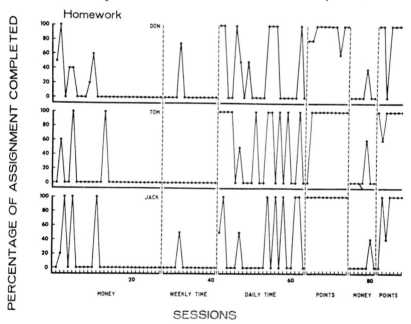

Figure 29. Percent of homework assignment completed by each boy under each of several conditions.

(one session) each day. The 3 hours were not consecutive, nor the time of day consistent. Responses were registered on a silent counter which appeared to be unnoticed by the youth.

Response Definition

It was necessary to differentiate between "ain't" used in normal conversation and the "ain'ts" used is discussions about the incorrect responses. Thus, "ain'ts" used as verbs were considered responses, while "ain'ts" employed as nouns or other parts of speech were not recorded.

Conditions

Baseline. No contingencies were placed on the youth's responses.

Correction. The correction procedure consisted of either house-parent's interrupting the boy's conversation, informing him of his error, suggesting an appropriate alternative, and requiring the youth to repeat the sentence using the correction. The house-parents corrected the mistake in a matter-of-fact manner. The subject's peers were also encouraged to assist in informing the boy of his errors.

Correction and Fines. This condition was identical to the previous phase except that a 20-point fine was levied on each response heard throughout the day. The "ain'ts" from each 3-hour session were recorded as above. Also, the total number of responses fined for the entire day was available by tallying the entries noted on the point card. Again, the other boys were told to inform the house-parents of any responses which occurred when they were not present. These responses were also fined.

Post Check. One month after the final session of the Correction and Fine condition the response was again recorded for five days (3 hours each day).

As can be seen in Figure 30, no effect was evident from the Correction condition but when the 20-point fine was made contingent on the youth's behavior, there was an immediate and consistent decline in the frequency of the inappropriate behavior, until, by the end of the second week, the response, "ain't," was eliminated. It was the impression of the house-parents that this effect was not accompanied by any noticeable decline in the youth's overall rate of speech. The dashed line in Figure 30 indicates the course of the decline in "ain'ts" recorded throughout each day during this condition.

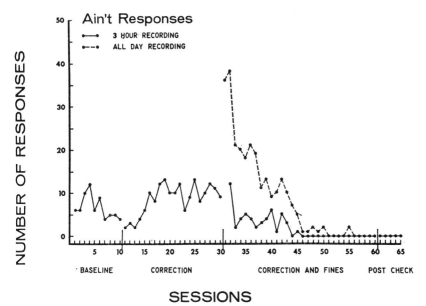

SESSIONS

Figure 30. Number of responses per day (3-hr session) for one youth un-der: 1) no consequences (baseline); 2) correction by the house-parents and other boys; and 3) correction and a 20-point fine for each response. Post checks of the behavior were taken 30 days later. The dashed line in-dicates the total number of responses for the entire day.

The Post Check condition, 30 days after the elimination of "ain'ts," revealed no trace of the response.

Observer reliability was recorded for over one-fourth of the ses-sions. The observer recorded data simultaneously with the primary recorder, but recording was independent. Agreement was never less than 93%, and the overall average was 99%.

DISCUSSION

The TOKEN ECONOMY (point system), which was designed to deal with a variety of social, self-care, and academic behaviors in the home-style treatment program for pre-delinquent boys, proved to be practicable, economical, and effective. The points seemed almost as convenient to administer as verbal consequences. In the series of experiments presented, the house-parents removed or presented points by requesting the youth's point card and recording the conse-quence. Subsequent to these studies, the youths themselves have per-formed the recording tasks equally well. The house-parents have

242 Clinical Studies in Behavior Therapy with Children, Adolescents and Their Families

simply instructed the boys to "take-off" or "give yourself" points. Cheating has not appeared to be a problem, possibly because of the extremely heavy fine if caught. The privileges for which the points were traded cost nothing, since they were all naturally available in the home as they would be in almost any middle-class home. Since the privileges could be purchased only for a week at a time, they were available over and over again as reinforcers, thus providing an almost unending supply.

The programs involving the point system successfully modifed aggressive verbal behavior, bathroom tidiness, punctuality, homework preparation, and poor grammar. The research goals remain of expanding the program to include more boys and more behaviors as well as developing means of transferring the newly established repertories to the natural contingencies of reinforcement. If these goals can be achieved, token reinforcement procedures should become a basic feature of home-style treatment programs for delinquents.

References

Ayllon, T. and Azrin, N. H.: The measurement and reinforcement of behavior of psychotics. *J Exp Anal Behav 2*, 357-383, 1965.

Berelson, B. and Steiner, G. A.: *Human behavior: an inventory of scientific findings*. New York: Harcourt, Brace & World, Inc., 1964.

Birnbrauer, J. C., Wolf, M. M., Kidder, J. D. and Tague, C. E.: Classroom behavior of retarded pupils with token reinforcement. *J Exper Child Psychology 2*, 219-235, 1965.

Bloch, H. A. and Flynn, F. T.: *Delinquency: the juvenile offender in America today*. New York: Random House, 1956.

Burchard, J. D.: Systematic socialization: a programmed environment for the habilitation of antisocial retardates. *The Psychological Record 17*, 641-476, 1967.

Burchard, J. D. and Tyler, V. O.: The modification of delinquent behavior through operant conditioning. *Behav Res Therapy 2*, 245-250, 1965.

Clark, M., Lachowicz, J. and Wolf, M. M.: A pilot basic education program for school dropouts incorporating a token reinforcement system. *Behav Res Therapy 6*, 183-188, 1968.

Cohen, A. K. and Short, J. F. Juvenile delinquency. In R. E. Melton and R. A. Nisbet (Eds.): *Contemporary social problems*. New York, Harcourt, Brace & World, pp. 77-126, 1961.

Cohen, H. L., Filipczak, J. A. and Bis, J. S.: Case project: contingencies application for special education. Progress Report, U.S. Department of Health, Education, and Welfare, 1965.

Glueck, S. and Glueck, E.: *Unraveling juvenile delinquency*. Cambridge, Mass., Harvard University Press, 1950.

McCord, W., McCord, J. and Zola, I. K.: *Origins of crimes: a new evaluation of the Cambridge-Sommerville youth study*. New York, Columbia University Press, 1959.

Powers, E. and Witmer, H.: *An experiment in prevention of delinquency: the Cambridge-Sommerville youth study*. New York, Columbia University Press, 1951.

Schwitzgebel, R. L.: *Street corner research: an experimental approach to juvenile delinquency*. Cambridge, Mass., Harvard University Press, 1964.

Slack, C. W.: Experimenter-subject psychology: a new method of introducing intensive office treatment for unreachable cases. *Ment Hyg 44*, 238-256, 1960.

Staats, A. W. and Butterfield, W. H.: Treatment of non-reading in a culturally deprived juvenile delinquent: an application of reinforcement principles. *Child Dev 36*, 925-942, 1965.

Thorne, G. L., Tharp, R. G. and Wetzel, R. J.: Behavior modification techniques: new tools for probation officers. *Federal Probation*, June 1967.

Wetzel, R.: Use of behavioral techniques in a case of compulsive stealing. *J Consult Psychol 30*, 367-374, 1966.

Wolf, M. M., Giles, D. J. and Hall, R. B.: Experiments with token reinforcement in a remedial classroom. *Behav Res Therapy 6*, 51-64, 1968.

Chapter 3

BEHAVIORAL CONTRACTING WITHIN THE FAMILIES OF DELINQUENTS*

RICHARD B. STUART

A NY INTERVENTION PROGRAM intended for use with delinquents must first define a specific subpopulation as a target group. Delinquents may be subdivided according to whether their predominant offenses are or are not classifiable as adult crimes, whether they are initial or chronic offenders, and whether or not they reside in environments replete with constructive resources which can be mobilized to their advantage. For many delinquents [e.g., for 24 per cent of the adolescent male wards of one Michigan county juvenile court (Huetteman, Briggs, Tripodi, Stuart, Heck and McConnell, 1970)], violations of parental authority and other uniquely juvenile offenses (e.g., possession of alcoholic beverages and failure to attend school) constitute the only "crimes" ever recorded. Many engage in chronically dysfunctional interactions with their families and schools, both of which settings contain the rudiments of effective behavioral controls.

A continuum of short- to intermediate-term dispositional goals is available for working with this group (see Table XVI). Ranging from maintaining the youth in his natural home environment, through a series of semi-institutional settings, to institutionalization

*From the *Journal of Behavior Therapy and Experimental Psychiatry*, 1971, 2, pp. 1-11. Reprinted by permission of the author and Pergamon Press, Ltd.

in correctional or psychiatric settings, the points along the continuum vary according to the extent to which they provide social structure and make use of natural forces of behavioral control in the community. Recent studies have shown that the more potent the influence of the natural environment throughout treatment, the greater the likelihood that behavioral changes will be maintained following treatment. For example, it has been shown that two groups of delinquents, who spent an average of 131·6 days in psychiatric settings or 91·8 days in correctional settings of every year that they were wards of the juvenile court, actually committed more offenses than another very similar group who were not institutionalized. (Huetteman *et al.*, 1970). Even stronger support of the need for community treatment is found in a large-scale review of many rehabilitation programs, which concluded with the finding that:

> . . . since severe penalities do not deter more effectively, and since prisons do not rehabilitate, and since the criminal justice system is inconsistent and has little quantitative impact on crime, the best rehabilitative possibilities would appear to be in the community (Harlow, 1970, pp. 33-34).

Community treatment for large numbers of delinquents will be possible only when techniques have been developed which (a) are effective, (b) require comparatively little time for administration, (c) can extend family influence to control behavior in a number of different situations, and (d) can be administered by para-professionals. It is suggested that behavioral contracting, to be described and illustrated in this paper, is one technique which meets each of these requirements and can be employed as a tactic in every instance in which efforts are made to strengthen the place of an adolescent in a natural, foster, or group home environment.

Rationale

At the core of the effort to use behavioral contracting to combat delinquency are two assumptions. First, it is assumed that the family plays a critical role in the etiology of delinquency when certain dysfunctional family interaction patterns coexist with a paucity of opportunities for acceptable performance in the community (Rodman and Grams, 1967) and when peer pressures are conducive to deviant behavior (Burgess and Akers, 1969). The family may function as a pathogen in two ways. First, the family may model and differentially reinforce patterns of antisocial behavior (Bandura and Walters, 1963). Second, the family may inadequately reinforce prosocial behavior in comparison with the reinforcement of antisocial behavior available in the community. Stuart (1970a) showed that the family of delinquents could be differentiated from the families of nondelinquents on the basis of their low rate of positive exchanges, while Patterson and Reid (1971) demonstrated that interactional patterns of coercion are more common within delinquent families than patterns of reciprocity.

The second assumption is that the family in many instances is a potentially powerful if not the only force available to aid the delinquent in acquiring prosocial responses. Over 15 years ago, Katz and Lazarsfeld (1955) clearly showed that in studies of attitude formation and change the family accounts for over two-thirds of the observed variance. Modern sociologists such as Schafer and Polk (1967) have shown that most social agencies, including schools in particular, are more oriented toward removing than rehabilitating the delinquent. Therefore it is essential to both eliminate the pathogenic elements of the family and to harness its vast power in order to mount constructive programs to aid delinquents.

Behavioral Contracts

A BEHAVIORAL CONTRACT is a means of scheduling the exchange of positive reinforcements between two or more persons. Contracts have been used when reciprocal patterns of exchange have broken down within families (Carson, 1969; Tharp and Wetzel, 1969) or in efforts to establish reciprocal exchanges from the outset in formal

TABLE XVI

CONTINUUM OF DISPOSITIONAL GOALS FOR THE TREATMENT
OF JUVENILE DELINQUENTS

— (1) Own home, strong controls
— (2) Own home, weak controls
— (3) Foster home, strong controls
— (4) Foster home, weak controls
— (5) Structured living situation, adults present
— (6) Unstructured living situation, adult monitoring
— (7) Group home (semi-institution)
— (8) Institution

relationships in therapeutic (Sulzer, 1962) and scholastic (Homme, Csanyi, Gonzales and Rechs, 1969) settings. Contracts structure reciprocal exchanges by specifying: who is to do what, for whom, under what circumstances. They therefore make explicit the expectations of every party to an interaction and permit each to determine the relative benefits and costs to him of remaining within that relationship (Thibaut and Kelley, 1959). Furthermore, by making roles explicit for family members, contracts enhance the likelihood that responsibilites will be met, and by postulating reciprocal exchanges within families, contracts contribute to interactional stability. Finally, because privileges and responsibilities are fairly well-standardized across families the execution of behavioral contracts in time-limited, high-pressure settings is quite feasible.*

Behavioral contracting with families rests upon four assumptions. First, it is assumed that:

> *Receipt of positive reinforcements in interpersonal exchanges is a privilege rather than a right.*

A privilege in this sense is a special prerogative which one may enjoy at the will of another person upon having performed some qualifying task. For example, states bestow driving privileges upon citizens who qualify for this privilege by passing certain performance tests and by driving with standard prudence. In contrast, a right implies undeniable and inalienable access to a prerogative. Furthermore, a right cannot be denied, no matter what an individual might do. In modern society there are virtually no rights beyond the right of the individual to think as he may choose. For example, people in a democratic society have the privilege to say what they think, but not to shout "fire" in a crowded theater no matter how hard it is to find a seat.

Within families it is the responsibility of one person to grant the privileges requested by another on a reciprocal basis. For example, an adolescent might wish free time—this is his privilege—and it is his parents' responsibility to provide this free time. However, the parents may wish that the adolescent attend school each day prior to going out in the evening—the adolescent's school attendance is their privi-

---

*Behavior Change Systems (3156 Dolph Drive, Ann Arbor, Michigan 48103) makes available behavioral contracting kits, including code book and computer compatible code forms in addition to standardized materials for use with clients.

lege and it is his responsibility to do as they ask. Privileges may, of course, be abused. Thus a parent might wish to know where his adolescent goes when he leaves home, but if the parents attack the adolescent when they learn of his plans, they have failed to meet their responsibility, i.e., use the information constructively. Thus, it is appropriate to consider as a part of the definition of a privilege the conditions for its appropriate use.

A second assumption underlying the use of behavioral contracts is:

Effective interpersonal agreements are governed by the norm of reciprocity.

A norm is a "behavioral rule that is accepted, at least to some degree, by both members of the dyad (Thibaut and Kelley, 1959, p. 129)." Norms serve to increase the predictability of events in an interaction, permit the resolution of conflicts without recourse to power and have secondary reinforcing value in and of themselves (Gergen, 1969, pp. 73-74). Reciprocity is the norm which underlies behavioral contracts. Reciprocity implies that "each party has rights and duties (Gouldner, 1960, p. 169)," and further, that items of value in an interchange must be exchanged on an equity or *quid pro quo* ("something for something [Jackson, 1965, p. 591"]) basis. Therefore, inherent in the use of behavioral contracts is acceptance of the notion that one must compensate his partner fairly for everything which is received, that is, there are no gifts to be expected within contractual relations.

A third principle basic to the use of behavioral contracts states that:

The value of an interpersonal exchange is a direct function of the range, rate, and magnitude of the positive reinforcements mediated by that exchange.

Byrne and Rhamey (1965) have expressed this assumption as a law of interpersonal behavior postulating that one's attraction to another will depend upon the proportion and value of positive reinforcements garnered within that relationship. In a similar vein, Mehrabian and Ksionsky (1970) have reviewed many years of social psychological research supporting the conclusion that: "Situations where affiliative behavior increases positive reinforcement . . . induce greater affiliative behavior (p. 115)."

In the negotiation of behavioral contracts, through a process of accommodation (Gergen, 1969, p. 73), each party seeks to offer to the other the maximum possible rate of positive reinforcement because the more positive reinforcements which are emitted, the more will be received. In this sense, each positive offered represents an individual's "investment" in a contract, and each privilege received represents "return on an investment." Therefore a good intrafamilial contract encourages the highest possible rate of mutual reinforcement as represented by the following diagram (Figure 31) in which CO_{FMA} implies the optimal choice for father, mother and adolescent, $CO_{F/MA}$ the optimal choice for father which the mother and adolescent will accept, etc., and k a value-determining constant.

$$CO_{FMA}=f\ [CO_{F/MA} +CO_{M/FA} +CO_{A/FM}]\ +k$$

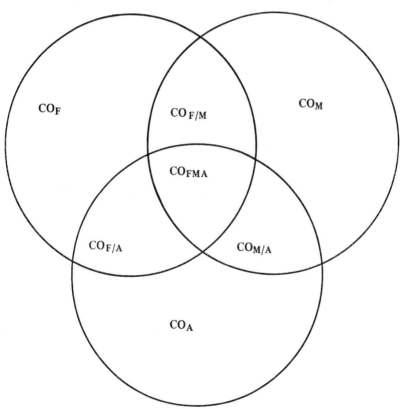

Figure 31.

The fourth and final assumption basic to the concept of behavioral contracting is:

Rules create freedom in interpersonal exchanges.

When contracts specify the nature and condition for the exchange of things of value, they thereby stipulate the rules of the interaction. For example, when an adolescent agrees that she will visit friends after school (privilege) but that she will return home by 6:00 p.m. (responsibility), she has agreed to a rule governing the exchange of reinforcers. While the rule delimits the scope of her privilege, it also creates the freedom with which she may take advantage of her privilege. Without this rule, any action taken by the girl might have an equal probability of meeting with reinforcement, extinction or punishment. If the girl did not have a clear-cut responsibility to return home at 6:00 p.m. she might return one day at 7:00 and be greeted warmly, return at 6:00 the next day and be ignored, and return at 5:30 the following day and be reprimanded. Only by prior agreement as to what hour would be acceptable can the girl insure her freedom, as freedom depends upon the opportunity to make behavioral choices with knowledge of the probable outcome of each alternative.

Just as contracts produce freedom through detailing reciprocal rule-governed exchanges, so must contracts be born of freedom, since coerced agreements are likely to be violated as soon as the coercive force is removed. Therefore effective behavioral contracts must be negotiated with respect to the following paradigm:

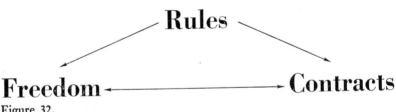

Figure 32.

Elements of Behavioral Contracts

Good behavioral contracts contain five elements. First, the contracts must detail the privileges which each expects to gain *after* fulfilling his responsibilities. Typical privileges used in behavioral contracts in the families of delinquents include free time with friends, spending money, choice of hair and dress styles and use of the family car for the adolescent. Second, good contracts must detail the responsibilities essential to securing each privilege. Again, in the families of delinquents, responsibilities typically include maintenance of minimally adequate school attendance and performance, maintenance of agreed-upon curfew hours, completion of household chores and keeping parents informed about the adolescent's whereabouts. Every effort is made to restrict privileges to prosocial behaviors and to keep responsibilities to a minimum. The former is necessary if the family is to effectively serve as an agent of social control. The latter is necessary because the parents of teenage children control comparatively few salient reinforcements and must use those which are controlled with sufficient care to maintain desired behavior. If the number of responsibilities is increased without comparable increase in the value of privileges offered, little or no reinforcement will be provided for the new responsibilities and they are unlikely to be met, weakening the general credibility of the contract.

As an added requirement, the responsibilities specified in a family contract must be monitorable by the parents, for if the parents cannot determine when a responsibility has been fulfilled, they cannot know when to properly grant a privilege. Therefore there are some things which are beyond the scope of behavioral contracts, such as where an adolescent goes when he is not at home or whom he sees as friends. The single exception to this rule is the possibility of using school attendance and performance as responsibilities. While it can be argued that classroom behavioral management is the primary responsibility of teachers (Stuart, 1970b), it is often not possible for a behavior modifier to gain access to *any* or all of an adolescent's teachers (Bailey, Phillips and Wolf, 1970), so he may be required to attempt to control behavior in school with reinforcements mediated in the home. When this is done, it is essential to arrange for systematic feedback to be provided by the teacher to the parent describing the teenager's attendance and performance in class. A simple card brought for a teacher's signature every day or week by the teenager is a sufficient and very practical means of securing this feedback (see Table XVII).

The third element of a good behavioral contract is a system of sanctions for failure to meet responsibilities. While in one sense the possibility of time out from privileges should be adequate to insure

TABLE XVII

SCHOOL PERFORMANCE CHART

Name of Student:————————————————— Date————————

In order to keep my parents posted on my progress in school, I am asking all my teachers to grade my work in all of my major subjects at the end of each class period. Would you please rate my performance as: A = excellent, B = above average, C = average, D = below average, E = failing. PLEASE USE INK and initial any corrections. THANK YOU.

Subject	Attendance	Homework	Tests and/or class discussion	Signature

the completion of responsibilities, there are obviously periods in the course of family life when this is not the case. At all times, behavior is under multiple contingency control (Stuart, 1970c), and in certain instances it is more reinforcing to violate the contract and to forfeit a subsequent privilege than to garner the rewards of adhering to the terms of the contract. At these times the existence of sanctions may tip the balance of a behavioral choice toward compliance with contractual obligations. Furthermore, sanctions have an added advantage: they provide the aggrieved party with a temperate means of expressing his displeasure. In families without explicit or understood behavioral contracts, the failure of a child to meet curfew is often met with threats of long-term "grounding." Faced with the threat of not being permitted to go out for weeks on end, the teenager is often persuaded to violate his contract even further and remain out later because the magnitude of the penalty is fixed and not commensurate with the magnitude of his violation.

When sanctions are built into the contract, they may be of two types. One is a simple, linear penalty such as the requirement that the adolescent return home as many minutes early the following day as he has come in late on the preceding day. The second type of sanction is a geometric penalty which doubles or triples the amount of make-up time due following contract violations. It is probably best to combine both types of sanctions, making certain that lateness does not reach a point of diminishing return when it would actually be impractical for the adolescent to return home at all because he would incur no greater penalty for continued absence.

The fourth element in a good behavioral contract is a bonus clause which assures positive reinforcement for compliance with the terms of the contract. Much behavior control within families consists of "negative scanning" (Stuart, 1969) or the EXTINCTION of positive responding (by ignoring it) coupled with the severe punishment of negative responding. The effect of this punishment is, of course, to strengthen negative behavior as a consequence of the facts that attention follows negative behavior and does not follow positive responses (Madsen, Becker, Thomas, Kosar and Plager, 1968). To counteract this, bonuses calling for permission to remain out longer than usual, extra money or extraordinary privileges such as the opportunity to have a party or to take a trip with friends are built into contracts as contingencies for extended periods of near-flawless compliance with contractual responsibilities.

When behavioral contracts are well executed, each member of the family is assured of receiving the minimum level of positive reinforcement (privileges) necessary to sustain his participation in the interaction. Furthermore, each party to the agreement is provided with a means of responding to contract violations and each is reinforced for long chains of desirable responses. The contract is not complete, however, unless a means is also built in for keeping track of the rates of positive reinforcements given and received. This is accomplished through feedback systems which serve two functions. First, they cue each individual as to how to respond in order to earn an additional inducement. Second, they signal each person when to reinforce the other. Furthermore, the provision of feedback in this context also sets the occasion for positive comments which themselves strengthen prosocial behavior. The exchange of feedback is facilitated by the use of a behavioral monitoring form calling for each person to check off the fulfillment of his own responsibilities (which includes provision of the privileges of the others).

Illustration

A behavioral contract constituted the primary treatment procedure in the management of a 16-year-old girl who was referred to the Family and School Consultation Project by the local juvenile court. At the time of referral, Candy Bremer* had been hospitalized as an inpatient at a local psychiatric hospital following alleged promiscuity, exhibitionism, drug abuse and home truancy. Associated

*Pseudonym

with these complaints was an allegation by her parents that Candy engaged in chronically antagonistic exchanges within the family and had for a year done near-failing work in school. Owing to the cost of private psychiatric care, the parents sought hospitalization at state expense by requesting that the juvenile court assume wardship. After initiating this action, the parents were informed by a court-appointed attorney representing their daughter that the allegations would probably not stand up in court. The parents accordingly modified their request to a petition that the court place Candy on the consent docket affording quasi-ward status without termination of parental rights.

At the time of referral, Mr. and Mrs. Bremer were 64 and 61 years old respectively, and both were physically ill—Mr. Bremer suffering from emphysema and Mrs. Bremer from a degenerative bone disease in her hip. Both holding college degrees, Mr. Bremer performed scholarly work at home on a part-time basis while Mrs. Bremer worked as a medical secretary. Candy, the third of their three children, was 20 years younger than her oldest sister. The Bremers resided in a very small ranch-type home which lacked a basement, so privacy could only be found in the bedrooms.

Initially, Mr. and Mrs. Bremer wished to maintain virtually total control over Candy's behavior. They were reluctantly willing to accept her at home but established as conditions that she adhere to a punishing curfew which allowed her out of the home for periods averaging two to three hours per summer day. Great effort was expended to convince the parents of the need to modify their expectations and to modify a continuous chain of negative interactions. However, when both of these failed, it was decided to execute a behavioral contract anyway, because the problems expected at home seemed less negative than the probable consequences of continued institutionalization and because it was hoped that a more realistic contract could be effectuated as time progressed. Within three weeks of the start of the contract, Candy was reported to be sneaking out of her bedroom window at night, visiting a local commune and returning home before dawn. It was found that over a 24-day period there were eight major contract violations, and the probability of an extended series of days of contract compliance was quite small* (see Figure 33). While it was deemed vital to introduce more privileges for Candy, it seemed imprudent to do this as a contingency for her having violated her contract in the past. Finally it was decided to do two things. A new contract, which was far more permissive, was introduced (see Table XVIII), accompanied by a new monitoring sheet (see Table XIX), but a new court order was requested and granted which proscribed Candy from entering communes. Candy was made to understand that,

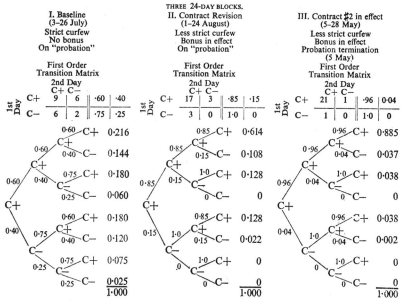

Figure 33. Candy Bremer–Curfew Maintenance Three 24-Day Blocks.

*These and subsequent data were evaluated using a Markovian chain designed to make predictions of future behavior based upon observation of past behavior in 24-day blocks. For an extended discussion of this procedure, see Kemeny, Mirkil, Snell and Thompson (1959). In simplified form, the analysis is completed through the following *steps*: (1) write the series of dichotomous observations as a series of +, — notations (+ — — + + — +, etc.); (2) count the number of + +, + —, — + and — — sequences, recording the totals in a 2 X 2 table; (3) compute the proportion of + + vs + — and — + vs — — sequences and enter these decimals in the appropriate cells of a 2 × 2 table; (4) draw as many Markovian tree forms as needed following the illustration in Table XVII; (5) for each + +, + —, — +, and — — series, write in the proportions obtained in step 3; (6) multiply all such entries in each series. CHECKS: (a) entries at each pair of branching alternatives (C + <) must total

$$0\cdot6\ \text{C}+$$
$$0\cdot4\ \text{C}-$$

1·00 (0·6 + 0·4). (b) The probability of all series must total 1·00.

Interpretation. The obtained values may be interpreted as the probability that each series, (e.g. + + — —) will occur, relative to all other series, assuming constant conditions.

should she be found in either commune, not she but the commune members would be liable to prosecution for contributing to the delinquency of a minor as they had been officially informed of the limitation placed upon Candy's activities.

As seen in Figure 33, this modified contract was quite effective, increasing the rate of compliance to the contract terms to a very respectable high rate. When court wardship was terminated and the contract was the sole behavioral prosthesis, Candy's behavior actually continued to improve.

TABLE XVIII
BEHAVIORAL CONTRACT

PRIVILEGES	RESPONSIBILITIES
General	
In exchange for the privilege of remaining together and preserving some semblance of family integrity, Mr. and Mrs. Bremer and Candy all agree to	concentrate on positively reinforcing each other's behavior while diminishing the present overemphasis upon the faults of the others.
Specific	
In exchange for the privilege of riding the bus directly from school into town after school on school days	Candy agrees to phone her father by 4:00 p.m. to tell him that she is all right and to return home by 5:15 p.m.
In exchange for the privilege of going out at 7:00 p.m. on one weekend evening without having to account for her whereabouts	Candy must maintain a weekly average of "B" in the academic ratings of all of her classes and must return home by 11:30 p.m.
In exchange for the privilege of going out a second weekend night	Candy must tell her parents *by 6:00 p.m.* of her destination and her companion, and must return home by 11:30 p.m.
In exchange for the privilege of going out between 11:00 a.m and 5:15 p.m. Saturdays, Sundays and holidays	Candy agrees to have completed all household chores *before* leaving and to telephone her parents once during the time she is out to tell them that she is all right.

In exchange for the privilege of having Candy complete household chores and maintain her curfew

Mr. and Mrs. Bremer agree to pay Candy $1.50 on the morning following days on which the money is earned.

Bonuses and Sanctions

If Candy is 1–10 minutes late

she must come in the same amount of time earlier the following day, but she does not forfeit her money for the day.

If Candy is 11–30 minutes late

she must come in 22–60 minutes earlier the following day and does forfeit her money for the day.

If Candy is 31–60 minutes late

she loses the privilege of going out the following day and does forfeit her money for the day.

For each half hour of tardiness over one hour, Candy

loses her privilege of going out and her money for one additional day.

Candy may go out on Sunday evenings from 7:00 to 9:30 p.m. and either Monday or Thursday evening

if she abides by all the terms of this contract from Sunday through Saturday with a total tardiness not exceeding 30 minutes which must have been made up as above.

Candy may add a total of two hours divided among one to three curfews

if she abides by all the terms of this contract for two weeks with a total tardiness not exceeding 30 minutes which must have been made up as above and if she requests permission to use this additional time by 9:00 p.m.

MONITORING

Mr. and Mrs. Bremer agree to keep written records of the hours of Candy's leaving and coming home and of the companions of her chores.

Candy agrees to furnish her parents with a school monitoring card each Friday at dinner.

_____

_____

_____

TABLE XIX
BEHAVIORAL CONTRACT: MONITORING FORM.

	1/17	2/18	3/19	4/20	5/21	6/22	7/23	8/24	9/25	10/26	11/27	12/28	13/29	14/30	15/31	16/—
Chores:																
Set table, etc.																
Dishes, kitchen, etc.																
Bathroom																
Vacuum, FR, LR, halls																
Cat boxes																
Other:																
Other:																
Curfew:																
Time leave afternoon																
Phone after school																
Time arrive home from school in afternoon																
Time leave in evening																
Destination approved																
Time return in evening																
Time leave afternoon																
Lateness																
Lateness made up																
Bonus Time.																
Bonus 1 earned																
Bonus 1 spent																
Bonus 2 earned																
Bonus 2 requested																
Bonus 2 spent																

Days of Month

Discussion

Behavioral contracting served as a very useful means of structuring a constructive interaction between Candy and her parents. By removing from the realm of contention the issues of privileges and responsibilities, the eliciters of many intrafamilial arguments were eliminated. When fights did occur, they tended to be tempered by the options available through the contract. The contract itself cannot account for a change in Candy's behavior; but the contract apparently served to assure the use of privileges such as free time and money as contingencies in the truest sense of the term.

The process of negotiating a contract through accommodation of each other's wishes (Gergen, 1969) might have been characterized as an "experience in form" by John Dewey. It appears to have laid the groundwork for a more effective interaction and in this case was adequate in and of itself. In other instances, it is likely that behavioral contracting could profitably be supplemented with interaction training for the parents, tutoring or vocational guidance for the adolescent or financial assistance for the family. The decision about which additional techniques should be employed is discretionary, but it is suggested that behavioral contracting be made a part of every plan to improve the interaction between an adolescent and his parents.

References

Bailey, J., Phillips, E. and Wolf, M.: Home-based reinforcement and the modification of pre-delinquents' classroom behavior. *Proceedings of the 78th Annual Convention of the American Psychological Association*, Vol. 5, 751-752 (Summary), 1970.

Bandura, A. and Walters, R. H.: *Social Learning and Personality Development*. Holt, Rinehart & Winston, New York, 1963.

Burgess, R. L. and Akers, R. L.: A differential association-reinforcement theory of criminal behavior. In *Delinquency, Crime and Social Process* (Edited by Cressey, D. R. and Ward, D. A.) Harper & Row, New York, 1969.

Byrne, D. and Rhamey, R.: Magnitude of positive and negative reinforcements as a determinant of attractions. *J Pers Soc Psychol 2*, 884-889, 1965.

Carson, R. C.: *Interaction Concepts of Personality*. Aldine, Chicago, 1969.

Gergen, K. J.: *The Psychology of Behavior Exchange*. Addison-Wesley, Reading, Massachusetts, 1969.

Gouldner, A. W.: The norm of reciprocity: A preliminary statement. *Amer Soc Rev 25*, 161-178, 1960.

Harlow, E.: Intensive intervention: An alternative to institutionalization. *Crime and Delinquency Literature 2*, 3-46, 1970.

Homme, L., Csanyi, A. P., Gonzales, M. A. and Rechs, J. R.: *How To Use Contingency Contracting in the Classroom.* Research Press, Champaign, Illinois, 1969.

Huetteman, M. J., Briggs, J., Tripodi, T., Stuart, R. B., Heck, E. T. and McConnell, J. V.: A descriptive comparison of three populations of adolescents known to the Washtenaw County Juvenile Court: Those referred for or placed in psychiatric hospitals, those placed in correctional settings, and those released following hearings. Unpublished manuscript, Family and School Consultation Project, Ann Arbor, Michigan, 1970.

Jackson, D. D.: Family rules. *Arch Gen Psychiat 12*, 589-594, 1965.

Katz, E. and Lazarsfeld, P. F.: *Personal Influence.* Free Press, Glencoe, Illinois, 1955.

Kemeny, J. G., Mirkil, H., Snell, J. L. and Thompson, G. L.: *Finite Mathematical Structures.* Prentice-Hall, Englewood Cliffs, New Jersey, 1959.

Madsen, C. H., Jr., Becker, W. C., Thomas, D. R., Kosar, L. and Plager, E.: An analysis of the reinforcing function of "sit down" commands. In *Readings in Educational Psychology* (Edited by R. K. Parker). Allyn and Bacon, Boston, 1968.

Mehrabian, A. and Ksionsky, S.: Models of affiliative behavior. *Psychol Bull 74*, 110-126, 1970.

Patterson, G. R. and Reid, J.: Reciprocity and coercion: Two facets of social systems. In *Behavior Modification in Clinical Psychology* (Edited by C. Neuringer and J. Michael). Appleton-Century-Crofts, New York, 1971.

Rodman, H. and Grams, P.: Juvenile delinquency and the family: A review and discussion. In President's Commission on Law Enforcement and Administration of Justice, Task Force on Juvenile Delinquency, *Task Force Report: Juvenile Delinquency and Youth Crime.* Washington, D.C.: U.S. Government Printing Office, 1967.

Schafer, W. E. and Polk, K.: Delinquency and the schools. In President's Commission on Law Enforcement and Administration of Justice, Task Force on Juvenile Delinquency, *Task Force Report: Juvenile Delinquency and Youth Crime.* Washington, D.C.: U.S. Government Printing Office, 1967.

Stuart, R. B.: Operant-interpersonal treatment for marital discord. *J Consult Clin Psychol 33*, 675-682, 1969.

Stuart, R. B.: Assessment and change of the communicational patterns of juvenile delinquents and their parents. In *Advances in Behavior Therapy, 1969* (Edited by R. D. Rubin). Academic Press, New York, 1970a.

Stuart, R. B.: Behavior modification techniques for the education technologist. In *Proceedings of the National Workshop on School Social Work, 1969-70* (Edited by R. C. Sarri). National Association of Social Workers, New York, 1970b.

Stuart, R. B.: Situational versus self control in the treatment of problematic behaviors. In *Advances in Behavior Therapy. 1970* (Edited by R. D. Rubin). Academic Press, New York, 1970c.

Sulzer, E. S.: Research frontier: Reinforcement and the therapeutic contract. *J Counsel Psychol 9*, 271-276, 1962.

Tharp, R. G. and Wetzel, R. J.: *Behavior Modification in the Natural Environment.* Academic Press, New York, 1969.

Thibaut, J. W. and Kelley, H. H.: *The Social Pyschology of Groups.* J. Wiley, New York, 1959.

Section VI

THERAPY BEHAVIOR WITH FAMILIES

SECTION VI IS OF PARTICULAR INTEREST TO THE CURRENT AUTHORS BECAUSE OF THEIR INVOLVEMENT IN FAMILY THERAPY. READINGS HERE INCLUDE EARLY WORKS (ENGELN, ET. AL. AND O'LEARY, ET. AL.) RELATED TO THE USE OF PARENTS AS THERAPISTS FOR THEIR OWN CHILDREN. OTHER ARTICLES DEMONSTRATE THAT PARENTS CAN SERVE AS THERAPEUTIC BEHAVIOR MANAGERS FOR SPECIFIC PROBLEMS, SUCH AS DYSLEXIA AND ASTHMA. PERHAPS THESE ARTICLES REPRESENT A NEW AND GROWING FORM OF FAMILY THERAPY. SOME READERS MAY QUESTION THE APPROPRIATENESS OF STUART'S ARTICLE RELATED TO MARRIAGE THERAPY. HOWEVER, IN THE MAJORITY OF CASES, SUCCESSFUL RESOLUTION OF THE PARENTS' DIFFICULTIES IS A SINE QUA NON FOR LASTING FAMILY TREATMENT.

Chapter 1

MODIFICATION OF A DEVIANT SIBLING INTERACTION PATTERN IN THE HOME*

K. DANIEL O'LEARY, SUSAN O'LEARY *and* WESLEY C. BECKER

Introduction

THERE HAVE BEEN MANY DEMONSTRATIONS in clinic settings of the application of a functional analysis of behavior to children's disorders (Ferster, 1967a, 1967b; Lovaas *et al.*, 1965; Wahler *et al.*, 1965; Wolf *et al.*, 1964). However, applications of behavioral principles in the home have been limited (Hawkins *et al.*, 1966; Williams, 1959). With the increasing emphasis on the diagnosis and modification of behavior *in situ*, it is probable that in the future, behavior therapists will concentrate on the stimulus situations in which the problem behavior is most likely to be emitted. Ultimately it is the parental environment which must maintain the child's behavior, and behavior reinforced in the clinic will be extinguished if parents do not provide the contingencies to maintain them. On the other hand, if behavior extinguished in the clinic receives parental attention, it is likely that the problem behavior will be quickly reinstated. Therefore, direct modification of children's behavior by parents under a clinician's guidance would seem to be a very useful approach.

*From *Behavior Research and Therapy*, 1967, 5, pp. 113-120. Reprinted by permission of Maxwell International Microforms Corporation.

This case study demonstrates the application of a set of procedures selected to produce efficiently behavior change in two deviant siblings. The procedures combined prompting, shaping, and instructions to increase cooperative behavior. This behavior was reinforced initially by M & M candies and later by points which could be exchanged for small toys. In the latter half of the study, time out from positive reinforcement (TO) was used to weaken some deviant behavior which was not reduced by the reinforcement of the incompatible cooperative behavior. TO was in the form of an isolation period (Hawkins *et al.*, 1966; Wolf *et al.*, 1964). Because of the exploratory nature of the application of these procedures in the home, the interactive behavior of two boys was first brought under control by the experimenter. Later this control was transferred to the boys' mother.

Subjects

A six-year-old boy, Barry A., and his three-year-old brother, Jeff, were the two subjects in this study. Both parents are university faculty members, and they have a third son who is two years old.

Psychiatric history

Barry had been under psychiatric treatment for two years and was described by his psychiatrist as "seriously disturbed." He was reported to be extremely hyperactive, aggressive, and destructive. His EEG was symmetric and within normal limits. Although it was not possible to give him an intelligence test, the psychiatrist felt that his intelligence was within normal limits. He was diagnosed as an "immature, brain-damaged child with a superimposed neurosis," although the nature and cause of his brain damage could not be specified.

Parental report

According to Mr. and Mrs. A., Barry fought with his brother whenever they were alone. He damaged toys and furniture. He had temper tantrums and failed to follow parental instructions. Shortly before Barry was referred to our research unit, he had thrown a rock through a neighbor's window. He roamed away from home, and he would occasionally enter strangers' houses.

Mrs. A. reported that the boys angered her by screaming, yelling, and hurting each other when they were alone in the basement playroom. Consequently, an observer and the experimenter watched interaction of the two boys when they played in the basement. From these observations it was quickly learned that there was a great deal of commanding behavior by Barry. If Jeff did not follow these commands, he would be coerced physically and often thrown on the floor. They would break each other's toys or constructions, and this would lead to further fighting. From the experimenter's observations in the home it appeared that parental attention was largely contingent upon high intensity undesirable responses. Since Mrs. A. usually remained upstairs while the boys were in the basement playroom, only the screaming, yelling, and fighting which could be heard easily received any attention.

On the basis of initial impressions made from the home observations it was decided to focus on the frequency of three general CLASSES OF BEHAVIOR: deviant, cooperative, and isolate. The deviant behavior consisted of kicking, hitting, pushing, name-calling, and throwing objects at each other. The cooperative behavior was asking for a toy, requesting the other's help, conversation, and playing within three feet of one another. Isolate behavior was designated as the absence of verbal, physical, or visual interaction between the boys.

Procedures and Results

The treatment was divided into four stages: the first baseline period, the first experimental period, the second baseline period, and a second experimental period. Observation and treatment occurred approximately three times per week extending from November to March (sickness and vacations precluded some observations).

Base period I

In order to assess inter-observer reliability, the observer and the experimenter made observations on five occasions during the baseline period. The observer and the experimenter sat three feet apart so that it was not possible for one observer to detect the symbols recorded by the other. Observations were made on a 20-second rate, 10-second-rest basis. Total observation time was approximately 30 minutes each day. The reliabilities were calculated by dividing the number of perfect agreements by the number of different responses observed. A perfect agreement was the presence of the same observed behavior for both raters in a 20-second interval. The average reliability calculated thus was .78. Using two raters, the proportion of agreement in the three general classes of behavior can also be calculated by dividing the smaller score by the larger (Hawkins *et al.*, 1966). Calculated thus, agreement on deviant responses ranged from 0.92 to 1.00 with a mean of 0.95. Agreement on cooperative responses ranged from 0.85 to 1.00 with a mean of 0.92. Agreement on isolate behavior was 1.00.

The experimental arrangement and the absence of a third trained observer made it difficult to obtain reliability checks after the first baseline period. While the failure to obtain reliability checks somewhat weakens the value of these data, the high level of initial reliabilities clearly demonstrates that the coding system could be objectively applied. The reported data are all based on the observations of the same observer.

Base period observations were made only when Mrs. A. was not in the playroom. She was, however, allowed to come down to the playroom to discipline the children as she saw fit, since the observers did not talk or interact with the children. Such times were simply excluded from the observations.

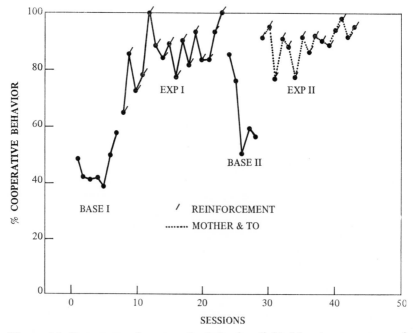

Figure 34. Percentage of cooperative behavior divided by the percentage of deviant and cooperative behavior.

During the first baseline period (Figure 34), the frequency of co-operative behavior divided by the total frequency of cooperative and deviant behavior yielded percentages ranging from 39 to 57 per cent with a mean of 46 per cent. Although the percentage of cooperative behavior on the graph shows a slight rise, the percentage of coopera-tive behavior calculated on the basis of cooperative, deviant, and iso-late behavior was actually declining. However, it was decided to graph only cooperative behavior as a percentage of cooperative be-havior plus deviant behavior because our experimental operations were aimed at changing the topography of whatever interaction oc-curred, and isolate behavior is not an interaction.

Experimental period I

During the first two days of the experimental period, cooperative responses emitted by either child were continually reinforced by the experimenter who put an M & M candy in the child's mouth and simultaneously said "Good." The cooperative responses which were reinforced were any instance of verbal utterances such as asking for a toy, requesting the other's help, and saying "Please" and "Thank You." On the third and fourth day the experimenter alternately REINFORCED APPROXIMATELY EVERY SECOND OR FOURTH COOPERATIVE RESPONSE. On the fifth day the boys were instructed that they would receive an M & M if they asked each other for things, if they said "Please" and "Thank you," if they answered each other's questions, and if they played nicely together, e.g. building things together, pull-ing each other in the wagon, taking turns, and carrying out a request. These instructions were repeated on all succeeding days of the ex-perimental periods, and the children were prompted by the experi-menter as he felt necessary throughout the study.

The token reinforcement system was also introduced on the fifth day. The boys were told that in addition to getting M & M's, CHECKS would be put on the blackboard for cooperative behavior and re-moved for deviant behavior. The blackboard was divided in half by a chalk line to designate separately the checks for Barry and Jeff. When a check was received for one or both boys the experimenter would tell them who was receiving a check. Checks could be ex-changed for BACK-UP REINFORCERS, which consisted of candy bars, bubble gum, caps, kites, comic books, puzzles, and other small toys. Frequent discussions were held with the boys' parents in order to ensure that the toys would indeed serve as reinforcers. The total cost of the token system throughout the treatment procedure was $10.67.

A procedure was used for each child in which the number of checks needed to receive the reinforcer was continually increased. On the twelfth day of the token system the use of M & M's was discontinued, but a back-up reinforcer was always present. However, there were some days when one or the other of the boys did not receive enough checks to obtain a back-up reinforcer. Initially, when the boys did not receive a reinforcer, they cried, screamed and had violent temper tantrums. The experimenter simply ignored this behavior and instructed Mrs. A. to do likewise. The purpose of increasing the number of checks to receive a reinforcer was to permit transition to greater DELAY OF REINFORCEMENT without disruption and in order to maintain the high percentage of cooperative behavior.

The amount of cooperative play was greatly increased during this period (Figure 34). As contrasted with the mean percentage of cooperative play during the first baseline of 46 per cent, the mean percentage of cooperative play during the first experimental period was 85 per cent.

Base period II

During the second base period, in which the experimenter was absent and only the observer present, the amount of cooperative play gradually declined to a level similar to that of the first baseline (50 per cent). This drop in the percentage of cooperative responses demonstrates that the experimenter could utilize instructions, prompts, and a token reinforcement system to control the children's behavior. As in the first base period, mother could intervene as she thought necessary.

Experimental period II

With the reinstatement of the experimental procedures the amount of cooperative behavior increased markedly. Two days after the second experimental period started, when the boys had resumed their prior percentage of cooperative responding, Mrs. A. was instructed to run the token system exactly as the experimenter had done with two additional features. On the second day a PUNISHMENT PROCEDURE TO was made contingent upon kicking, hitting, pushing, name-calling, and throwing objects at each other. On the sixth day, a stretch out of the token system was begun, requiring points to be earned over several days for pay off. As can be seen in Figure 34, when the second experimental period was terminated, the delay of reinforcement was three days.

To assist Mrs. A. in learning what to do, two hand signals were used by the experimenter to indicate when Mrs. A. was to administer token reinforcers or the punishment procedure. During the second experimental period, the experimenter gradually faded into the background so that Mrs. A. was able to execute the procedures without signals from the experimenter.

Although the percentage of deviant behavior was relatively low during the first experimental period, occasional fights which ended in yelling and screaming occurred and were very disruptive. Since giving and removing checks was not powerful enough to eliminate all of the deviant behavior, a punishment procedure called time out from positive reinforcement (TO) was instituted (Ferster and Appel, 1961). The TO procedure consisted of isolating either of the children in the bathroom for the deviant behavior listed above. Everything which could easily be removed was taken from the bathroom so that the boys had little opportunity to amuse themselves. After some initial resistance upon being taken to the bathroom, both boys accepted the TO without much argument. They had to remain in the bathroom for at least five minutes. In addition, they had to be quiet for a period of three minutes before they were allowed to come out. This latter requirement ensured that termination of TO was contingent upon behavior which the mother wished to strengthen (being quiet on request) and permitted TO to function both as a punisher for behavior which led to TO and a negative reinforcer for behavior which terminated TO.

During the first three days of the TO procedure, TO was used approximately once a day for each child. It was used at most four times a day, and during the last four days of the experimental period it was used only once for Jeff. The decreasing frequency of the need for TO is indicated in the cumulative record of Figure 35.

As can be seen in Figure 34, this combination of procedures under mother's control produced high cooperative behavior (90 per cent) during the second experimental period.

The application of the TO procedure was restricted to the ex-

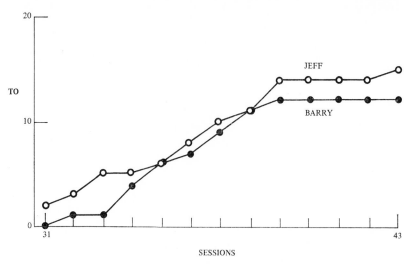

Figure 35. Cumulative frequency of TO.

perimental hour initially, but following the ninth session of the second experimental period (session 40) when the percentage of cooperative play seemed relatively stable, Mrs. A. was allowed to use TO at other times. In addition, following session 40 the minimum amount of time the children had to stay in the bathroom was increased to eight minutes. The number of times TO was used outside the experimental session fell from three times per day to less than one time every other day over approximately one month. As can be seen in Figure 35, TO was not needed in the experimental session after day 40.

Discussion

As mentioned previously, cooperative behavior was represented as a percentage of deviant plus cooperative since our manipulations were aimed at changing the topography of whatever interactions occurred. From a graph of isolate behavior as a percentage of isolate, cooperative and deviant behavior (Figure 36), it can be seen that the changes produced during the first experimental period were not due to a change in the amount of isolate play. That is, the experimental manipulations did not greatly reduce all interactions at the same time that cooperative interactions were made stronger.

The rise in isolate play during the second experimental period was probably the result of fewer prompts being used by Mrs. A.

than by the experimenter. This increase in isolate play was not interpreted as a particularly undesirable outcome because the topography of their interactions had changed markedly. Our aim to reduce the frequency of the hitting, kicking, pushing, name-calling, and throwing objects and to increase cooperative interactions. Had we been concerned about a decrease in the frequency of interactions *per se*, we could have manipulated the contingencies in order to maintain a high level of interaction.

The drop in cooperative play during the second baseline could be attributed to the discontinuance of the token reinforcement system, the instructions, or the prompts. The physical absence of the experimenter during the second baseline period may also have been related to the changes in the behavior observed. Because of the severity of the boys' problems and parental concerns, it was impossible to introduce the experimenter, instructions, prompts, token and back-up reinforcers systematically. Consequently, the relative contributions of each aspect of the treatment cannot be here assessed. Furthermore, Jeff's increasing verbal repertoire probably helped maintain cooperative play as the study progressed. Other equally unknown factors may have accounted for the behavioral changes observed.

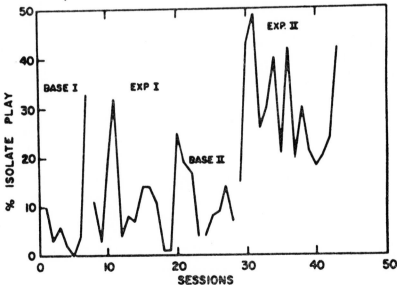

Figure 36. Percentage of isolate behavior divided by the percentage of deviant, cooperative, and isolate behavior.

Thus, this study represents a demonstration rather than an experimental analysis.

It should be made clear that the application of the set of procedures used in this study did not eliminate all deviant behavior. Barry sporadically emitted rough behavior at school and because of his disruptive outbursts at school, he will be placed in behavior modification class. Nonetheless, Barry's parents and teacher reported that he progressed markedly during the year. The incidents of hitting and kicking were greatly reduced. He will now ask for things rather than grab them and an anecdotal report indicates that he plays well with a neighbor's child.

The experimental phase of this study was not designed to reprogram the boys' entire environment, but reprogramming could be accomplished in many ways. Following the experimental phase of our work, Mr. and Mrs. A. were instructed to continue the use of TO for hitting, kicking, and pushing. Some of Barry's other behavior, such as his infrequent but repetitive head turning and occasional wild arm swinging, were simply to be ignored. Formerly, Barry had been under a great deal of AVERSIVE CONTROL and the parents were strongly advised to stop spanking Barry.

As mentioned previously, it was evident from parental report and home observation that many of Barry's low intensity responses had been extinguished by his parents. However, disruptive behavior of high intensity received attention from both parents and this attention likely reinforced such behavior. In order to reverse this condition, both parents were advised to respond to the children when they were behaving appropriately, not only when they were misbehaving. The importance of praise and affection in maintaining appropriate behavior was repeatedly emphasized. In order to establish and reinforce more appropriate behaviors, Barry now receives a penny each time he makes his bed, and he has been saving this money for small toys.

Barry's eneuretic problem was eliminated with the use of a commercially produced alarm device. The alarm is connected to a bed pad, and the alarm rings whenever the child urinates on the pad. Barry had worn diapers every night prior to the use of the alarm device, and he had a long history of failures in attempting to arrest the bedwetting. Consequently, both Barry and his mother were given as much understanding of the treatment process as possible, a realistic appreciation of the possibility of cure and the demands which the treatment procedures would place upon them. Following Lovibond's account (1964), it was emphasized that about one-third of children whose bedwetting is arrested, start wetting again and have to use the device a second time. Thus complete treatment was thought of as requiring the use of the device on two occasions. Records of the treatment were kept, and within seven weeks of starting the treatment Barry was completely dry. A three month follow-up indicated that there was no relapse.

The fact that this boy, who had been diagnosed "brain damaged," could behave as well as he did astonished his parents. Such evidence should make one very hesitant to use such labels as "brain damaged." Like autism and mental retardation, the label "brain damaged" implies concepts and assumptions which generate attitudes of futility. Bijou's (1965) comment with regard to autism and retardation seems equally important concerning brain damage.

> "These disturbances, like other forms of psychological behaviors, are undoubtedly determined by multiple conditions—social, physical, and organismic—and, as such, call for not a dismissing label but a challenge for analysis."

The need for further exploration of behavior therapy techniques with children is great. It has been demonstrated that reinforcement techniques are effective in shaping cooperative responses in both normal and schizophrenic children (Azrin and Lindsley, 1956; Hingten *et al.*, 1965). However, the study reported here is one of the few demonstrations of behavior modification in the home, and our techniques were devised to meet clinical and research needs as the study progressed. It is evident, however, that the principles of behavior modification can be utilized readily by a parent to change a child's behavior.

References

Azrin, H. H. and Lindsley, O. R.: The reinforcement of cooperation between children. *J Abnorm Soc Psychol 52*, 100-102, 1956.

Bijou, S. W.: Experimental studies of child behavior, normal and deviant. In *Research in Behavior Modification* (Eds. Krasner, L. and Ullmann, L. P.) Holt, Rinehart & Winston, New York, 1965.

Ferster, C. B.: An operant reinforcement analysis of infantile autism. *Am J Psychother* (In press.)

Ferster, C. B.: Operant reinforcement in the natural milieu. *Excep Child* (In press.)

Ferster, C. B. and Appel, J. B.: Punishment of Ss responding in matching to sample by time out from positive reinforcement. *J Exp Anal Behav 4*, 45-56, 1961.

Hawkins, R. P., Peterson, R. F., Schweid, E. and Bijou, S. W.: Behavior therapy in the home: amelioration of problem parent-child relations with the parent in a therapeutic role. *J Exp Child Psychol 4*, 99-107, 1966.

Hingten, J. N., Saunders, B. J. and Demeyer, M. K.: Shaping cooperative responses in early childhood schizophrenics. In *Case Studies in Behavior Modification* (Eds. Ullmann, L. P. and Krasner, L.). Holt, Rinehart & Winston, New York, 1965.

Lovaas, I., Schaeffer, B. and Simmons, J.: Experimental studies in childhood schizophrenia: building social behaviors in autistic children using electric shock. *J Exp Study Personality 1*, 99-109, 1965.

Lovibond, S. H.: *Conditioning and Enuresis*. Macmillan, New York, 1964.

Wahler, R. G., Winkel, G. H., Peterson, R. F. and Morrison, D. C.: Mothers as behavior therapists for their own children. *Behav Res & Therapy 3*, 113-124, 1965.

Williams, C. D.: The elimination of tantrum behavior by extinction procedures. *J Abnorm Soc Psychol 59*, 269, 1959.

Wolf, M. M., Risley, T. and Mees, H.: Application of operant conditioning procedures to the behavior problems of an autistic child. *Behav Res & Therapy 1*, 305-312, 1964.

Chapter 2

BEHAVIOUR MODIFICATION TECHNIQUES APPLIED TO A FAMILY UNIT— A CASE STUDY*

RICHARD ENGELN, JOHN KNUTSON, LINWOOD LAUGHY *and* WARREN GARLINGTON

M ANY STUDIES HAVE DEMONSTRATED the effectiveness of the techniques of operant conditioning in altering the behaviour of children in the laboratory and in the home (Baer, 1962; Williams, 1959; Madsen, 1965; Hart *et al.*, 1964). Most of these studies have dealt with relatively simple behaviours and involved the manipulation of reinforcement contingencies by an expert therapist from outside the family. A few recent studies have attempted to extend the application of these techniques to a purely clinical situation dealing with complex global behaviours. The emphasis in these situations has been on enhancing generalization, by training the parents to function as social reinforcers.

Meyer and Gelder (1963) and Berkowitz and Zigler (1965) have noted that the success of behaviour therapy is to a large extent determined by the relationship developed between the "therapist" and the patient. The parents are already established as the significant people in the child's life before he is brought into the clinic for

*From the *Journal of Child Psychology and Psychiatry*, 1968, 9, pp. 245-252. Reprinted by permission of Maxwell International Microforms Corporation.

therapy. Furthermore, the undesirable behaviour usually happens at home rather than at the clinic, and therefore the parents are the only ones present to control the consequences of that behaviour. Wahler *et al.* (1965) trained the mothers in three cases to be good behaviour therapists, by having them interact with their children in a playroom setting and using signal lights to reinforce them, when they reinforced the children appropriately. Russo (1964) trained mothers to function as good behaviour therapists by having them watch a therapist interact with their children in a playroom, then have the mothers go into the playroom with the therapist and child and gradually take over the role of the therapist as he gradually withdrew from the interaction. Straughan (1964) used a similar technique to help both the mother and child gain awareness of the relation between the child's behaviour and the mother's behaviour. The present study is a demonstration in one clinical case of the further extension of the focus of behaviour modification by involving the entire family unit, rather than just the identified child patient and the mother.

Presenting Problem

The Jacksons were a working-class family who lived in a rural logging environment. Mr. Jackson was a sawmill worker. He found the home situation so aversive that he tried to spend as little time there as was necessary. He rarely responded to the children, except to strike them or yell at them when they irritated him. To appease his children, he would often promise to take them on some of his hunting or fishing trips, but then sneak out early in the morning before they had awakened. Mrs. Jackson was an extremely obese woman who had previously spent some time in the state mental hospital. She felt grossly inadequate in dealing with her husband and her children.

Mrs. Jackson came to the clinic seeking assistance for relieving the behaviour problems of her six-year-old son, Jacky. He was the second oldest of her four children. At the time of referral, Mrs. Jackson was concerned that she would become seriously depressed by the home situation and that Jacky would do irreparable damage to himself or to others.

The major complaint expressed was that no one could in any way control Jacky's behaviour. He would not respond to any demands of the parents or of his kindergarten teacher. When he did not want to do as he was told, violent temper tantrums, involving hyperactivity, swearing, and aggressive attacks, were likely to occur. On several occasions, he left home for hours at a time. Extended crying jags and screaming spells were also very frequent responses to commands or requests made by adults. When upset he would seek out a special pillow which seemed to calm him down. Associated with this extreme disobedience was a large amount of apparently unprovoked aggression. This would be directed toward his siblings, neighbourhood children, and children he had never seen before, even if they were older and bigger than he was. On one occasion, he became angry with his two-year-old sister, seized a butcher's knife, and made menacing moves towards her. Although he did not injure her, he clutched the knife until his knuckles were white and his body trembled; it was very difficult for his mother to remove the knife from him. On another occasion, he climbed out of the window of their parked car and began to strike another child, whom Mrs. Jackson believed to be a total stranger. Thefts were also quite prominent in his behaviour, as Jacky often stole small amounts of money and many knives from the home.

Mrs. Jackson reported that the entire small town in which they lived had knowledge of Jacky's reputation, and most families refused to permit him or his brothers to come on to their property. Because of this, rock-throwing battles were frequent between the Jackson boys and the neighbouring children. The school had refused to accept Jacky into the first grade unless he received some treatment.

Method

After an intake interview with the mother, the Jackson family was seen weekly for almost 11 months. A total of 27 one-hour sessions was held. Due to vacation periods and inclement weather the weekly schedule could not always be met. They lived about 150 miles from the clinic so each visit required a three-hour drive each way.

Three therapists were involved in working with the Jackson family. Therapist *A* worked with Mrs. Jackson, initially gaining information about the reinforcement contingencies operating in the home, and later attempting to explain the basic concepts of operant conditioning as they might be applied to her child. A short paper* ex-

*This paper was written by Mrs. Anne Hastings for use in the clinic.

plaining these principles in lay terminology was given to her. Therapist *B* worked with Jacky in a playroom setting, observing his behaviour, and establishing himself as a strong SOCIAL REINFORCER. Following six unstructured playroom sessions, a decision was made to concentrate on compliance behaviour: obeying commands given by an adult. The following paradigm was designed so that the opportunity for compliance was frequent during the sessions. Therapist *B* would say "Jacky" and record whether *S* made eye contact with him, as a measure of attention. This was followed by a command to perform some small manipulation with the toys in the playroom, e.g. "Put the blocks in the cupboard." The commands were given in a conversational tone and occurred every 90 seconds. Eye contact and obeying commands had to occur within 15 seconds for the response to be considered correct. Initially eye contact and compliance were treated as independent responses, but after four sessions, commands were made CONTINGENT on eye contact. Therapist *B* and an observer who was viewing through a one-way mirror, independently recorded the responses during these sessions. Therapist *C* visited the Jackson home, observing the reinforcement contingencies operating there and establishing a relationship with Mr. Jackson. This relationship was facilitated by the therapist's ability to become involved in the activities of Mr. Jackson (e.g. dressing a deer); as a result, Mr. Jackson, initially hostile towards outsiders, developed an interest in the behaviour modification programme.

After a baseline session, the treatment sessions began. Therapist *B* reinforced both eye contact and compliance, independently, with candy and social stimuli, such as attention, smiling, and praise. Inattention or lack of compliance resulted in a WITHDRAWAL OF ALL SOCIAL STIMULI FOR 60 SECONDS; therapist *B* terminated his interaction with *S* by looking away and refusing to respond to him. As the percentage of correct responses increased, the candy was placed on an INTERMITTENT SCHEDULE (approximately VR3) while social reinforcement was maintained on a CONTINUOUS SCHEDULE. Still later, eye contact and compliance were handled as a chain; commands were omitted unless eye contact had been obtained, and reinforcement occurred only at the end of the chain when the commands were obeyed.

While therapist *B* worked with Jacky in the playroom, therapist

A and Mrs. Jackson observed through the one-way mirror. Techniques of behaviour modification were explained as they occurred, and Jacky's behavioural changes dramatically emphasized their effectiveness to Mrs. Jackson. Jacky did not know he was being observed.

After six sessions, eye contact and compliance were being elicited virtually 100 per cent of the time with therapist *B*. At this time, Mrs. Jackson entered the playroom with therapist *B* and Jacky. During a 10-minute period, she would give five to 10 commands to Jacky and would reinforce appropriate behaviour, and initiate extinction when inappropriate behaviour occurred. Therapist *B* would then continue working with Jacky while therapist *A* would give Mrs. Jackson feedback on her behaviour in the playroom. Initially, she was very inept, and consequently could not maintain the desired behaviour in her son. However, as she became more accustomed to the situation, she became efficient in administering contingent reinforcement, and effective in controlling her son's behaviour.

As Mrs. Jackson learned the principles and application of reinforcement and extinction in behavioural control, she established a programme within the home. Therapists *A* and *C* served as resources to aid in its implementation. Mrs. Jackson used gummed stars, which could be exchanged for various toys and treats, to reinforce obedience and completed chores about the home. Extinction was used to reduce undesirable behaviour (e.g. temper tantrums, fighting and disobedience). As the programme became established in the home the children were reinforced for intervals of time during which these undesirable behaviours did not occur.

During this same period of observation at the clinic and the star system at home, Mrs. Jackson began to report positive changes in Jacky's behaviour both at home and at school. However, as Jacky's behaviour improved, his older brother Fred, who had displayed little problem behaviour previously, became more aggressive and disobedient both at home and at school. Mrs. Jackson reported an increase in fights between the boys and a total lack of cooperative behaviour. At this time Fred was introduced to the therapy programme at the clinic.

For four sessions, therapist *B* worked with the two boys separately, reinforcing eye contact and compliant behaviour. In addition, if both boys did well in the playroom and while waiting in the recception room, they were reinforced with a trip to the animal lab. When eye contact and compliance were occurring virtually 100 per cent of the time in both boys, therapist *B* began working with them together in the playroom, differentially reinforcing cooperative behaviour between them by using attention and praise as reinforcers. They were reinforced for working together when carrying out a command, or for any other spontaneous cooperation they might show during a session. Initially, cooperation was only sporadic, partly because Jacky discovered that he could make Fred angry by not cooperating, and thus losing the reinforcement for both of them. This problem was solved by changing the reinforcing operations so that the boys would be reinforced independently. Two large cardboard counters were installed high on the wall and labelled with the boys' names. The rules were set so that a cooperative response gained each boy three points. If only one boy was willing to cooperate, he earned one point and the other boy earned none. If either of the boys was overly-aggressive during a session, he was punished by losing five points. "Aggression" was interpreted liberally with normal horse play not penalized. If enough points had been earned during a session, the boys could spend them on some after-session activity, such as a visit to the animal lab, or an ice cream cone. The number of points required was raised each session, and the boys responded with more and more cooperative behaviour. Mrs. Jackson's youngest son, Mark, sat in the reception room waiting for the other boys to finish. If he waited quietly, he was also rewarded by being allowed to participate in the after-session activity.

Mrs. Jackson continued to observe, and therapist *A* continued his encouragement and explanations of what was going on. She reported that cooperative behaviour at home was improving.

Due to the encouragement and urging of therapist *C*, Mr. Jackson made two trips to the clinic to watch the boys in sessions when they were working together. His wife reported he was very impressed with their behaviour. Following these visits, he agreed to cooperate in the programme his wife had started in the home. Mrs. Jackson reported that he became an active participant in the home programme, and at least one area of communication was opened up between them.

Results and Discussion

The first change was the frequency of eye contact and compliance shown by Jacky during the playroom sessions. In the baseline session prior to treatment, 48 commands were given. Eye contact was obtained 43 per cent of the time, and compliance was obtained on 49 per cent of the trials. During the first session in which these responses were reinforced, both eye contact and compliance were obtained 62 per cent of the time. Ignoring Jacky when he did not make the appriate responses appeared to be very aversive to him. At first during these "time-out" periods, he would try to attract the therapist's attention, sulk, or become aggressive, throw objects around the room, and push the therapist. This was gradually replaced either by quiet play or by patiently waiting until the "time-out" period was over. The second reinforcement session produced 46 per cent eye contact and 61 per cent compliance. There were three distinct parts to this session; a period of 100 per cent responding was followed by a period of extreme negativism in which Jacky withdrew and refused to have anything to do with the therapist, which in turn was followed by another period of 100 per cent responding. A third session resulted in 85 per cent responding; but the fourth session resulted in another demonstration of negativism, 10 per cent responding. From this point on in treatment, compliance was obtained virtually 100 per cent of the time.

These data emphasize that Jacky's improvement in performance was anything but gradual and smooth. He was aware of the contingencies involved. During the first session, he said, "All I have to do to get some candy is to do what you tell me." But the improvement in behaviour was hindered until he had learned that "time-outs" could not be influenced by unacceptable behaviour.

When Fred was brought into the programme, he emitted eye contact and compliance almost 100 per cent of the time from the first session. He was already aware of the contingencies involved and had met the therapist often because of Jacky's participation in the programme. The importance of the therapist's relationship with the boys was emphasized by Fred's refusing the candy reinforcement and working entirely for the praise and interaction from the therapist. The fact that almost no shaping was necessary with Fred tends to validate his mother's statement that he was much more obedient than was Jacky.

When the boys were brought into the playroom together, there was some initial competition for the therapist's attention, and some aggression toward each other. These behaviours gradually extinguished as working together was reinforced. When points were given for working together, the boys initially competed to see who could get the most points. On one occasion, Fred earned enough points for a trip to the animal lab; but Jacky didn't. Jacky cried vociferously, and Fred did not enjoy his reward. Later, during another session when Fred had more points than Jacky, he stated that he wasn't going to do anything more until Jacky had caught up with him in points. Another example of this developing cooperation occurred when the boys were painting. Only one of the two paint brushes was usable so they took turns using the good brush.

Mrs. Jackson's initial attempts as a social reinforcer were very cold, and her attempts to provide physical events as reinforcements were very unrealistic. At one time, her promises of reinforcement were so far removed from the behaviour that it lost its effect. She promised the boys a trip to the zoo in a distant city some time in the summer if they were good. At first, she could not understand the concepts of operant conditioning even though they had been explained to her in detail; she could learn this only through repeated experience and observations of concrete situations.

The changes which had occurred in the family when treatment was terminated, included improvement both in the home and at school. The parents, of course, might well be presenting a biased report, but they represent the only source of information concerning the home. Both Mr. and Mrs. Jackson reported that the extremely aggressive behaviour which Jacky was showing a year ago had been markedly reduced. He infrequently displayed any unprovoked aggression toward the other children. He did have a quick temper and, if provoked, would fight back. This is not necessarily inappropriate behaviour, especially in the area where he lives. The cooperation training had been carried over into the home and was reported to be quite successful as Jacky and Fred worked or played together much of the time. Both boys obeyed their parents much more readily and the parents had learned to be more consistent in rewards and punishments. An incidental but important change occurred in the parents' relations. In working together to solve the children's behaviour problems, Mrs. Jackson reported that they had begun to communicate more than before. She felt the general marital situation had improved.

The principal of the boys' school was contacted for his impressions of their behaviour. He stated that both boys had improved considerably both in the classroom and on the playground. He added, however, that they still had a long way to go. Because of their previous behaviour and reputation, especially in Jacky's case, many potential playmates would have nothing to do with them. He stated that they will both have a long rough road ahead of them for the next couple of years, but their future looks promising.

Treatment sessions were terminated in late May, 1967. In late September the principal of the boys' school and each of their teachers were contacted to ascertain how the changes reported during treatment were holding up in the school. The principal stated that he had had no reports of classroom problems, but he reiterated his previous statement that the boys, especially Jacky, would have rough going because of their well-established reputation as trouble-makers in the community.

Fred's teacher reported: ". . . he seems to be happy, does his work reasonably well, and is cooperative in the classroom." She had had but one complaint about his behaviour on the playground but that was not serious.

Jacky's teacher gave essentially the same report. She said: ". . . he has adjusted to the children in the room and they to him very nicely. He can stand in line for a drink and await his turn. He seems to be playing with the rest at recess. There has been absolutely no tattling on him from the playground, so I know he has not been giving any trouble."

Therapist C revisited the home on 31 October. He observed a number of request-compliance sequences between Mrs. Jackson and the boys, although compliance was carried out in a somewhat "unruly" manner. He reported that, according to the mother, Jacky now has a number of friends and is doing well in school. Mr. Jackson was not home during this visit, but Mrs. Jackson reported that the communication between them which seemed to be developing in the spring had disappeared and Mr. Jackson had returned to his previous uncommunicative self.

The major gain reported by therapist *C* is that Mrs. Jackson now feels "on top of the situation" and able to deal much more effectively with the children. She believes, however, that nothing has really changed in her relationship with her husband.

Summary

A systematic programme of therapy was carried out with a family unit. The initially identified patient was a young boy, age 6, whose extremely aggressive behaviour towards other children had left him isolated from potential friends and caused fear in the community that he would seriously injure someone. Before a programme of 27 contacts, based on operant conditioning principles, was completed, the boy's mother, father, and an older brother were all closely involved. The following steps in therapy were systematically carried out:

1. Systematic reinforcement of (a) eye contact and (b) compliance with a command in the clinic playroom.
2. Concurrent training of the mother in the relevant principles, through observation of the therapist's behaviour and by discussion.
3. Training of mother in the playroom in reinforcement and extinction of her son's compliant behaviour.
4. Establishing in the home a programme of systematic reinforcement of the boy and his older brother.
5. Establishing cooperation between the boys in the playroom by making reinforcement for both boys contingent on such behaviour.

Reports from the parents indicated that behaviour changes in the direction of increased compliance and cooperation occurred in the home. A report from the school principal indicated that marked changes occurred in both boys' classroom and playground behaviour in the direction of greater cooperation and contact with other boys. The principal was less optimistic about the boys' next few years because of the intense negative feeling that had developed toward, especially, the younger boy because of his previous behaviour. A 4-6 month follow-up revealed that behaviour in the school continued to be acceptable. The home situation had deteriorated as far as interaction between the parents was concerned, but the mother reported that compliance and cooperation from the children continued for the most part.

References

Baer, D. M.: Laboratory control of thumbsucking by withdrawal and re-presentation of reinforcement. *J Exp Psychol 5*, 525-528, 1962.

Berkowitz, H. and Zigler, E.: Effects of preliminary positive and negative interaction and delay conditions of children's responsiveness to social reinforcement. *J Pers Soc Psychol 2*, 500-505, 1965.

Hart, B. M., Allen, K. E., Buell, J. S., Harris, F. R. and Wolf, M. M.: Effects of social reinforcement on operant crying. *J Exp Child Psychol 1*, 145-153, 1964.

Madsen, C. H.: Positive reinforcement in the toilet training of a normal child: a case report. In *Case Studies in Behavior Modification* (Edited by Ullmann, L. P. and Krasner, L.) pp. 305-307. Holt, Rinehart and Winston, 305-307, 1965.

Meyer, V. and Gelder, M. G.: Behaviour therapy and phobic disorders. *Br J Psychiat 109*, 19-28, 1963.

Straughan, J. H.: Treatment with child and mother in the playroom. *Behav Res Ther 2*, 37-41, 1964.

Walker, R. G., Winkel, G. H., Peterson, R. F. and Morrison, D. C.: Mothers as behavior therapists for their own children. *Behav Res Ther 3*, 113-134, 1965.

Williams, C. D.: The elimination of tantrum behavior by extinction procedures. *J Abnorm Soc Psychol 59*, 259, 1959.

Chapter 3

PARENTS AS BEHAVIOR THERAPY-TECHNICIANS IN TREATING READING DEFICITS (DYSLEXIA)*

DAVID RYBACK *and* ARTHUR W. STAATS

IN 1963 IT WAS SUGGESTED that parents must be considered to be the trainers of their children. "Whether the parent intends to or not, he manipulates many conditions of learning that will determine to a large extent the behaviors the child will acquire. As long as the child's behavioral development consists of innumerable training experiences, the parent has many of the controlling variables in his hands and cannot relinquish them regardless of his philosophy of child development . . . Faced with a training task of such imposing responsibilities, it would seem that the parent would need an understanding of the principles of behavior by which children learn . . . This suggests that the parent could be an active participant in arranging circumstances to produce most effectively an abundant, rich, adjustive, behavioral repertoire using a minimum of aversive stimulation and a maximum of positive reinforcements . . ." (Staats, 1963, pp. 412-413.)

Since this behavioral analysis of parent-child interactions, a number of studies have extended learning principles to childhood behavior problems, employing the parent as trainer or behavior thera-

*From the *Journal of Behavior Therapy and Experimental Psychiatry*, 1970, *1*, pp. 109-119. Reprinted by permission of the author and Pergamon Press, Ltd.

pist. Wahler, Winkel, Peterson and Morrison (1965) worked with mothers in the clinic and taught them to discriminate target behaviors of their children and to respond according to certain CONTINGENCIES. In a subsequent step the mothers discriminated without cues from the experimenter but received feed-back on their accuracy. The behaviors dealt with were commanding vs. co-operative behavior.

In their work with parent-child relationships, therapists have in several cases also moved out of the clinic and into the home setting. Russo (1964) demonstrated that parents can serve as trainers in both home and clinical settings, while Straughan (1964) conducted the therapy sessions at home. Straughan worked with the child in a play-room and served as a model while the parent observed. In a similar fashion, Rickard and Munday (1965) served as models in shaping non-stuttering in a nine-year-old while the mother observed. Subsequent to this, the mother acted as a model while the father observed. Similar modeling techniques were used by Ryback (1966) in training parents in the shaping of speech behaviors in mute schizophrenic children.

Walder (1966) and Wetzel, Baker, Roney and Martin (1966) have also used parents to treat their autistic children. Other behavior problems which have been treated by parents as trainers include emotional disturbances (Andronico and Guerney, 1967), destructive behaviors (O'Leary, O'Leary and Becker, 1967), aggressive behavior (Zeilberger, Sampen and Sloane, 1968), hyperactivity in the classroom (Patterson, 1965a) and at home (Hawkins, Peterson, Schweid and Bijou, 1966), school phobia (Patterson, 1965b) and excessive scratching (Allen and Harris, 1966). Zeilberger *et al.*, have generally concluded that "the most efficient way to modify deviant behavior may be to change the reactions of the natural milieu to that behavior" (1968, p. 47).

Of all the studies dealing with parents as subprofessional behavior modifiers only one deals with language training although this study (Ryback, 1966) lacked precise criteria for measuring behavior changes. All other studies involved behaviors that could be altered in a relatively brief period of time. However, many deficits of human behavior are usually overcome only on the basis of learning over lengthy time periods (Staats, 1969). Simple instructions to reinforce or not reinforce a behavior will not suffice in such cases. It would seem necessary to develop, through research, methods and procedures for the standard application of behavioral principles in the treatment of complex cognitive deficits. It would be important to demonstrate that complex behavior therapy procedures could be successfully employed by the parent, under the supervision of the psychiatric or psychological profession.

One cognitive deficit that has been of perennial concern to medicine and psychology is the failure to learn to read normally, a deficit called dyslexia, displayed by a considerable percentage of children. Staats began the study of reading learning and of token-reinforcer methods for treating dyslexia in 1959 and has continued this work in a series of studies (Staats, Finley, Minke and Wolf, 1964; Staats, Minke, Finley, Wolf and Brooks, 1964; Staats, Staats, Schutz and Wolf, 1962). (His token-reinforcer system has spread widely, see Ayllon and Azrin, 1969). Part of this project has involved the development of methods by which subprofessional personnel, under professional supervision, could successfully treat children who had severe problems of learning to read (Staats and Butterfield, 1965; Staats, Minke, Goodwin and Landeen, 1967a; Staats, Minke and Butts, in press).

The purpose of the present experiment was to determine whether the same set of methods and materials could be successfully utilized by parents in the treatment of their own children's cognitive deficits. The behavioral deficit of dyslexia is ordinarily not easily treated and requires long-term treatment efforts by professionals. This study is the first to test the possibility that behavioral methods, when made standard and explicit, can be employed by the parent in individual treatment of complex behavioral deficits.

Method

Subjects and parents

One child was selected from the University of Hawaii Laboratory School. Three were chosen from the waiting list for the Reading Clinic at the University of Hawaii. These children were chosen from a population of students described as poor readers on the basis of standard achievement tests and teacher referrals. Final selection for participation in the experiment was on the basis of a 100-word test developed from the reading material. All children reading fewer than 80 out of the 100 words but no less than 20 were selected for the experiment.

S_1 was a 13-year-old boy of Japanese descent, an only child and had been diagnosed as mentally retarded by the State Psychologist of the Department of Public Instruction as well as by a clinical psychologist in private practice. S_1 was in a special non-graded class because of his learning difficulties and read 43 out of the 100-word test. At the onset of the program, Parent$_1$ had recently quit her job as librarian because of somatic manifestations of tension. She was unaware of the source of her tension since events in her life, including her marriage, were satisfactory. A 41-year-old woman, P_1, was below average in arithmetic and spelling skills, but was very superior in reading skills according to the Wide Range Achievement Test (WRAT) by Jastak, Bijou and Jastak.

S_2 was an 11-year-old fifth-grade girl of Caucasian descent; the oldest of four children, her siblings were nine and one-half, seven and four years old. S_2 had been diagnosed as an emotional problem by a clinical psychologist as well as by her teachers, her reading problem was thought to stem from her emotional problems. She read 61 words on the 100-word test. Parent$_2$ was a 31-year-old housewife. One of P_2's chief concerns during the experimental period was an ailing mother who made sporadic demands on her and this was sometimes a drain on her energy. P_2 was well below average in arithmetic, spelling and reading skills.

S_3 was a ten and one-half-year-old fifth-grade boy of Hawaiian descent; the second of four children, his siblings were eleven and one-half, eight and one-half and seven years old. He had been described by the Department of Education as a learning disability and he had been diagnosed by a pediatrician, on the basis of neurological tests, as a learning disability with minimal cerebral dysfunction. He read 50 words on the 100-word test. Parent$_3$ was a 31-year-old clinic clerk at a hospital near her home. She was above average in arithmetic and spelling skills and was at a superior level in reading skills.

S_4 was an eight and one-half-year-old third-grade boy of Hawaiian descent; the youngest of four children, his siblings were 12, 11 and ten years old. No problems were reported other than his learning disabilities and a heart ailment. He read 29 words on the 100-word test. Parent$_4$ was a 41-year-old woman who worked as a cashier at a cafeteria. P_4 was below average in her arithmetic, spelling and read-

TABLE XX

WIDE RANGE ACHIEVEMENT TEST SCORES OF PARENTS

Sub-test	$Parent_1$	$Parent_2$	$Parent_3$	$Parent_4$	Mean
Reading					
Grade level	16.5	7.9	14.4	7.7	11.62
Percentile	99.4	34	96	37	60.60
Spelling					
Grade level	10.8	6.5	12.0	5.8	8.77
Percentile	77	19	84	23	50.75
Arithmetic					
Grade level	6.7	7.1	10.1	5.3	7.30
Percentile	23	25	63	12	30.75
Derived IQ	114.0	90.3	115.7	88.7	102.2

ing skills. The parents were given the Wide Range Achievement Test and the results are summarized in Table XX.

The combined income of each family ranged from $11,000 to $15,000 per annum. Each mother had completed a high school education while two fathers had completed high school, one had completed eighth grade and one had completed a year of college. The IQ's of the mothers ranged from 89 to 116, as the Table indicates, on the estimated scores which were derived from the WRAT results by averaging the Reading, Arithmetic and Spelling Standard Scores.

Training materials

The stimulus materials and procedures employed in the study have been described in detail elsewhere (Staats and Butterfield, 1965; Staats et al., 1967a), and a manual further elaborates the techniques of recording the data and supervising the therapy-technicians (Staats, Van Mondfrans and Minke, 1967b). The procedures and token-reinforcer system will be called herein the Staats Motivation-Activating Reading Technique (SMART), based upon the evidence that the procedures ensure continuous motivation of the child throughout a complex training program. The materials are based upon the Science Research Associates Reading Laboratory. These stories are graded and involve a somewhat controlled introduction of new words in each lesson. The present methods require a list made of all of the new words added in each story, beginning with the first story. The training for each lesson thus begins with the individual presentation to the child of the new words to be learned, printed on 5 × 8 inch cards. Each new word is presented as a stimulus; if the child cannot read the word he is PROMPTED. The children learn to read each word to a criterion of one correct unprompted reading, each word being deleted from the series as criterion is reached. Following this the paragraphs of the story are read by the child (the story is printed on 8½x11 inch paper). The child is PROMPTED on any words he cannot read, and the paragraph is re-read, if necessary, until it is done perfectly. Following the reading each paragraph of the story to criterion, the child is presented with the whole story to read silently.

The S.R.A. stories also include questions in each of the stories to test the comprehension. Thus, following the silent reading of the story the child is presented with the questions. Whenever a question is missed the child rereads the relevant paragraph in the story and responds to the question again.

Thus, each lesson consists of the following phases: The Individual Word Learning Phase, the Oral Paragraph Reading Phase, the Silent Reading Phase and the Comprehension Question Phase. A Vocabulary Review is presented following every 20 lessons, to test the extent to which the words previously learned in those lessons have been retained. The test thus occurs several weeks following for most of the words.

Token-reinforcer system

The motivational system consists of token-reinforcers of different value. The tokens are plastic discs of three different colors. A blue token is worth one-tenth of a cent (or one point on the graph of reinforcement accrual described below), a white token is worth one-fifth of a cent or two points), a red token is worth one-half cent (or five points). The daily recording of the child's progress is demonstrated to him with positive comment and approval from the parent. The parents were instructed in the use of positive social reinforcement and in avoiding the use of disapproval of any kind, including urging to do well, or to do better.

The child received in exchange for his tokens, when a sufficient number had been accrued, a cash account with the parent by which the child could purchase any item of his choice limited only by the amount of money he earned to date. The child had the opportunity of purchasing inexpensive items such as candy bars (within the customs of the family) as well as more expensive items. For the latter he would have to save his accumulating tokens for a longer period.

The different values of tokens were presented contingent upon the child's reading behaviors. According to plan the higher value reinforcers were delivered contingent upon the most valuable behaviors, thus, for example, the child was reinforced more heavily for reading a word correctly in his first attempt than after prompted learning trials and he was reinforced more highly for correctly answering the comprehension questions than for the silent reading itself (to ensure that the silent reading had occurred). However, the child was reinforced for all of his effortful behaviors in the reading task.

Behavior recording

The major source of data for the present type of study consists of the effects of the training upon the behavior of the subject during the extended experimental period. This methodology calls for a detailed recording of the stimuli presented to the subject and his responses to those stimuli. Thus, every single word stimulus presented to the child was recorded as was the response to that stimulus. When the paragraph reading task was presented each response to a word stimulus was recorded. If the child missed a word more than once this was also recorded. The number of token-reinforcers received was recorded, and so on. For these purposes data sheets (see Staats *et al.*, 1967b) were employed by the parents. Part of the training of the parents consisted of instruction in how to perform the recording duties.

Parent training and supervision

The training of parents involved approximately four hours. During this time they received a demonstration of the procedures by *E* (the first author) and were given a basic outline of the procedures. Then detailed instructions concerning the administration of the procedures and the collection of data were given. Questions were handled as they arose. Finally, the parents were given actual practice in administering the materials, taking turns playing the role of the child.

During the first couple of weeks, direct supervision of parents' participation was periodically maintained in the manner described (Staats, *et al.*, 1967b). Following this, *E*'s supervision was phased out gradually until the parents were working on their own except for the review tests which were administered by *E*.

One of the central aspects of *E*'s supervision of the parents' behaviors in the training situation involved the use of a checklist (see Staats *et al.*, 1967b). This checklist related to two aspects of the parents' behaviors: firstly, to the mechanics of the therapy-technicians' task and, secondly, to the more subtle concerns of the behavior modification training techniques. On the one hand some checklist items called attention to such things as filling out the data sheets, recording time, writing down words missed for later review, counting tokens, filling out the token graph and so on. On the other hand the checklist contained items referring, for example, to the parent's pause in presenting single word stimuli before prompting, to re-presenting the missed words, delivering tokens, presenting paragraphs until the child had them entirely correct, use of pointing to direct the child's attention, checking occasionally on child during silent reading, correcting comprehension questions and having child reread relevant paragraphs in case of error, and so on. There were additional items that directed attention to aspects of the parents' training characteristics and to the behavior of the child; for example, to the parent watching to see if the child looked at the word when repeating it after prompting or if the child practiced interfering rehearsals in trying to learn the words, giving positive social reinforcement and avoiding any negative social reinforcement (especially on errors), and so on. Besides the specific check list *E* observed the quality of the training in general—especially with respect to insuring the absence of any negative social reinforcement, either direct or implied. When any procedures were erroneously handled or when the training included undesirable elements, corrective measures were immediately discussed with the parent following the session.

Half-hour group meetings of the parents and *E* were held at the end of the first, third and eighth weeks of the program to discuss any problems which may have arisen, technical or otherwise, and to discuss the motivation of the children as well as the parents' own motivation.

Testing materials

The 100 item single word reading test consisted of words randomly selected from the universe of 4253 words of the reading materials. Twenty words were selected from each of the five grade levels (1.2, 1.7, 2.3, 3.0, 4.0). The words were presented individually on 3 × 5 inch cards and had to be correctly pronounced for receipt of credit. Two alternate forms of the test were developed. The words of these were matched for difficulty according to the Thorndike-Lorge word count (Thorndike and Lorge, 1944), and across reading grade levels. One form of the test was used as a pre-test and the other as a post-test. The original form was also administered as an additional post-test. Evidence has shown the 100-word test to be a valid indicator of Ss' performance on the SMART (Staats *et al.*, 1967b; 1969).

The Wide Range Achievement Test (WRAT) (Jastak, Bijou and Jastak, 1965) was employed to characterise the academic achievement of each of the parents working with the children. The Diagnostic Reading Scales (Spache, 1963) were individually administered before and after the behavior therapy training procedures.

Results and Conclusions

Over a 5- to 7-month period, four mothers administered the Staats Motivation-Activating Reading Technique (SMART) to their children. During this period, Ss made many reading responses. They cooperated in the experiment with good attention and diligent work habits. The production of this type of behavior for such children in training conducted by the parent is of primary significance in itself. That is, it is only with procedures that yield such attention and work responses that the thousands of learning trials for complex learning can occur.

In this context it is interesting to consider the number of learning trials that did occur. That is, the total number of words the child read in the various types of training (including the comprehension and review tests) were tabulated as the training progressed. In the present study, the four Ss made an average of 74,730 single word reading responses during an average of 51.25 hours of training. During 65 hours of training, S_1 made 82,466 single word reading responses; during 50 hours of training, S_2 made 71,244; during 55 hours of training, S_3 made 95,906; and during 35 hours of training, S_4 made 49,303 single word reading responses. CUMULATIVE RECORDS of the words read over the period of training are depicted in Figure 37.

As Figure 37 shows, the reading rates of the four Ss accelerated positively over the training sessions, although the acceleration was slight for S_2. This acceleration in response rate may be considered

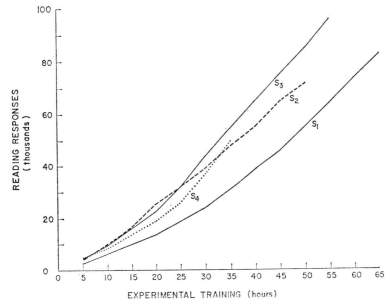

Figure 37. Cumulative number of single word reading responses as a function of the time in experimental training.

typical in these procedures since it has already occurred with a number of subjects (Staats *et al.*, 1967a, 1969). The typical curve is like that of S_1 and S_3 where an early acceleration is shown followed by a high linear response rate. These results indicate the high quality of the children's attention and work behaviors during training, resulting in the many learning trials, a prerequisite for any complex skill acquisition. It should also be noted that the acceleration occurred even though the reading material became increasingly difficult and was extended over a long period.

Before reading each story, Ss were presented with individual cards for all the words in that story which had not been previously presented. When these words were presented, Ss read a certain proportion correctly, the other words being missed on first presentation. The missed words were considered to be new words. Records were kept of the number of words the children missed on first presentation, the number of these words which were then later missed in the oral reading of the paragraphs, as well as the number of words originally missed that the Ss could not read on the review tests presented at a later time. S_1 learned 910 new words; S_2 learned 591; S_3 learned 1040; and S_4 learned 450 during training.

Although the Ss missed these new words on initial presentation, they were given training trials on these words and then read them again in the oral reading of the paragraphs. The number of errors made on this second presentation provided a measure of short-term retention of the words that had been previously learned. Thus, S_1 retained 576 (about 63 per cent) of these words during the Oral Reading Phase; S_2 retained 504 (about 85 per cent); S_3 retained 917 (about 88 per cent); and S_4 retained 431 (about 94 per cent). These results indicate that the criterion of one correct unprompted trial in the original vocabulary-learning phase produced considerable learning when the words were read in context.

A measure of long-term retention was obtained by individually presenting the words that had been first learned in the preceding 20 lessons. This test was given 10-15 days after training occurred. The training included the previous single word presentations of the words as well as the reading of the words in context both orally and silently. In addition, however, many new additional words had been learned in the interim. According to this measure, S_1 retained 478 of the 910 words (53 per cent) on the long-term retention test; S_2 retained 404 of the 591 words (68 per cent); S_3 retained 585 of the 1040 words (56 per cent) and S_4 retained 340 of the 458 words (74 per cent). These results indicate that the children covered a considerable amount of reading material, that they learned to read a large number of new words whether presented individually or in context and that even after a considerable intervening period they retained a good proportion of what they learned.

The 100-word reading test was administered to the Ss at the onset of the program and an alternate form of the test was administered at the termination of the program. Subject$_1$ made an increase of 31 per cent on the post-test over the pre-test, while S_2, S_3, and S_4 made increases of 44 per cent, 66 per cent and 224 per cent respectively. The pre-test mean was 45.75 while the post-test mean was 85.75. A one-tailed correlated t test indicated a significant increase at the 0.01 level of probability.

The results of the original form of the 100-word test, when administered at the completion of the program, were very similar to those of the alternate form. Subjects 1-4 scored 89, 86, 87 and 95, respectively, on the original form, as compared with the results on the other post-training form of the test, as shown in Table XXI. Thus, the two forms were very similar and may be considered to be representative samples of the universe of 4253 words. In the comparison of the two post-training tests three of the four scores deviate by four points or less. Only one score deviates as much as 11 points.

In addition to the above, the Spache Diagnostic Reading Scales were administered both at the onset and termination of the program. The pre- and post-test results are also shown in Table 38. On the Word Recognition subtest (in which Ss read single words aloud) the pre-test mean score indicated a 4.5 grade reading level (GRL), an increase significant at the 0.05 level. On the Instructional subtest in which Ss read stories aloud, the pre-test mean score indicated at 2.6 GRL while the post-test mean score indicated a 4.5 GRL, an increase significant at the 0.005 level. On the Independent subtest in which Ss read silently and were tested for comprehension, the pretest mean score indicated a 3.0 GRL while the post-test mean score indicated a 4.7 GRL, an increase significant at the 0.025 level. For all Ss and in all subtests save one (Word Recognition for S_3), an increase of at least one grade level was obtained on the independent, standardized test. These are very important findings because they indicate that the training is not only specific to the particular materials involved. The children showed consistent increases on the standardized test—and the increases were larger than expected on the basis of the length of training involved.

One aspect of the SMART concerns the RATIO OF REINFORCERS to reading responses. The procedures were designed to reduce progressively the number of reinforcers given per reading response as the training progresses or, conversely, to require more reading responses per unit of reinforcement. Demonstration that this is possible in a long-term training program "is in part an answer to the question whether the use of extrinsic reinforcers in training will produce a child who is dependent upon these reinforcers" (Staats and Butterfield, 1965, p. 941). Figure 38 shows the ratio of reinforcers to the number of reading responses over the course of the training. The results support the earlier demonstrations in that the ratio of reinforcers to reading responses can be seen to decrease as a function of

TABLE XXI

PRE- AND POST-TEST RESULTS IN READING ABILITY

Subject	Time of administration	Spache Diagnostic Reading Scales Reading Grade Level			100-Word test	
		Word recognition	Instructional level	Independent level	Score	Gain (%)
S_1	Pre	2.8	2.5	2.5	43	81
	Post	4.5	4.5	4.5	78	
S_2	Pre	3.8	3.0	3.75	61	44
	Post	5.0	4.5	5.0	88	
S_3	Pre	3.3	2.75	3.5	50	66
	Post	3.5	4.5	4.5	83	
S_4	Pre	2.3	2.25	2.25	29	224
	Post	5.0	4.5	5.0	94	
	t	2.786	11.719	4.434	4.655	
	p	$<.05$	$<.005$	$<.025$	$<.01$	

number of training sessions. This is especially interesting in light of the acceleration in rate of reading responses as shown in Figure 37.

The mean cost of the reinforcers per child was $18.34. Subject$_1$ earned $17.36, S_2 earned $18.79, S_3 earned $20.89 and S_4 earned $16.32. Training of the parents took merely four hours. Since the parents were trained in a group setting, the average time for training was one hour per parent. Hence, the cost of reinforcers required in the SMART and the expenses of training parents were minimal. In addition, of course, there was time involved in the supervisory visits. However, these totaled roughly five hours per parent. Much of this could probably be shortened. It is quite evident that widespread medical or psychological treatment is not possible with a ratio of one highly-trained professional per child. The present methods, and their extension to other areas, could offer a method of extending treatment to larger numbers of children—with greater economy than is presently possible.

Discussion

This study is the fourth in a sequence of experiments demonstrating the application of the Staats Motivation-Activating Reading Technique. Previous studies have involved children in the 14- to 16-year age range. The present study showed the procedures to work effectively with four children whose ages averaged 10.7 years.

One reason for which many, if not most, professionals are unwill-

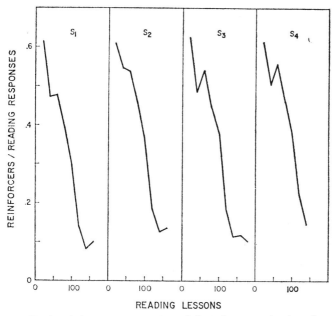

Figure 38. Ratio of the monetary value of the tokens received to the number of reading responses made as a function of the number of lessons read.

ing to venture into the area of parent-child therapeutic interaction is that the previous history of the dyadic interplay between child and parent may prevent the therapist's approach from being effective. Thus, the customary parent-child interaction in the context of complex skill acquisition is apt to be aversive for both participants. This situation is even more likely to occur with the child who has learning problems (or emotional, social, or cognitive problems). Any training program to be successfully conducted by the parent must overcome these past experiences of both parent and child.

In this context it is important to discuss the types of problems the various children treated with the SMART have had, in addition to reading deficits. In the previous experiments in which training was conducted by non-professional therapy-technicians (although not by parents) the children included a minority group juvenile delinquent, children from special classes for the retarded, children with emotional problems and ghetto black children who were severe educational problems. A number of these children were disturbed and delinquent children. In the present study the children's problems—mental retardation, emotionally disturbed, and cerebral dysfunction—would indicate the children to present serious treatment cases. Despite the severity of the diagnoses, the children responded well and the acquisition of reading skills did take place. Thus, utilizing the present procedures, it appeared that parents could serve as therapists for their children in an area in which only specialized professionals would ordinarily become involved.

As a side interest two of the siblings of the experimental Ss were given the pre- and post-tests at the same time that they were administered to the experimental Ss. S_2's nine and one-half-year-old sister obtained a pre-test score of 80 and a post-test score of 84 on the matched versions of the 100-word reading test, and this despite the fact that she had special tutoring in reading by a retired remedial reading specialist throughout the duration of her sister's SMART program. During this time, S_2 attained a 44 per cent increase on the post- over the pre-test. On the Spache Diagnostic Reading Scale, S_2's sister obtained scores of 4.5, 4.0 and 4.5 on both pre- and post-test scores of the three subtests. Again, no progress was shown. Although S_2 was a year ahead of her sister in school, she was quite a bit behind her sister in reading level at the beginning. But by the termination of the SMART administration, S_2 had caught up with her sister as indicated by the pre- and post-tests.

In a similar fashion S_3's eight and one-half-year-old brother, a third grader who also had a severe reading disability, was given the pre- and post-tests. Although S_3 attained a 66 per cent increase on the post- over the pre-test of the 100-word reading test, his younger brother, who received no help during this time, scored seven and 11 on the pre- and post-tests respectively. On the subtests of the Spache Diagnostic Reading Scales the control sibling scored 1.6, 1.0 and 1.5 on the pre-test while scoring 1.8, 1.0 and 2.0 on the post-test, again indicating very little gain during the six-month period. These results are important in providing some partial control data, and are also interesting methodologically. That is, use of siblings in this manner can be seen to have general implications for providing controls in behavior modification where one employs relatively few children.

It should be noted that despite the instruction of the parents, a problem in the training interaction did occur with the P_1S_1 dyad. Thus, P_1 sometimes inadvertently punished S_1 whenever he made a reading error. This was not done by what she said (merely a prompt of the erred response) but rather by how she said it; that is, with an annoyed, disappointed tone of voice. The parent was informed about this problem and the procedures were improved. This indicates the advantage of having professional supervision in some cases as was also shown in one of 18 therapy-technicians in an earlier study (Staats *et al.*, 1967a). It may be suggested, however, that sub-doctoral professionals can also be trained in the techniques and provide the supervision.

In conclusion, the importance of the present research findings lies in the fact that the SMART can be used by parents to teach their own children who have learning disabilities or other problems that result in cognitive deficits. Moreover, it is not necessary that the parents have previously had any special training nor that they be above average in intelligence, nor, for that matter, that they be educated beyond high school. Thus, the four parents with only four hours training in the SMART administration and subsequent supervision (notably in the one case) were able to successfully administer the materials. Moreover, training was administered in the everyday context of ongoing family demands on the mothers, in the homes of the respective families, while two of the mothers were holding full-time jobs. Even the very busy parent can administer the SMART with success if motivated and able to read.

References

Allen, K. E. and Harris, F. R.: Elimination of a child's excessive scratching by training the mother in reinforcement procedures. *Behav Res & Therapy 4*, 79-84, 1966.

Andronico, M. P. and Guerney, B., Jr.: The potential application of filial therapy to the school situation. *J Sch Psychol 6*, 2-7, 1967.

Ayllon, T. and Azrin, A. H.: *The Token Economy: A Motivational System for Therapy and Rehabilitation.* Appleton, New York, 1969.

Hawkins, R. P., Peterson, R. F., Schweid, E. and Bijou, S. W.: Behavior therapy in the home: amelioration of problem parent-child relations with parent in a therapeutic role. *J Exp Child Psychol 4*, 99-107, 1966.

Jastak, J. F., Bijou, S. W. and Jastak, S. R.: Wide Range Achievement Test. Wilmington, Delaware: Guidance Associates, 1965.

O'Leary, K. D., O'Leary, S. and Becker, W. C.: Modification of deviant sibling interaction pattern in the home. *Behav Res & Therapy 5*, 113-120, 1967.

Patterson, G. R.: An application of conditioning techniques to the control of a hyperactive child. *Case Studies in Behavior Modification* (Eds. L. P. Ullmann and L. Krasner), pp. 370-375. Holt, New York, 1965a.

Patterson, G. R.: A learning theory approach to the treatment of the school phobic child. *Case Studies in Behavior Modification*. (Eds. L. P. Ullmann and L. Krasner), pp. 279-285. Holt, New York, 1965b.

Rickard, H. C. and Munday, M. B.: Direct manipulation of stuttering behavior: an experimental-Clinical approach. *Case Studies in Behavior Modification*. (Eds. L. P. Ullmann and L. Krasner), pp. 268-274. Holt, New York, 1965.

Russo, S.: Adaptations in behavioral therapy with children. *Behav Res & Therapy 2*, 43-47, 1964.

Ryback, D.: M&M's and behavior modification. *J Council Except Child 16*, 3-7, 1966.

Ryback, D.: Cognitive behavior modification: Motivated learning reading treatment with parents as therapy-technicians. Unpublished doctoral dissertation, University of Hawaii, 1969.

Spache, G. D.: Diagnostic Reading Scales. California Test Bureau, 1963.

Staats, A. W.: (with contributions by C. K. Staats), *Complex Human Behavior*. Holt, Rinehart and Winston, New York, 1963.

Staats, A. W.: *Learning, Language, and Cognition*. Holt, Rinehart and Winston, New York, 1968.

Staats, A. W.: Development, use and social extensions of token-reinforcement systems. Paper presented at the *Conference on Progress in Behavior Modification*. Honolulu, 1969.

Staats, A. W. and Butterfield, W. H.: Treatment of nonreading in a culturally deprived juvenile delinquent: an application of reinforcement principles. *Child Dev 36*, 925-942, 1965.

Staats, A. W., Finley, J. R., Minke, K. A. and Wolf, M. M.: Reinforcement variables in control of unit reading responses. *J Exp Anal Behav 7*, 139-149, 1964a.

Staats, A. W., Minke, K. A. and Butts, P.: A token-reinforcement remedial reading program administered by black instructional-technicians to backward black children. *Behav Ther*, In press.

Staats, A. W., Minke, K. A., Finley, J. R., Wolf, M. M. and Brooks, L. O.: A reinforcer system and experimental procedure for the laboratory study of reading acquisition. *Child Dev 35*, 209-231, 1964b.

Staats, A. W., Minke, K. A., Goodwin, W. and Landen, J.: Cognitive behavior modification: 'motivated learning' reading treatment with subprofessional therapy technicians. *Behav Res & Therapy 5*, 283-299, 1967a.

Staats, A. W., Staats, C. K., Schutz, R. E. and Wolf, M. M.: The conditioning of reading responses utilizing 'extrinsic' reinforcers. *J Exp Anal Behav 5*, 33-40, 1962.

Staats, A. W., Van Mondfrans, A. P. and Minke, K. A.: *Manual of administration and recording methods for the Staats 'Motivated Learning' Read-*

ing Procedure. Wisconsin Research and Development Center for Cognitive Learning, Madison, 1967b.

Straughn, J. H.: Treatment with child and mother in the playroom. *Behav Res & Therapy 2,* 37-41, 1964.

Thorndike, E. L. and Lorge, I.: *The Teacher's Word Book of 30,000 Words.* Columbia University, New York, 1944.

Wahler, R. G., Winkel, G. H., Peterson, R. F. and Morrison, D. C.: Mothers as behavior therapists for their own children. *Behav Res & Therapy 3,* 113-124, 1965.

Walder, L. O.: Teaching parents to modify the behaviors of their autistic children. Paper presented at the meeting of the American Psychological Association, 1966.

Wetzel, R. J., Baker, J., Roney, M. and Martin, M.: Out-patient treatment of autistic behavior. *Behav Res & Therapy 4,* 169-177, 1966.

Wolf, M. M., Giles, D. K. and Hall, V. R.: Experiments with token reinforcement in a remedial classroom. *Behav Res & Therapy 6,* 51-64, 1968.

Zeilberger, J., Sampen, S. E. and Sloane, H. N., Jr.: Modification of a child's problem behaviors in the home with the mother as therapist. *J Appl Behav Anal 1,* 47-53, 1968.

Chapter 4

OPERANT TREATMENT OF ASTHMATIC RESPONDING WITH THE PARENT AS THERAPIST*

JOHN T. NEISWORTH *and* FLORESE MOORE

A PPLYING EMPIRICALLY BASED principles and strategies, behavior therapies are increasingly promoting the feasibility and desirability of using the home as the setting and parents as the agents for child therapy. This is in contradistinction to traditional approaches that employ hypothetical models, clinical settings, and highly trained personnel.

A growing number of successful studies dealing with various child problems is demonstrating the economy of time and professional effort of behaviorally based therapies. Representative of such studies are those of Williams (1959), O'Leary, O'Leary and Becker (1967), and Zeilberger, Sampen, and Sloane (1968) dealing generally with parental treatment of disruptive or aggressive child behaviors. Lal and Lindsley (1968), and Conger (1970) provide examples of somatic problems responsive to therapy conducted by mothers. Results and descriptions of training groups of mothers as reinforcement therapists are reported by Lindsley (1966), and Hirsch (1968).

The problem of interest in this study, asthma, has received much attention from psychoanalytic perspectives but rarely has asthma been

*From *Behavior Therapy*, 1972, 3, pp. 95-99. Reprinted by permission of the Journal and the author.

conceived of as an operant (see review by Hirt, 1965). Turnbull (1962) has summarized previous research that views asthma as a learned response. Most of this research, however, has employed a respondent rather than operant paradigm. While asthma-like responses can be respondently conditioned, extinction rapidly occurs in the absence of UCS, and it is suggested that operant reinforcement could account for maintenance and amplification of respondently or organically produced asthmatic responses. While this study does not investigate the origin of asthmatic responses in a child, it does report successful treatment through operant procedures.

History and Diagnosis

The patient, a seven-year-old boy, was the oldest of two sons of American parents who resided in Japan until the patient was 18 months old. At the age of six months, the boy was diagnosed as asthmatic; he was frequently hospitalized for periods of 1-4 weeks. Doctors stated that his condition would probably improve upon the family's return to the United States. However, by the age of two the patient continued to display repeated asthmatic attacks (coughing, wheezing, abrupt inspiration) which required frequent visits to the hospital emergency room for immediate relief. From the ages of two to seven years, the boy was seen almost monthly by a specialist due to continued severity of the problem. Various medications were administered and dietary restrictions imposed in an effort to ameliorate the condition.

Results of the various medical attempts were questionable; the child still had frequent attacks and visits to hospital emergency rooms remained necessary.

By the time it was suggested that the child might be helped by behavior therapy, a pattern of parental concern and continued attention to the problem had been well established. Typically, the mother would caution the child not to overexert himself, not to eat certain foods, and to be sure to take his medicine. She described the child as "nervous" and reported that emotional upsets or excitement precipitated the child's attacks. Of particular concern were the child's prolonged wheezing and coughing at bedtime. Further investigation revealed that both medicine and sympathetic attention were given especially during the bedtime asthmatic episodes.

After exposure to operant conditioning rationale and treatment procedures, the mother herself suggested that the child's problem might well be conceived of in operant terms and treated accordingly. She analyzed her own behavior towards the child and suggested that it might be supporting or aggravating the problem. Specifically, it was hypothesized first, that asthmatic responding was being maintained or amplified by the presentation of verbal and tactile attention (as well as medicine) during or immediately after a seizure, and second, that behavior incompatible with coughing, wheezing, and generally "being sick" was not being reinforced. A schedule of differential reinforcement for being "sick" as opposed to being well seemed to be operating.

Intervention and Results

In addition to the case history, and prior to any systematic changes in the contingencies related to asthmatic behaviors, data were collected for 10 days to provide a baseline (Fig. 39). It was decided to record only nighttime in-bed responding since this was the occasion of most intense behavior; further, it was not possible to obtain accurate daytime data. Due to the nature of the responses and data collection restrictions, duration rather than frequency was chosen as the response measure. Coughing, wheezing, gasping, and similar responses lacking in discreteness and often overlapping in occurrence made frequency counts difficult. Response time, however, was relatively easy to record. All data were collected each evening in the home of the child by the junior author.

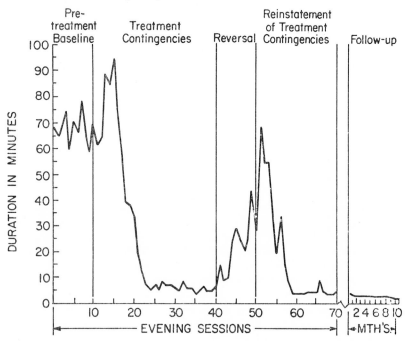

Figure 39. Duration of bedtime asthmatic responding as a function of contingency changes.

Immediately following the baseline phase, two systematic treatment strategies were initiated. First, based on the hypothesis that parental attention to the problem was reinforcing the behavior, an extinction procedure was employed. The parents agreed to discontinue all attention and administrations of medicines during bedtime asthmatic attacks. The child was put to bed with the usual affectionate interactions between parents and child. Once the bedroom door was closed, however, no further interaction occurred until morning.

Because extinction procedures often require extended use, it was decided to implement an additional strategy; REINFORCEMENT OF INCOMPATIBLE BEHAVIOR. Specifically, the child was told he could have lunch money (instead of taking his lunch to school) if he coughed less frequently on a given night than the night before. This contingency permitted reinforcement for even slight improvements in the behavior, making reinforcement highly probable and progress easy.

It can be seen from Fig. 39 that the initial effect of the intervention program was to increase the duration of coughing and wheezing. (We have frequently found this initial inflation of behavior on an extinction schedule). However, after seven days the effects of treatment became noticeable; by Day 23 the behavior reached a low that remained somewhat stable.

To provide further evidence of the efficacy of the treatment contingencies, the parents reluctantly agreed to reversal procedures. Specifically, attention and medication again were given during the brief asthmatic episodes. (Lunch money, however, was not withdrawn, i.e., the child received money on a noncontingent basis.) As Fig. 39 shows, response duration increased quickly and climbed towards baseline intensity. At this point, the parents urged a return to the treatment contingencies. This was done, resulting again in an initial increase in response duration followed by a drop to a stable new low of about 5 min. As a follow-up, the parents periodically were requested to time bedtime coughing. This reminded the parents of the need to continue the new contingency arrangements and provided follow-up data. During 11 months of such follow-up inquiries and data, the problem remained at essentially the treatment low (between two-seven minutes).

Discussion

The systematic management of two simple contingencies resulted in a drastic reduction in the duration of nighttime asthmatic responding in a seven-year-old boy. Withholding of attention during coughing and wheezing and "payment" for reduction of such responding successfully and quickly effected changes that years of medical treatment alone could not. Reinstatement of the original cough-attention contingency relationship produced a return to prolonged asthmatic episodes. Minimal responding was again established upon restoration of treatment contingencies. An 11-month follow-up failed to reveal any appreciable increment in the child's nighttime asthmatic attacks. Indeed, the parents reported that daytime coughing also sharply declined and pediatrician's reports indicated a general improvement in health. This study, which adds to the growing literature that stresses the crucial role of "therapy" conducted by parents, does not purport to obviate "organic" factors in the etiology or maintenance of asthmatic responses. Rather, it pinpoints the dramatic role that environmental contingencies may have in the amplification and attenuation of the problem.

References

Conger, J. C.: The treatment of encopresis by the management of social consequences. *Behav Therapy 1*, 386-390, 1970.

Hirt, M. L.: *Psychological and allergic aspects of asthma*. Springfield, Thomas, 1965.

Hirsch, I. S.: Training mothers in groups as reinforcement therapists for their own children. *Dissertation Abstracts 28*, (11-B), 4-156, 1968.

Lal, H. & Lindsley, O. R.: Therapy of chronic constipation in a young child by rearranging social contingencies. *Behav Res Therapy 6*, 484-485, 1968.

Lindsley, O. R.: Parents handling behavior at home. *Johnstone Bulletin 9*, 27-36, 1966.

O'Leary, K. D., O'Leary, S., and Becker, W. C.: Modification of a deviant sibling interaction pattern in the home. *Behav Res Therapy 5*, 113-120, 1967.

Turnbull, J. W.: Asthma conceived as a learned response. *J Psychomatic Res 6*, 59-70, 1962.

Williams, C. D.: The elimination of tantrum behavior by extinction procedures. *J Abnorm Soc Psychol 59*, 269, 1959.

Zeilberger, J., Sampen, S. and Sloane, H. N.: Modification of a child's problem behaviors in the home with the mother as therapist. *J Appl Behav Anal 1*, 47-53, 1968.

Chapter 5

OPERANT-INTERPERSONAL TREATMENT FOR MARITAL DISCORD*

RICHARD B. STUART

THE OPERANT-INTERPERSONAL APPROACH to marital treatment rests on three assumptions concerning the character of marital interaction. First, it is assumed that the exact pattern of interaction which takes place between spouses at any point in time is the most rewarding of all of the available alternatives. This implies that the interaction between spouses is never accidental; it represents the best balance which each can achieve between individual and mutual rewards and costs (Thibaut & Kelley, 1959, p. 12). Thus when a husband consistently fails to leave his friends in order to spend time with his wife, it may be concluded that his friends offer greater relative rewards than his wife.

The second assumption is that while the specifics may vary for each couple, most married adults expect to enjoy reciprocal relations with their partners. Reciprocity has the general sociological connotation that "each party has rights and duties [Gouldner, 1960, p. 169]" and the specific behavioral connotation that each party to an interaction should dispense social reinforcement at an equitable rate (Patterson & Reid, 1967, p. 1). In effect, a quid pro quo or "something for something" arrangement underlies suc-

*From the *Journal of Consulting and Clinical Psychology*, 1969, 33, pp. 675-682. Reprinted by permission of the author and the American Psychological Association.

cessful marriage (Jackson, 1965, p. 591). The exchange of rewards in marriage may be viewed as a quasi-legal contract affording distinct safeguards to each partner. Whenever one partner to a reciprocal interaction unilaterally rewards the other, he does so with the confidence that he will be compensated in kind in the future. For example, if the husband agrees to entertain his wife's parents for a weekend, he does so with the expectation that his wife will accompany him on a weekend fishing trip at some time in the future.

Reciprocity develops as a consequence of a history of POSITIVE REINFORCEMENT. There is extensive empirical support for the proposition that ego will be more attracted to alter and will reinforce alter more if he has been positively reinforced by alter (Bachrach, Candland, & Gibson, 1961; Brewer & Brewer, 1968; Byrne, 1961, 1962; Byrne & Nelson, 1965; Homans, 1961; Komorita, Sheposh, & Braver, 1968; Newcomb, 1955; Pruitt, 1968).[3] When disordered marriages are evaluated in light of this reinforcement-attraction hypothesis, it is seen that each partner reinforces the other at a low rate and each is therefore relatively unattractive to and unreinforced by the other.

TABLE XXII

[3]Byrne and Rhamey (1965) have postulated a law of attraction magnitude which takes the following form:

$$A_x = m \left(\frac{\Sigma (PR_x \times M)}{\Sigma (PR_x \times M) + \Sigma (NR_x \times M)} \right) + k,$$

. . . [where] X is a positive linear function of the sum of the weighted positive reinforcements (Number × Magnitude) received from X divided by the total number of weighted positive and negative reinforcements received from X [p. 887].

The third assumption is that in order to modify an unsuccessful marital interaction, it is essential to develop the power of each partner to mediate rewards for the other. In support of this assumption, it can be shown that individuals will be more positively attracted to each other when each has been successful in influencing the other to comply with his wishes (Thibaut & Kelley, 1959, p. 124; Thibaut & Riecken, 1955). Conversely, it can be shown that when one party to an interaction fails in his influence attempts, he becomes "SOCIALLY BANKRUPT" (Longabaugh, Eldred,

Bell, & Sherman, 1966, p. 87) as he lacks the resources needed to control the other's behavior; failing to gain control through positive strategies, he resorts to negative means of control.

In successful marriage, both partners work to maximize mutual reward while minimizing individual costs. A reciprocal exchange of potent social reinforcement is established in which each partner controls sufficient rewards to compensate the other for the rewards which are expected or received from him. In an unsuccessful marriage, both partners appear to work to minimize individual costs with little apparent expectation of mutual reward. In an effort to trim costs, few positive rewards are dispensed; positive reinforcement, as a strategy of behavioral control, is replaced by negative reinforcement (removal of an aversive event following the expected response).

Either or both of two broad patterns of behavioral control, coercion and withdrawal, are likely to emerge in unsuccessful marriages. In COERCION, one member seeks to gain positive reinforcement from the other in exchange for negative reinforcement (Patterson & Reid, 1967). As an example, a husband might wish his wife to express greater affection; following the failure of his amorous advances, he might become abusive, accusing his wife of anything from indifference to frigidity, abating his criticism when he receives the desired affection. The three flaws in this approach are: first, to the extent that he makes himself unpleasant, he is less likely to receive affection; second, to the extent that he is abusive or accusing, he debases his wife's affection and simultaneously reduces its reinforcing properties for himself; and third, to the extent that her affection is offered in compliance to his demand, it will appear to be appeasement rather than a gesture of genuine affection (Haley, 1963, 1967).

The withdrawal which is likely to occur in unsuccessful marriages is analogous to one of several strategies available in a prisoner's dilemma game:

> If the structure of the situation is such that (*a*) the reward is small, (*b*) terminating the interaction is made difficult, and (*c*) the retaliatory response must take a form which is identical to the disliked other's harmful behavior, then cognitive consistency principles would lead one to expect an increase in ill will, but no retaliatory behavior [Swingle, 1966, p. 270].

Retalitory behavior might require the husband to match his wife's actions; but to the extent that he devalues his wife for so behaving, consistency would demand that he behave otherwise. Withdrawal has the advantage of denying satisfaction to his wife while at the same time creating a situation requiring her to continue to behave assertively. Thus it is a low-risk tactic of control. The reinforcement for approach behavior on the wife's part would be termination of the husband's withdrawal. At the same time that the husband is withdrawn from his wife, however, he may also find other social and nonsocial reinforcers in his cronies, mistress, or can of beer.

Based on this formulation, the operant-interpersonal approach seeks to construct a situation in which the frequency and intensity of mutual positive reinforcement is increased. The effect of positive reinforcement in inducing positively "biased SCANNING [Janis & Gilmore, 1965]," or searching for assets rather than liabilities in the spouse, has been well demonstrated, particularly when the positive reinforcement is large and is offered under positive sponsorship (Elms & Janis, 1965, p. 53). It is anticipated that this positive scanning will replace negatively biased attitudes, making positive responding more likely. Positive responses, in turn, are intended to augment the range and importance of social reinforcement mediated by each spouse for the other, leading to reestablishment of successful interaction patterns.

Treatment Considerations

Operant-interpersonal treatment occurs in four orderly steps. The first step requires training the couple in the logic of the approach, consisting of two self-evident premises. The first premise is that the impressions which each spouse forms of the other is based on the behavior of the other. Accordingly, when one changes his behavior, there are corresponding changes in the other's impressions and expectations of him. Spouses who lose sight of this typically attribute marital difficulty to the personality of the other. For example, the wife who believes that her husband "is passive" implicitly suggests that her husband's personality must change before the marital disturbance can be overcome. Conversely, the wife who believes that her husband "behaves passively" need only find ways to modify her behavior (as she is in control of his actions) in order to modify his problematic responses.

This leads to the second premise, which asserts that in order to change interaction in a marriage, each partner must assume initiative in changing his own behavior before changes can be expected in his spouse. The typical couple is "locked into" problematic patterns of interaction as long as each requires a change in the other prior to changing his own behavior. If coercion and withdrawal are in fact basic problematic processes in discordant marriages, then spontaneous behavior change is highly unlikely to occur, as the response cost is too great and the potential reward too small.

Clients benefit from an explanation of the logic of the approach for at least two reasons. First, such explanations may help to free each spouse from his inaccurate and negatively biasing prejudices. Second, when each spouse is fully aware of the logic of the treatment, he can participate more fully in effective therapeutic planning and execution (Stuart, 1967).

The second step in treatment consists of asking each spouse to list the three behaviors which he would most like to accelerate in the other. This task is often subject to four difficulties. First, couples tend to begin by listing requests for decelerating negative behaviors, which may be expected in view of the fact that much of their interaction prior to seeking treatment has been negative. The difficulty with attempting to decelerate behavior is that its attainment would require the use of aversive stimuli or extinction paradigms, and the typical unhappy couple is already disproportionately committed to these negative strategies. Second, each spouse is likely to phrase his "three wishes" in molar rather than molecular units, and many of these are likely to be formulated in preverbal terms. For example, a husband is likely to list the request that his wife "act more feminine." "Feminine" is a modifier which is subject to varied interpretation and which may modify a wide range of behaviors. These molar requests must be reduced to specifics which include description of the desired behavior, its rate, and the context in which it is expected to occur. Third, each spouse is likely to proclaim that the other should "know what I want—if I have to tell him, then he is not as sensitive to me as he should be." Many unhappily married couples share the naïve expectation that their spouse should be clairvoyant, and it is therefore often necessary to stress the need that each must communicate his wishes to the other in order to increase the probability that they will be gratified. The fourth obstacle in this apparently simple listing of behavior change objectives is concerned with the punctuation of the behavioral chains. It has been observed that each spouse is likely to describe each unit of his own behavior as sandwiched between two negative actions on the part of his spouse (Watzlawick, Beavin, & Jackson, 1967, pp. 54-59). These three element CHAINS (other-negative, self-positive, other-negative) obscure the true interaction, as the speaker omits reference to his stimulation of the other's initial negative actions.

The third step in the treatment calls for transcription of the three wishes of each as headings on a Behavior Checklist which is posted at some convenient point in the house. Each spouse is asked to record the frequency with which the other performs the act which he desires. While monitoring undoubtedly influences the rate of occurrence of each set of responses, this exercise does provide a crude base line against which to evaluate change.

The fourth step consists of working out a series of exchanges of desired behaviors. The typical couple complains of a "lack of communication," which is a euphemism for a failure to reinforce each other. On closer analysis, this complaint is frequently seen as a reference to low-rate conversational and sexual behavior. This communication gap is overcome in the fourth step by arranging for each partner to compensate the other for the behaviors which he identified as socially reinforcing to him.

In marriages which have not dissolved reciprocity into coercion or withdrawal, a simple exchange of behaviors is effective. Couples are asked to accelerate desired behaviors on an equal basis. For example, one husband complained that his wife failed to greet him at the door, that she did not straighten the family room in anticipation of his return home from work, and that meals were rarely ready on time. His wife complained that he failed to spend sufficient time with the children (it was agreed that 30 minutes before bed was sufficient), failed to take her out for an occasional movie, and failed to pay attention to meals when they were well prepared. Accordingly, each of these behaviors was restated as a positive (e.g., greet husband at door) and was listed on the Behavior Monitoring Form. Each person recorded the frequency with which the other completed the desired behavior. When these behaviors were accelerated at a sufficient rate, other goals were added.

In marriages in which reciprocity appears to be essentially absent, a TOKEN ECONOMY has proven successful. Where reciprocity fails, couples tend not to trust each other. It is therefore important to arrange for some immediate form of reinforcement. Tokens are an ideal media for such reinforcement because (*a*) they are given immediately, (*b*) they can be redeemed for the specific consequences which the recipient deems desirable at that point in time, (*c*) they are concrete and unambiguous, (*d*) the giving and receiving of tokens is customarily associated with positive social interchange, and (*e*) they permit an exchange of behaviors which are not contiguous. Token systems have been used effectively in a wide range of settings (e.g., mental hospitals—Atthowe & Krasner, 1968; classrooms—Clark, Lachowicz, & Wolf, 1968; and institutions for delinquents—Tyler & Brown, 1967), and extension of this technique to marital treatment appears warranted.

Illustration and Results

Four couples have used the token system to modify each other's behavior. Individuals ranged in age from 24 to 52 and in education from high school diploma to doctorate. The couples were married for from three to 23 years and had a maximum of two children. Each of the couples sought treatment as a last-ditch effort prior to obtaining a divorce. In each instance, the wife listed as her first wish that her husband converse with her more fully, or at least that he not "close me out of his life even when he is at home." Considerable discussion was often necessary to identify what intensity level of conversation was positively reinforcing to the wife, and this was made clear and rehearsed during the treatment sessions. The wife was then instructed to purchase a kitchen timer which she could carry with her about the house. She was instructed to set the timer as soon as her husband entered and to give him one token when the bell rang after each hour in which he conversed at the criterion level. If he failed to behave at the criterion level by the end of the first 30 minutes of each hour, she had to notify him of this and offer constructive suggestions, cueing him as to how his performance could be improved upon. If she failed to do this, he had to be given a token even if he failed to perform adequately. If he so requested, at the half-hour cue time, the timer could be reset so that he could earn a token during the next hour (so that he waited 60 rather than 90 minutes before being rewarded).

The criterion level for conversation is naturally a negotiable factor. No one could be expected to talk to his wife constantly; if for no other reason, his children would not allow it. Therefore, conversational tokens can be earned for a wider range of responses ranging from intense conversation at one extreme to the wife's feeling free to interrupt her husband with a question at agreed intervals at the other extreme.

While tokens may have some intrinsic reinforcing properties in their own right (in addition to being associated with positive social

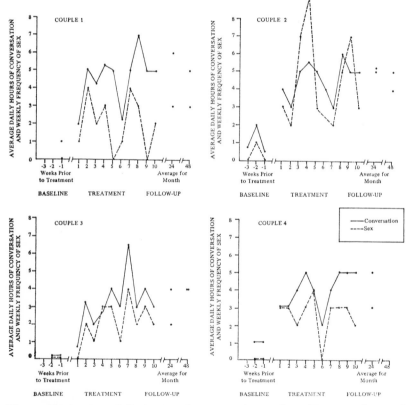

Figure 40. Average daily hours of conversation and weekly rate of sex of our couples—before, during, and after operant marital therapy.

responses when they are offered), they become more powerful when they function as contingencies for some other event. With the four couples cited, tokens were redeemable at the husband's request from a menu stressing physical affection. A different menu was constructed for each couple which took into account the baseline level of sexual activity, the desired level of sexual activity, and the number of hours available for nonsexual (in this instance conversational) interchange. Each of these couples had sex less than once per week (ranging from once in the year prior to treatment to once in the week prior to treatment), each desired sex an average of three times per week, and each had approximately five hours together on weeknights and 14 hours on weekends, making a total of approximately 52-54 hours per week. Accordingly, husbands were charged three tokens for kissing and "lightly petting" with their wives, five tokens for "heavy petting," and 15 tokens for intercourse. (These behaviors were not rehearsed during treatment sessions).

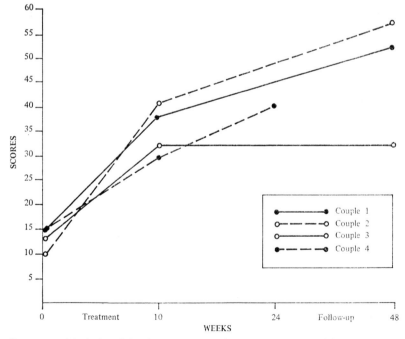

Figure 41. Marital satisfaction assessment inventory scores of four couples--before, at last session, and at follow-up of operant marital treatment.

Tokens earned and spent were recorded on the Behavior Checklist, which also provided data for continued graphing of interactional behavior. The performance of each of these couples is represented in Figure 40, where it will be seen that the rates of conversation and sex increased sharply after the start of treatment and continued through 24- and 48-week follow-up periods.

At the start of treatment, at the conclusion of regularly scheduled interviews, and at the time of follow-up, each spouse was asked to complete a brief inventory measuring the extent of his own and his perception of his spouse's satisfaction in and commitment to the marriage. This inventory was adapted from the work of Farber (1957). The results are depicted in Figure 41 where it can be seen that the rate of reported satisfaction increased in association with the reported behavioral changes. These changes enabled the couples to become more similar to nonclinic families on this dimension (Levinger & Breedlove, 1966, p. 369).

With each of these couples, all therapeutic sessions were held jointly. Sessions were held during the first four, the sixth, eighth, and tenth weeks, for a total of seven sessions. When it is considered that these couples were each on the brink of filing for divorce, this could be considered relatively inexpensive treatment. Follow-up contacts were held by phone or by mail, and all data, including that collected during sessions, were based on self-report.

Discussion

The therapeutic recommendations of alternative courses of behavior are consistent with Goldiamond's (1966, p. 118) recommendation to his patients that: "If he wished his wife to behave differently to him, then he should provide other stimuli than the ones which produced the behaviors he did not like." Each spouse was directed in specific modifications of his own behavior in an effort to modify the behavioral environment in which his partner's behavior occurred. The antecedents for changed behavior were probably twofold: therapeutic recommendations exercised some discriminant stimulus control as did the expectation of changes in the behavior of the spouse. The therapist suggested that each party engage in behaviors which had doubtless been requested, cajoled, and demanded by each party countless times before. As therapeutic directives, these new requests were differentiated from the old in two important respects. First, they were clarified. Second, they were removed from the context of coercive demands in which granting the request would have been tantamount to reinforcing dysfunctional patterns of negative reinforcement. In addition, the treatment was characterized to each couple as a "game" in which each would be able to modify the general rules of the relationship so that positive rather than negative strategies would pay off.

It is impossible to isolate which aspects of this complex treatment approach carry the weight of the observed change. Behavioral rehearsal and the manipulation of social reinforcers were the objectively identified variables but other observers would undoubtedly stress other factors as well. One technical point of particular importance is the fact that at no time was an attempt made to "FADE" (or slowly remove) the behavior modification system, replacing it with more natural processes of behavioral control (Krasner, 1965, 1966). Indeed, continued reliance on the therapeutic techniques as a means of programming and evaluating each other's behavior could result in considerable gain with low cost. In fact, one characteristic of an ideal therapeutic technique might be that it is transferable to the natural environment without change.

This pattern of treatment is likely to be challenged on two counts. Some critics will charge that the therapeutic strategies of this approach are "trivial" because they are based on "superficial" changes in behavior. Two counterarguments should be stressed. First, the only data which are available to the therapist as a scientist are observable behaviors, and it is at the level of behavior that changes must be sought (Skinner, 1953). Second, it must be stressed that these were the changes sought by the clients and were therefore in accord with the therapeutic contract. To have sought other goals would have meant ignoring the presenting complaints.

In response to the triviality argument, it is also relevant to cite the data concerning the level of marital satisfaction. However, these must be considered to be "soft data" as they are based on global self-ratings such as "How committed are you to stay in this marriage?" and "What proportion of time spent with your spouse would you consider to be 'fully satisfying'?" It is impossible to determine exactly what degree of meaningfulness can be attributed to answers to such questions and they should, at best, be interpreted as indications of trend.

References

Atthowe, J. M., Jr. and Krasner, L.: Preliminary report on the application of contingent reinforcement procedures (token economy) on a "chronic" psychiatric ward. *J Abnorm Psychol 73*, 37-43, 1968.

Bachrach, A. J., Candland, D. K. and Gibson, J. T.: Group reinforcement of individual response experiments in verbal behavior. In I. A. Berg and B. M. Bass (Eds.), *Conformity and deviation*. New York: Harper, 1961.

Brewer, R. E. and Brewer, M. B.: Attraction and accuracy of perception in dyads. *J Pers Soc Psychol 8*, 188-193, 1968.

Byrne, D.: Interpersonal attraction and attitude similarity. *J Abnorm Soc Psychol 62*, 713-715, 1961.

Byrne, D.: Response to attitude similarity-dissimilarity as a function of affiliation need. *J Pers 30*, 164-177, 1962.

Byrne, D. and Nelson, D.: Attraction as a linear function of proportion of positive reinforcements. *J Pers Soc Psychol 1*, 659-663, 1965.

Byrne, D. and Rhamey, R.: Magnitude of positive and negative reinforcements as a determinant of attraction. *J Pers Soc Psychol 2*, 884-889, 1965.

Clark, M., Lachowicz, J. and Wolf, M.: A pilot basic education program for school dropouts incorporating a token reinforcement system. *Behav Res Therapy 6*, 183, 1968.

Elms, A. C. and Janis, I. L.: Counter-norm attitudes induced by consonant versus dissonant conditions of role-playing. *J Exper Res Pers 1*, 50-60, 1965.

Farber, B.: An index of marital integration. *Sociometry 20*, 117-134, 1957.

Goldiamond, I.: Self-control procedures in personal behavior problems. In R. Ulrich, T. Stachnik, and J. Mabry (Eds.), *Control of human behavior*. Chicago: Scott, Foresman, 1966.

Gouldner, A. W.: The norm of reciprocity: A preliminary statement. *Am Soc Rev 25*, 161-178, 1960.

Haley, J.: *Strategies of psychotherapy*. New York: Grune & Stratton, 1963.

Haley, J.: Marriage therapy. In H. Greenwald (Ed.), *Active psychotherapy*. New York: Atherton Press, 1967.

Homans, G. C.: *Social behavior: Its elementary forms*. New York: Harcourt, Brace & World, 1961.

Jackson, D. D.: Family rules. *Archives of General Psychiatry 12*, 589-594, 1965.

Janis, I. and Gilmore, J.: The influence of incentive conditions on the success of role playing in modifying attitudes. *J Pers Soc Psychol 1*, 17-27, 1965.

Komorita, S. S., Sheposh, J. P. and Braver, S. L.: Po :r. th :e c' wer, and cooperative choice in a two-person game. *J Pers Soc Psychol 8*, 134-142, 1968.

Krasner, L.: Operant conditioning techniques with adults from the laboratory to "real life" behavior modification. Paper presented at the meeting of the American Psychological Association, Chicago, September 1965.

Krasner, L.: The translation of operant conditioning procedures from the experimental laboratory to the psychotherapeutic interaction. Paper presented at the meeting of the American Psychological Association, New York, September 1966.

Levinger, G. and Breedlove, J.: Interpersonal attraction and agreement: A study of marriage partners. *J Pers Soc Psychol 3*, 367-372, 1966.

Longabaugh, R., Eldred, S. H., Bell, N. W. and Sherman, L. J.: The interactional world of the chronic schizophrenic patient. *Psychiatry 29*, 78-99, 1966.

Newcomb, T. M.: *Social psychology.* New York: Holt, Rinehart & Winston, 1955.

Patterson, G. R. and Reid, J.: Reciprocity and coercion: Two facets of social systems. Paper presented at the meeting of the Institute for Research in Clinical Psychology, Lawrence, Kansas, April 1967.

Pruitt, D. G.: Reciprocity and credit building in a laboratory dyad. *J Pers Soc Psychol 8*, 143-147, 1968.

Skinner, B. F.: *Science and human behavior.* New York, Macmillan, 1953.

Stuart, R. B.: *Guide to behavior modification.* Unpublished manuscript, University of Michigan, 1967.

Swingle, P. G.: Effects of the emotional relationship between protagonists in a two-person game. *J Pers Soc Psychol 4*, 270-279, 1966.

Thibaut, J. W. and Kelley, H. H.: *The social psychology of groups.* New York, Wiley, 1959.

Thibaut, J. W. and Riecken, H. W.: Some determinants and consequences of the perception of social causality. *J Pers 24*, 113-133, 1955.

Tyler, V. O., Jr. and Brown, G. D.: Token reinforcement of academic performance with institutionalized delinquent boys. Paper presented at the meeting of the Western Psychological Association, San Francisco, May, 1967.

Watzlawick, P., Beavin, J. H. and Jackson, D. D.: *Pragmatics of human communication: A study of interactional patterns, pathologies and paradoxes.* New York, Norton, 1967.

Section VII

BEHAVIOR THERAPY WITH THE SEVERELY DISTURBED CHILD

SECTION VII FOCUSES ON CHILDHOOD SCHIZOPHRENIA AND AUTISM, TWO PARTICULARLY VEXING PROBLEMS FOR CHILD CLINICAL PROFESSIONALS. REAMS HAVE BEEN WRITTEN REGARDING THE NATURE OF THESE DISORDERS AND REGARDING PROPER TREATMENT FOR THESE PATHETIC EXAMPLES OF THE HUMAN CONDITION, BUT PROGRESS HAS BEEN MINIMAL. HOWEVER, IN THE RECENT PAST, BEHAVIOR THERAPY HAS MADE CONTROVERSIAL BUT IMPORTANT ADVANCES IN BOTH THE CONCEPTUALIZATION OF AND TREATMENT OF THESE CHILDREN. OUR FOUR OFFERINGS REPRESENT A SAMPLING OF RELATIVELY RECENT WORK IN THIS MOST IMPORTANT AREA.

Chapter 1

A BEHAVIORAL STRATEGY FOR LANGUAGE TRAINING OF A CHILD WITH AUTISTIC BEHAVIORS*

STEPHEN I. SULZBACHER *and* JANIS M. COSTELLO

T HE CASE OF TEDDY illustrates the strategy of the experimental analysis of behavior in treating the communication deficits of a child with autistic behaviors. The speech clinician coordinated the efforts of parents, teacher, and psychologist to generate and maintain appropriate behavior of the child in various settings. Consistently applying the same procedures to the child's behavior at school, at home, and in the clinic is of critical importance in maintaining and generalizing newly acquired vocal responses and nonvocal behavior to all areas in the child's environment (Lovaas, 1968).

The experimental analysis of behavior (Skinner, 1938, 1957), sometimes called operant conditioning or behavior modification, is characterized by an emphasis on objective definition and quantification of the behaviors selected as targets for precisely programmed and recorded procedures (Ayllon and Azrin, 1968). Holland (1967) and Brookshire (1967) present some of the basic behavioral principles; individual techniques for a variety of problems are described by Kerr, Myerson, and Michael (1965), Lovaas, Berberich, Perloff, and

*From the *Journal of Speech and Hearing Disorders*, 1970, 35, pp. 256-276. Reprinted by permission of the author and the Journal.

Schaeffer (1966), Baer, Peterson, and Sherman (1967), Risley and Wolf (1967), Schell, Stark, and Giddan (1967), Stark, Giddan, and Meisel (1968), and Hingtgen and Churchill (1969). In their recent monograph, Girardeau and Spradlin (1970) bring together a number of studies to provide a systematic framework within which the clinician may analyze and develop explicit speech and language procedures.

Case History

Teddy was born after a full-term pregnancy and his birth history was essentially normal. His acquisition of gross motor skills followed a somewhat delayed pattern, and medical reports, when Teddy was six, listed several "soft" signs of neurological dysfunction. Multidisciplinary evaluations between ages four and five indicated a poor prognosis with diagnoses of mental retardation, infantile autism, organic brain damage, emotional disturbance, and arrested hydrocephalus. Reports consistently described bizarre and stereotyped behavior, and special skills of the "idiot savant" type in relation to reading and spelling. Teddy's younger brother and sister are both normal. With regard to speech development, the mother reported that Teddy talked at the age of six months and began demonstrating peculiar reading and spelling skills before his fourth birthday. These skills included reading and spelling words that appeared on television, which Teddy spent a great deal of time watching.

Although a psychologist and an audiologist found Teddy untestable at the age of four, he was recommended for diagnostic therapy in a delayed language group. After several months this therapy was discontinued when he failed to interact with peers or clinicians, cried, and spent much of the time gesturing to himself in front of a mirror. The only speech noted during these sessions was "g'bye," "bye-bye," and "bridge."

A year later, as Teddy was approaching his sixth birthday, he was seen for individual speech and language instruction at a clinic in another city. Again, attempts at formal testing were not successful. This clinician described Teddy's speech pattern as "indiscriminate whining and jargon," poor articulatory movements, and inability to imitate isolated consonant and vowel sounds. Receptive and expressive language skills were described as "very primitive." It was noted that he demonstrated his unusual ability to read written symbols and numbers, although he could not demonstrate any association of meaning to them.

A psychological reevaluation shortly before the beginning of the present program suggested a pattern of behavior "somewhat similar to that seen two years earlier, although . . . more responsive to the environment . . . unresponsive to verbal stimuli from other people." An increase in echoic behavior and hyperactivity was noted. At this time it was discovered that he had a bilateral conductive hearing loss of 30 dB, re: ASA, but no remedial action was taken.

Diagnostic and Baseline Procedures

Teddy was six years, five months old at the beginning of the program. Pre-treatment probes of Teddy's behavior included the Peabody Picture Vocabulary Test, Leiter International Performance Scale, Templin-Darley Articulation Test administered imitatively, and video tapes of his performance with adults and other children on an informal series of social, preschool, and language tasks.

However, major emphasis in diagnosis, as well as during treatment, was on the continuous measurement of changes in objectively defined target behaviors. A behavior is objectively defined when its frequency of occurrence can be counted or when its presence or absence is evident to any observer. A TARGET BEHAVIOR is a specific response or set of responses that is selected for change. Some target behaviors occur in excess (for example, jargon) and the goal of treatment is deceleration of frequency of occurrence. A second kind of target behavior is one that does not occur often enough or at all (for example, speaking in complete sentences) and the goal is acceleration or increase of occurrences of the behavior. During clinic sessions, observers made continuous measurement of changes in target behaviors; video tapes of five sessions at regular intervals confirmed the relative accuracy of data kept by the clinician. Similarly, the mother and teacher kept records of the effects of treatment variables in the home and school. These records formed the basis for changes in treatment procedures and for decisions to begin treatment of new target behaviors.

On the basis of the case history and presenting complaints, three overall, long-range goals for Teddy's treatment were formulated: (1) deceleration of certain undesired vocal and nonvocal behaviors; (2) acquisition of the language and social skills required for success in school; and (3) generalization of these skills to Teddy's environment away from the clinic.

Prelanguage Target Behaviors

Teddy's treatment will be presented in chronological order. During the first five months of treatment, Teddy was scheduled for 20-minute sessions, five times a week. He was brought to the speech clinic in a state of mild food deprivation (about seven hours). It was necessary to establish reliable control over Teddy's vocal and nonvocal behavior before actual speech or expressive language training could be effective. Two target behaviors were specified as the initial goals of therapy: (1) to teach Teddy to look at the clinician (eye contact) in response to vocal requests and (2) to decelerate behaviors inappropriate to learning—jargon, leaving his chair, and making faces and gestures.

Teaching Eye Contact. Before this tactic was initiated, Teddy had a rate of looking at people which was near zero. He would even hold his hands up to the side of his head like blinders to avoid eye contact while walking down the hall with someone. The procedures instituted during the initial sessions with Teddy were limited to establishing reliable responding to the command "Teddy, look at me." This stimulus was presented approximately 20 times during each 20-minute session; if Teddy responded within five seconds, the clinician said, "Good!" or, "Good boy, Teddy!" and immediately gave him a piece of candy.

Although Teddy never responded to the request during the first two sessions, the curve of Figure 42 shows rapid rise of correct response during sessions three-eight, followed by considerable variation as it slowly approaches 100 per cent. It is reasonable to assume that at least some of the variability can be attributed to the addition of new procedures in later sessions. New procedures were always introduced at the beginning of a session so that these presumably more difficult tasks preceded the familiar, presumably more reinforcing, tasks during any given session. This ordering is an application of the PREMACK PRINCIPLE (Homme, et al., 1963; Premack, 1959), which states that performance on a nonpreferred task can be enhanced by programming the opportunity to perform a more preferred task immediately after the successful completion of the first task.

Activities during the initial sessions consisted mainly of blocks,

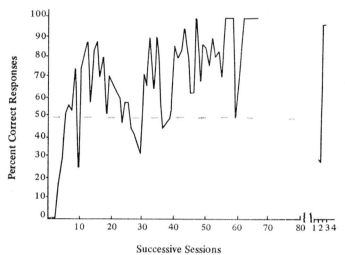

Figure 42. Percentage of correct responses to the command "Teddy, look at me."

puzzles, and other manual tasks. An observer recorded the frequency of Teddy's looking at the clinician without the clinician requesting him to do so. The data presented in Figure 43 show that this behavior occurred only after the fourth session. Until the twenty-first session all of these spontaneous glances were

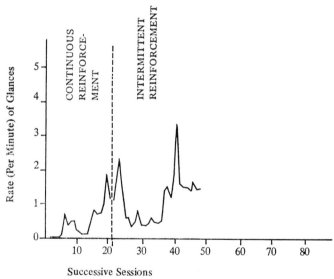

Figure 43. Teddy's average rate of spontaneously glancing at the clinican.

reinforced with verbal praise and candy. After the twenty-first session, candy was dispensed irregularly for both spontaneous and requested glances.

As part of GENERALIZATION of treatment from clinic to home, Teddy's mother was asked to record his eye contact at home. Her data indicated spontaneous glances occurred at home at a frequency greater than 90 per day. These data were obtained with the intent of being used as a baseline against which to evaluate the effects of generalization procedures for eye contact at home. Since the data indicated a high baseline frequency, it was unnecessary to institute any specific procedures in this instance.

Decelerating Inappropriate Behaviors. Figure 44 shows the total number of minutes per 20-minute session that the observer noted Teddy to be behaving inappropriately. In this case, inappropriate behavior was defined as (1) speaking jargon; (2) not staying in his chair during therapy; or (3) looking in, or making faces in, the one-way mirror occupying a sizeable portion of one wall of the therapy room. These behaviors were labeled as a single target because they formed a class incompatible with the terminal behaviors pinpointed for speech and language training. For the first 50 sessions a TIME-OUT procedure was used to decelerate these behaviors. Whenever the clinician observed Teddy engaging in any one of these behaviors, she would remove the materials being used, turn her face toward the floor, and remain motionless until Teddy was no longer emitting the inappropriate behavior, thus putting him on time-out from positive reinforcement. Since the inappropriate behavior persisted, on the fifty-first session, "No!" and "Sh!" were introduced as consequences of the inappropriate behaviors in an alternative attempt to further decelerate them. By comparison with the baseline of the initial 50 sessions, the data show the latter consequences were effective.

It should be noted at this point that the data in Figures 42, 43 and 44 were collected concurrently and the same numbers refer to the same successive sessions in each of these figures. Strictly speaking, the effects of these procedures have not been demonstrated independently of each other. However, it can be said that the overall goal of decelerating Teddy's undesired behavior and accelerating his visual attending to the clinician was achieved after the combined application of these procedures.

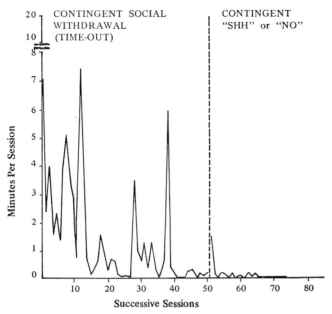

Figure 44. Total time per 20-minute session spent in inappropriate behavior (jargon, out of seat, or looking in mirror).

Teaching Expressive Language

A program was designed to teach Teddy specific language skills which educators as well as speech clinicians, consider important. Three language skills commonly required in kindergarten and first grade, as well as on psychological tests, are color, picture, and object naming. It is crucial that language training of the preschool child be coordinated with the objectives of the local school if successful generalization of the child's behavior to that environment is to be achieved.

Naming Colors, Pictures, and Objects. On initial trials many cues were provided to reduce the likelihood of an incorrect response. As Teddy continued to respond correctly, the CUES WERE SYSTEMATICALLY REMOVED until the desired correct response could be reliably obtained under a variety of training situations. One procedure used was to establish imitative naming by presenting Teddy with an object and the verbal stimulus, "Say ———." After several successes, the stimulus object was presented with the verbal stimulus, "What's this? Say ———." The pause between the question and the word *say* was gradually increased until "What's this?" was sufficient to elicit a correct response. With those objects to which Teddy did not respond appropriately, a situation which occurred very infrequently, the clinician provided an IMITATIVE MODEL which was gradually faded out (e.g., yellow . . . yell . . . ye . . .). The consequences for correct responses were the same as those used previously to establish looking behavior. Verbal praise and candy were presented immediately following a correct response. At the end of the five-month series of sessions, Teddy reliably named colors with the pictures and objects on which he had been trained, as well as some on which he was not trained. It is likely that he knew the names of some of these items previously, but the critical behavior achieved in these sessions was that he would now reliably name them on command.

Teaching Functional Language. The technique used in this phase of Teddy's training illustrates the adaptability in the behavioral strategy to utilize capabilities that are unique to the individual patient and enable the clinician to achieve more efficiently the desired behavior. In view of Teddy's unique ability to "read," a tactic similar to the common television teleprompter was employed. The clinician held up a sign on which was printed MAY I HAVE A COOKIE and held up a cookie. When Teddy read the sign, he was given the cookie. After this response occurred reliably, other objects were substituted for cookie and another sign reading MAY I HAVE ————, was substituted. When his response became appropriate to this situation, a blank card and the object to be requested were held up and Teddy would then repeat the phrase and the name of the object appropriately. After the initial training with cookies, Teddy almost always used the phrase appropriately with other objects for which he had a name on the first trial.

Since the intent was to teach responses that would be functional, the choice of target behaviors was often based on pinpointing responses occurring frequently in the repertoires of normal children and teaching them to Teddy. The flash-card technique was thus extended to include conversational sequences and phrases like "Thank you," "You're welcome," etc. Teddy quickly learned to associate the correct response to a variety of conversational cues but would sometimes recite his repertoire of responses when presented with an unfamiliar cue.

Extending Treatment to the Home

Since one of the long-range goals of this treatment was to modify Teddy's behavior in his total environment, regular conferences with his mother were instituted during the first month of treatment. These sessions occurred once or twice weekly throughout the time Teddy was being seen at the clinic. The strategy used in the clinic for selected target behaviors, with frequency of occurrence as the basic measure of change, was also applied in helping the mother extend treatment at home.

Teddy engaged in a number of disruptive behaviors at home that were INCOMPATIBLE with establishing generalization of Teddy's new language skills to the home. As a first step the mother was asked to list for the clinic team the problems she felt were most troublesome. Her most pressing concerns were: (1) Teddy would bounce and rock at high frequency throughout the day, often beginning before dawn. He had broken several chairs and the couch by bouncing on them and we observed him bouncing with such violence that the vibrations were felt throughout the house. (2) Teddy frequently turned the knobs on the family color television set, causing concern by the parents about damage to the color control system. (3) Teddy was not toilet trained.

There can be no question that these problems are appropriate for treatment through a speech clinic if behaviors learned in the clinic are to carry over to the home. The speech clinician is wise to obtain consultation from other professional disciplines; a coordinated program can treat the whole child in his whole environment and not merely isolated behaviors (Ayllon and Azrin, 1968).

Toilet Training and Disruptive Behaviors. After visiting the home and consulting with the parents, we instructed the mother in how to collect data on the behaviors of concern to her. Modification procedures for toilet training and disruptive behaviors were discussed with the mother and it was decided to set aside a chair in the utility area of the kitchen to be Teddy's time-out chair, and the parents agreed to keep that corner of the kitchen empty except for the chair and a small kitchen timer. The chair faced the kitchen and there were no physical restraints to keep Teddy from leaving the chair. It was agreed that the time-out contingency would be 15 minutes in the chair, where Teddy could do as he wished, except that if he left the chair, he would be told to return and the timer would be reset for 15 minutes. A notebook to record Teddy's progress was kept on top of the refrigerator near the chair. This notebook also contained a behavioral prescription specifically outlining the procedures to be employed:

Procedures

I. Whenever Teddy is found to have dirty underpants:
1. Be firm and friendly;
2. Tell him those are his only underpants;
3. Wash them in his presence and return them to him damp;
4. Insist he put them on;
5. Make sure he keeps them on for half an hour; be firm, even if he has a tantrum;
6. If he keeps them on for half an hour, and he doesn't dirty them during this time, replace the damp underpants with dry ones and praise him for keeping clean for that time;
7. If he takes them off, make him put them on again. Keep your eye on him and be quick to catch this, particularly for the first week.

II. Whenever Teddy bounces:
1. Tell him once and only once to stop;
2. If he bounces again, take him to the utility area and tell him he may not jump around anywhere in the house except in that chair. Let him know he must stay in the chair for 15 minutes until the timer rings.
3. Make him stay in the chair, forcibly if necessary, particularly for the first week; remember to reset the timer if he gets up.

III. Record keeping:
1. Record every instance of underpants washing;
2. Record every instance of sending Teddy to the utility room;
3. Record every instance of resetting the timer if Teddy gets out of his chair.

IV. Be friendly but firm. Let Teddy know things have changed. It will be necessary for you to spend a great deal of time on this for the first week, but after that you will find that Teddy will not require as much attention, if you have been consistent and systematic in carrying out the program. It should not be necessary to scold or punish Teddy. You can even smile when you take him to the room to wash his pants, but never let him avoid the new rules.

V. Playing with TV set (note: this procedure was added after the bouncing behavior had subsided):

1. Send Teddy to the time-out chair whenever he is seen touching the control knobs of the television set.

2. Do not apply this contingency unless you actually see him do it. You should be prepared to assist him in changing channels when he indicates such a request, since the contingency applies to all knobs.

Figures 45, 46, 47 and 48 summarize the results of these procedures. Note that the numbering of days is the same, for comparison purposes, in Figures 45 and 46. As can be seen in Figure 45, frequency of bouncing or rocking, initially quite high, was reduced to zero in a matter of days. Figure 46 shows that Teddy quickly learned to remain in the time-out chair once he was put there. Note the brief disturbance in the uniformly zero frequencies on Figure 46 after three weeks of training not to bounce. This change occurred at the point when playing with the TV set was added as a target behavior. Figure 47 shows the reduction in frequency of TV knob turning behavior with the time-out chair consequence. The mother had been instruct-

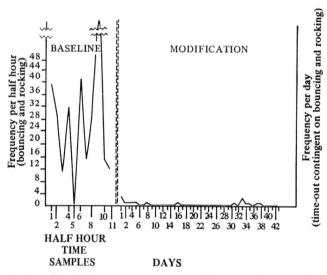

Figure 45. Baseline (left ordinate) and modification (right ordinate) frequencies of bouncing and rocking in the home. Note that the baseline measure was a series of half-hour time samples while during the modification period, total frequency per day was recorded.

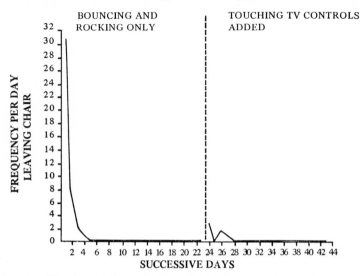

Figure 46. Number of times Teddy left the time-out chair without permission (after being put there for bouncing and rocking and, after the dotted line, for touching the TV controls).

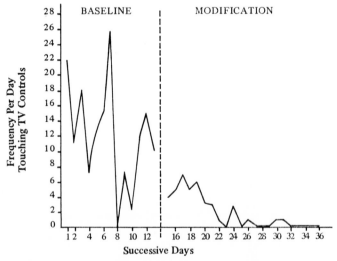

Figure 47. Baseline and modification frequencies of touching control knobs on the television set.

ed to collect data for baseline purposes on all the above behaviors before any new procedures were initiated.

During the time these procedures were being instituted in the

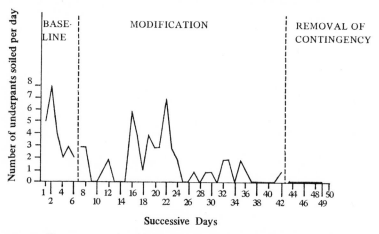

Figure 48. Frequency of soiling measured by counting the daily total of soiled underwear under three experimental conditions.

home, the mother was asked to bring her notebook every time Teddy came to the clinic for speech sessions. The clinician was careful to praise and reinforce the mother for maintaining consistent procedures at home and for keeping her records. At this time, Teddy was mastering the previously described language skills at the clinic and the mother was instructed to insist on the use of the new phrases at home as soon as each was learned. For example, Teddy was required to say, "May I have ————?" whenever he wanted more food at the dinner table. Since this generalization from the clinic to home was done one phrase at a time and procedures for use of new language skills were regularly reviewed with the mother, Teddy never required more than one or two prompts before he began using his new language ability at home.

The data in Figure 48 illustrate the application of a toilet training procedure and present an interesting paradox: a deceleration procedure failed to modify behavior, but the behavior did change in the desired manner when the procedure was discontinued. Although Teddy did not wet himself, he did frequently soil and this was a source of distress for the family. More important, however, was the fact that toilet training is a prerequisite for entry to most public school classes. Since the behavioral prescription in I above failed to produce results within a month, it was discontinued with the intent of obtaining a few days of baseline data before trying another procedure. Teddy used the toilet during this subsequent period of time and there were essentially no soiling or wetting accidents during the next four months over which data were collected.

The decision to record daily total soiled underwear rather than actual incidents was one of convenience for the mother. While multiple incidents could occur undetected in the same set of underwear, an accurate figure could be obtained for days on which no soiling occurred. This was the important datum.

Results of the Five-Month Language and Behavior Training

After five months of treatment, the initial behavioral objectives of treatment were achieved. Steps were taken to find an appropriate school placement for Teddy. It was decided to suspend clinic sessions for the summer months although the mother was still given assistance with the behavior and language program.

The Peabody Picture Vocabulary Test and the Leiter International Performance Scale, on which Teddy had been pretested five months earlier, were readministered. The relative changes in these test scores reflect the language emphasis of Teddy's training. Teddy's score on the Leiter, a nonlanguage performance test of intelligence, was unchanged from the pretest mental-age score, which was four years and three months. However, his language-age score on the Peabody increased from two years, three months, to four years, 10 months; and the Peabody IQ score, which was below limits at the beginning of treatment, increased to 80.

Treatment of Behaviors at School

The clinic team met with school officials in Teddy's district, who agreed to place Teddy, now seven years old, in a full-day primary special education class. Although formal instruction in the speech clinic was discontinued, the clinician agreed to continue consultation with the school and parents. Teddy's teacher reviewed the video tapes of Teddy's therapy sessions and discussed the clinic and home procedures with the clinician. At this point, the teacher naturally assumed the responsibility as Teddy's case manager and the speech clinician joined the psychologist in a consultant role.

Shortly after the beginning of school, Teddy's teacher reported two problems. When the teacher was not at the front of the class,

Teddy occasionally got out of his seat and imitated the teacher by repeating sentences she used with the class, such as, "Did everyone brush his teeth this morning?" and "It is story time now." In addition, Teddy went to other children during class time and initiated the conversational sequences he had been taught during his therapy sessions. These behaviors were disruptive to the class and had to be prevented.

When they analyzed the situation, Teddy's teacher and the clinician observed that many of these behaviors occurred when Teddy was out of his seat. Therefore, it was decided to institute a procedure to discourage Teddy's leaving his seat, thereby preventing the disturbing behaviors from occurring in class, but not decelerating those behaviors themselves, since vocal communication was desirable in Teddy's repertoire. Because the time-out chair had been useful at home, it was decided to apply the same tactic in the classroom. Whenever Teddy left his seat, the teacher instructed him to go and sit in the time-out chair in the corner of the classroom. Figure 49 shows effect of this contingency in reducing the frequency of Teddy's leaving his seat.

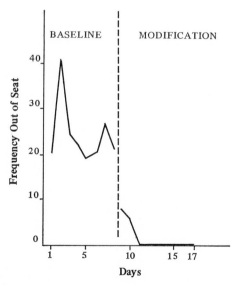

Figure 49. Number of times out of seat per day at school (baseline and modification conditions).

TABLE XXIII SUMMARY OF TRAINING TRIALS FOR SHAPING DESCRIPTIVE SENTENCES

At the break indicated (A) the clinician taught four new words, *lady, blouse, skirt, eyes*. B – trials; S – spontaneous response; I – imitated response; * – reinforced with candy.

Stimulus	4/11 B	4/13 1	4/13 2	4/13 3	4/18 1	4/18 2	4/18 3	4/20 1	4/20 2	4/20 3	4/25 1	4/25 2	4/25 3	5/2 1	5/2 2	5/2 3	5/9 1	5/9 2	5/9 3	5/11 1	5/11 2	5/11 3	5/11 4	5/11 5	5/11 6
face	S	S	S								S	S	S	S	S	S	S								
hair	S	S	S								S	S	S	S	S	S	S								
fingers	S			S								S	S	S	S	S	S								
dress	S	S	S	S	S																				
nose		S	S	S	S	S	S	S	S	S	S	S	S	S	S	S	S	S	S	S	S	S	S	S	
2 circles		S	S	S	S	S	S	S	S	S	S	S	S		S	S	S	S	S	S	S	S	S	S	
1 circle		S	S	S	S	S	S	S	S	S	S	S	S	S	S	S	S	S	S	S	S	S	S	S	
fingernail		S			S	S	S		S	S	S	S	S		S	S	S		S	S	S	S	S	S	
lips							S	S	S	S															
ears							S		S																
l-a-d-y							I																		
eyebrows					S*	S*	S*	I						S	S	S	S				S	S	S	S	S
lady's skirt																									
A																									
lady		I*	S*	S*	S	I	I	S	S	S*	S	S	S	S	S	S	S	S	S	S	S	S	S	S	
blouse		I*	I	I	S	I*	S*	S*	S*	S*	S	S	S	S	S	S	S	S	S	S	S	S	S		
skirt		I*	I	I	S*	S*	S*	S*	S*	S	S	S*	S*	S	S	S	S								
eyes		I*	S*	S*	S*	S	S	S	S	S	S	S*	S*	S			S								
I . . . see . . . a . . . lady.											I*														
I see a lady.											I*	S*	S*	I*	S*	S*									
I see a lady with . . . pretty . . . hair.														I*			I*								
I see a lady with pretty hair.																	I* S*	S*							
I see a lady with pretty hair and . . . brown . . . eyes.																	I*	S*		I*					
I see a lady with pretty hair and brown eyes.																				S	S	I*	I	S*	S*
I see a lady with pretty hair and brown eyes.																						I*	I*	I	S*
She's wearing a blouse.																								I*	S*

Subsequent Speech and Language Training

Teaching a Descriptive Response. Midway through the school year, Teddy returned to the clinic for speech instruction sessions to attack some of the specific inappropriate behaviors reported by the mother and teacher. Although Teddy was rapidly beginning to develop a large repertoire of vocal labels for pictures and objects, he was still not using functional conversational speech.

To approximate this skill, it was necessary to analyze what was different in Teddy's language behavior from that of a "normal" child. One striking difference was that he rarely used sentences, relying instead on his one-word repertoire. It was decided to expand this one-word labeling repertoire into a response chain that Teddy could use to provide a description in sentence form of a picture containing many objects. It should be pointed out that from the behavioral point of view a conversational response chain is an objectively defined skill that can be taught just as easily as simple one-word labeling.

The procedure for building a descriptive repertoire was presentation of a magazine picture with the instruction "Teddy, tell me about this picture. What do you see?" The arbitrarily determined terminal response (target behavior) required was, "I see a lady with pretty hair and brown eyes. She's wearing a blouse." Teddy's initial, unreinforced baseline responses consisted of pointing to and labeling *face, hair,* and *dress*; that is, single-word responses. The order of teaching and the pattern of Teddy's responses on this task can be found in Table XXIII. The training was carried out over eight sessions, the first day being baseline. At least three trials were presented each session with intervening activities between these trials. Initially Teddy emitted single word responses accompanied by pointing. Besides the words Teddy emitted without training, the clinician taught four single words important to the terminal response. These are the words listed below the break indicated (A). In this table, S indicates a spontaneous response, i.e., emitted without a model from the clinician immediately preceding the response; I, an imitated response; and an asterisk (*) means that particular response was reinforced with praise and candy. It should be immediately obvious that the reinforcement schedule was intermittent, but that it maintained a high rate of responding. It is interesting to see the rapid acquisition of the phrases and sentences. On 4/25, Trial 2, the first connected speech stimulus was presented. Teddy did not imitate the phrase when it was presented as a whole, so each word was presented separately for him to imitate. He correctly repeated each word and was subsequently reinforced. Then the whole phrase was presented again and this time he imitated it correctly. On the next trial the entire phrase was emitted correctly and spontaneously as the first response. Another example of rapid learning was during Trial 1, 5/9, when the entire response "I see a lady with pretty hair" was emitted spontaneously and correctly after only one training trial seven days earlier. Response acquisition remained rapid and durable for the rest of the trials. These sessions were the first recorded incidents of Teddy emitting verbal responses of any significant length and can be seen as the beginning of conversational speech. At this time the teacher began a similar language activity in the classroom for the entire class, and thus further expanded Teddy's repertoire of verbal chains.

Teaching a Functional "Pivotal" Phrase. As a continuation of the program designed to teach Teddy to use more sentences, the emphasis was on responses that would be generally useful in his environment. It was decided that response such as "That's a ————" or "Those are ————," used with singular and plural nouns, would be likely to occur frequently enough that, if learned during formal language instruction, it might become functional in his home and school environment. The importance of grammatical syntax in developing normal language has been stressed by Gray and Fygetakis (1968).

The teaching program consisted of a series of probes to determine Teddy's REPERTOIRE at specified times. After instruction, a reprobe was conducted to measure the extent of Teddy's learning on the specific task and to yield information about the generalization of the responses he had added to his repertoire. The stimuli used were common objects.

A pretraining probe of 10 objects was used before teaching procedures for "That's a ————" were initiated. Teddy was presented with the stimulus, "Teddy, what's that?" followed by the model, "That's a car." He initially substituted b/th, but correct articulation was required throughout. After several presentations of the model, imitative cues were faded into PROMPTS where the clinician only whispered the /th/ sound and Teddy would follow this cue with the complete correct response. Rapidly even this prompt could be eliminated and Teddy would emit the correct response to the stimulus, "Teddy, what's that?"

Table XXIV illustrates the preteaching frequency of occurrence of "That's a," the responses for the four teaching trials, and the re-

TABLE XXIV

SUMMARY OF RESULTS OF LANGUAGE INSTRUCTION IN USE OF
A FUNCTIONAL "PIVOTAL" PHRASE IN SENTENCES

Training Sequence	No. Items	% Correct	Schedule of Reinf.
Preteaching Probe	10	20	DRO
"That's a"	10	0	DRO
Teaching Trials	10	90	crf
"That's a"	10	80	crf
	10	90	crf
	10	100	crf
Post-Teaching Probe			
"That's a"			
Original items	10	100	DRO
Novel items	5	80	DRO
Preteaching Probe	10	0	DRO
"Those are"	10	0	DRO
Teaching Trials	10	40	crf
"Those are"	10	90	crf
	10	100	crf
Post-Teaching Probe			
"Those are"			
Original items	10	100	DRO
Novel items	5	80	DRO
Preteaching Probe	120	2.5	DRO
Generalization			
Teaching Trials	60	1.7	DRO
Generalization	27	63	VR2
	28	93	VR2
	4	100	crf
	6	100	FR 2
	12	100	FR 3
	18	100	FR 4
	20	100	FR 5
	27	100	VR 12
Post-Teaching Probe			
Generalization	60	100	DRO

sponses on the post-teaching reprobe with original 10 objects and five new ones inserted randomly. Notice that reinforcement during training was continuous, but that during the pre- and post-teaching probes there was a DIFFERENTIAL REINFORCEMENT of other behavior (DRO); that is correct responses were never reinforced.

The same procedure was used for teaching "Those are" responses, with a new set of 10 plural objects. The data show that on the preteaching probes Teddy never emitted "Those are" responses, but that after three teaching trials with the 10 plural objects, he was using the phrase 100 per cent of the time. He maintained this rate on the post-teaching probe without reinforcement for correct responding.

It was then necessary to measure the generalization of these two newly learned responses. The stimuli were the 15 objects used in "That's a" training, now presented in both singular and plural form, and the 15 objects used in "Those are" teaching, also in both singular and plural form, for a total of 60 stimuli. A stimulus was placed on the table and Teddy was asked, "Teddy, what do I have here?" This question was a neutral stimulus that did not include prompts for "That" or "Those." Correct responses were not reinforced. Teddy emitted only three "Those are" responses and no "That's a" responses. Obviously, these responses had not generalized and more teaching was necessary.

Using again common objects, another 60-item probe was administered with differential stimuli, that is, "Teddy, what's that?" or "Teddy, what are those?" to see if these vocal stimuli provided cues for differential responding with "That's a" or "Those are." Since all but one of his responses were again single words, the vocal stimuli apparently did not have discriminative function for sentences. An analysis of this deficit suggested that the stimulus events that controlled Teddy's sentence responses were absent during the generalization probes. Since a reinforcement schedule also operates as a stimulus, it was postulatd that Teddy's sentence responding was specific to the continuous reinforcement schedule (crf) in force during the training segments. Therefore, the schedule was made gradually leaner over the next three sessions, beginning with candy reinforcement for 50 per cent of the trial (VR 2) until, at the end of the third session, Teddy got a candy reinforcer for only eight per cent of his correct responses (VR 12), while maintaining 100 per cent correct respond-ing. At this point the 60-object generalization reprobe was presented again with the neutral stimulus, "Teddy, what do I have here?" and with nondifferential reinforcement (DRO). Teddy emitted 100 per cent correct responses.

One might speculate, from these data, that the schedule of rein-forcement was a functional discriminative stimulus. It would follow from this finding that using candy as a consequence in other settings would enhance transfer of Teddy's newly acquired behavior, not necessarily because of the reinforcement value of the candy, but be-cause of its stimulus properties.

Current Status

At the completion of training "That's a" and "Those are" re-sponses, Teddy's speech instruction was discontinued. He was seven and one-half years of age at that time and did not have totally ac-ceptable "normal" language, but the effects of the training proce-dures were beginning to show in his ability to learn appropriate re-sponses quickly and in the spontaneous generalization of his responses.

It has been three and one-half years since the initiation of the treat-ment regimen described. Teddy at 10 years, zero months, has com-pleted three years of school. He has advanced rapidly, skipping the equivalent of one grade, and is currently in an intermediate-level (grades 4 and 5) special education class. Psychological testing in the school has confirmed the report of his teacher that his reading, spell-ing, and arithmetic skills are all at or above grade level. His final grades for the past school year in all subjects including social studies, science, and language arts were average or above. His grades for arts and crafts, general behavior, following directions, and using time were all satisfactory.

During the early treatment there had been several unsuccessful attempts to teach Teddy some play skills and appropriate social be-havior. Although Teddy would try out his responses on peers in these situations, his repertoire was not sufficient for him to maintain com-munication. Reports indicate during his first two years of school he still preferred to play alone at recess. During the last year, however, he began to acquire social skills appropriate for his age and routinely played with other children in school and in his neighborhood. His favorite game is baseball and he plays it well enough to be included in sandlot games in his neighborhood.

Teddy's language repertoire has greatly expanded and he now routinely converses in sentences in an essentially normal manner. His general articulation is what one would expect from a child his age. The only reported difficulty is that he occasionally speaks too fast when excited and must be told to slow down, but this is not uncommon for children his age. In a recent telephone conversation with his clinician, Teddy enthusiastically discussed in a factual and intelligent manner the progress of the major league baseball team in Kansas City, which he follows in the newspaper and on television.

Teddy will continue in his special education class for the next year and it is expected that he will enter a regular education program at the junior high school level. There is no question at the moment that this previously untestable child with grossly deviant autistic behavior can now look forward to a meaningful and productive role in society. It is gratifying to note that all the behaviors there were programmed for Teddy have remained in his repertoire, which has in turn expanded beyond the specifically programmed responses. The undesired behaviors that were initially decelerated have not reappeared nor have any instances been noted of other undesired behaviors being substituted for them.

Discussion

The question of which of the procedures in force was related to changes in Teddy's behavior cannot be answered with the data available on Teddy. However, the intent of this study was pragmatic: to demonstrate how procedures, whose effects on behavior have already been rigorously demonstrated (for example, Girardeau and Spradlin, 1970), can be applied clinically without sacrificing scientific rigor. Where a given behavioral effect is scientifically demonstrated to result from application of an objectively defined procedure under conditions A, B, and C, and the same effect occurs under a less precisely controlled condition D, the assumption of a lawful relationship is made more believable. The present study is dependent on the cited references for behavioral principles and seeks to extend the range of applicability of those principles.

Sidman (1960) has emphasized the importance of selecting an appropriate baseline. Certainly a continuous record of frequency of occurrence of the behavior to be modified provides the most convincing evidence against which to compare the frequency after a modification procedure has been introduced (e.g., Figures 47, 48, and 49). Figure 45 illustrates a situation where the cost in time and effort of obtaining a frequency count for the entire day was too high and an ideal baseline was not obtained. Because of the very high frequency of bouncing and rocking, Teddy's mother could not record this and still do her other daily work. Therefore, half-hour samples were prearranged to be taken at various times of day over the course of the week and the psychologist also took the same data at the home during two of these same periods as a reliability measure. The importance of teaching parents how to observe and record behavior at home cannot be overestimated. Not only does this provide accurate data for the professional, but it also involves the parent as an actively responding collaborator in treatment (Patterson and Gullion, 1969).

The use of the probe technique (Table XXIV) in the case where behavior is already under fairly precise control has several potential advantages over the more simple baseline procedure (Sidman, 1960). In addition to being less time consuming, this technique is more sensitive to subtle effects and led, in this case, to the discovery of the stimulus effect of the schedule of reinforcement on Teddy's ability to generalize his responses.

There can be no hiding the fact that the use of the data from the first few days of treatment as a basis for evaluating subsequent changes in behavior is an inferior practice (Figures 42 and 43). However, a baseline does not have to be a no-treatment condition. In Figure 44, behavior under one treatment condition is the baseline against which a second treatment effect is compared.

All the data presented from the clinic were recorded by the clinician (except Figure 43), but there was uniform agreement between the clinician and the observer who recorded the same data through a one-way window. By writing out the program tasks prior to each lesson, data recording was reduced to checking each item as correct or in error on the list of daily tasks. On those tasks for which Teddy received candy for each correct response, data recording was further simplified. A cup filled with only as many candies as the number of trials was prepared prior to the session. Wherever an error was made, the clinician put that candy into a second cup out of Teddy's sight. This procedure yielded a count of errors and was also a convenient way of ensuring that the correct number of trials were presented during each session. Time spent inappropriately was measured instead of frequency of inappropriate behavior only because it was easier to record. Starting and stopping a stopwatch to cumulate time did not interfere at all with other procedures.

It was fortunate that relatively few specific procedures were sufficient to enable Teddy to generalize his newly acquired behaviors to stimulus situations in his "outside" environment. The data in Table XXIV illustrates a technique for training a child to respond differentially to rather subtle stimulus cues.

The tactics described above did achieve the goals initially set for Teddy. He learned verbal labels and grammatical syntax, and was taught to use these skills at home and at school. By insisting on early generalizing of language and behavior training from the clinic to the home, it was possible to maintain the behavior learned through clinic techniques in the more natural conditions of the everyday world.

Acknowledgment

Parts of this study were presented at the 1967 Convention of the American Association on Mental Deficiency and the 1968 Annual Convention of American Speech and Hearing Association. The authors are grateful for the advice and support of Frederic L. Girardeau, William M. Diedrich, and James A. Sherman and the Bureau of Child Research of the University of Kansas. This work was supported in part by Grant Number 5 T1 MH-8262-03 from the National Institute of Mental Health. It was conducted while the authors were with the Bureau of Child Research and the Hearing and Speech Department, respectively, at the University of Kansas Medical Center.

Joyce Houser, Teddy's public school teacher, also contributed in large part to the success of Teddy's treatment, as did Ellen Shamasko, Teddy's speech clinician during the first part of the study. This manuscript was prepared with the help of Marcia Wallerstein and the support of Children's Bureau Project No. 413 at the Child Development and Mental Retardation Center of the University of Washington.

References

Ayllon, T. and Azrin, N: *The Token Economy*. New York, Appleton, 1968.

Baer, D. M., Peterson, R. F. and Sherman, J. A.: The development of imitation by reinforcing behavioral similarity to a model. *J Exp Anal Behav 10*, 405-416, 1967.

Brookshire, R. H.: Speech pathology and the experimental analysis of behavior. *J Speech Hearing Dis 32*, 215-227, 1967.

Girardeau, F. L. and Spradlin, J. E. (Eds.): A functional analysis approach to speech and language. *ASHA Monogr No. 14*, 1970.

Gray, B. B. and Fygetakis, L.: The development of language as a function of programmed conditioning. *Behav Res Ther 6*, 455-460, 1968.

Hingtgen, J. N. and Churchill, D. W.: Identification of perceptual limitations in mute autistic children. *Arch Gen Psychiat 21*, 68-71, 1969.

Holland, A. L.: Some applications of behavioral principles to clinical speech problems. *J Speech Hearing Dis 32*, 11-18, 1967.

Homme, L. E., deBaca, P. C., Devine, J. V., Steinhorst, R. and Rickert, E. J.: Use of the Premack principle in controlling the behavior of nursery school children. *J Exp Anal Behav 6*, 544, 1963.

Kerr, N., Meyerson, L. and Michael, J.: A procedure for shaping vocalizations in a mute child. In L. P. Ullmann and L. Krasner (Eds.), *Case Studies in Behavior Modification*. New York, Holt, 1965.

Lovaas, O. I.: Some studies on the treatment of childhood schizophrenia. *Res Psychother 3*, 103-121, 1968.

Lovaas, O. I., Berberich, J. P., Perloff, B. F. and Schaeffer, B.: Acquisition of imitative speech in schizophrenic children. *Science 151*, 705-707, 1966.

Patterson. G. R. and Gullion, M. E.: *A Guide for the Professional for Use with "Living with Children."* Champaign, Ill., Research Press, 1969.

Premack, D.: Toward empirical behavior laws: I. Positive reinforcement. *Psychol Rev 66*, 219-233, 1959.

Risley, T. R. and Wolf, M. M.: Establishing functional speech in echolalic children. *Behav Res Ther 5*, 73-88, 1967.

Schell, R. E., Stark, J. and Giddan, J. J.: Development of language behavior in an autistic child. *J Speech Hearing Dis 32*, 51-64, 1967.

Sidman, M.: *Tactics of Scientific Research*. New York, Basic Books, 1960.

Skinner, B. F.: *The Behavior of Organisms*. New York, Appleton, 1938.

Skinner, B. F.: *Verbal Behavior*. New York, Appleton, 1957.

Stark, J., Giddan, J. J. and Meisel, J.: Increasing verbal behavior in an autistic child. *J Speech Hear Dis 33*, 42-48, 1968.

Chapter 2

AVERSIVE CONTROL OF SELF-INJURIOUS BEHAVIOR IN A PSYCHOTIC BOY*

B. G. TATE *and* GEORGE S. BAROFF

Introduction

THERE HAVE BEEN MANY ATTEMPTS to explain self-injurious be-havior (Cain, 1961; Dollard *et al.*, 1939; Freud, 1954; Goldfarb, 1945; Greenacre, 1954; Hartmann *et al.*, 1949; Sandler, 1964). It has been labeled masochism, auto-aggression, self-aggression, and self-destructive behavior. The present authors prefer the term self-in-jurious behavior because it is more descriptive and less interpretive. Self-injurious behavior (SIB) does not imply an attempt to destroy, nor does it suggest aggression: it SIMPLY MEANS BEHAVIOR WHICH PRODUCES PHYSICAL INJURY TO THE INDIVIDUAL'S OWN BODY. Typi-cally SIB is composed of a series of self-injurious responses (SIRs) that are repetitive and sometimes rhythmical, often with no obvious reinforcers, and therefore similar to stereotyped behavior. Common types of SIB are forceful head-banging, face slapping, punching the face and head, and scratching and biting one's body.

A patient who emits SIRs at high frequency and/or magnitude is particularly difficult to work with because the behavior interferes with the production of more desirable responses and there is always the risk of severe and permanent physical injury, e.g. head and eye

*From *Behavior Research and Therapy*, 1966, 4, pp. 281-287. Reprinted by permis-sion of Maxwell International Microforms Corporation.

damage. Usually such patients must be physically restrained or maintained on heavy dosages of drugs. Lovaas *et al.* (1964), however, successfully employed punishment in the form of painful electric shock to dramatically reduce the frequency of SIRs in several schizophrenic children. Ball (1965) used the same technique with a severely retarded girl and achieved similar results.

The present paper describes two punishment procedures used to control SIB in a psychotic boy. In Study I, PUNISHMENT was withdrawal of human physical contact contingent on a SIR. In Study II, PUNISHMENT was response-contingent painful electric shock. Following a description of the subject, the procedures and results of Studies I and II are presented, followed by a report on related behavioral changes and a general discussion.

Subject

Sam was a nine-year-old, blind male who was transferred for evaluation and treatment on a research basis from an out-of-state psychiatric hospital to Murdoch Center, a state institution for the mentally retarded. At the age of five he was diagnosed as autistic and was hospitalized. For the next four years he received group and individual psychotherapy, and drug therapy with no long-term benefit. Drugs were used in an effort to control self-injurious behavior, screaming, and hyperactivity.

The SIB began at about the age of four and consisted of face slapping. By age nine, his SIB repertoire included banging his head forcefully against floors, walls, and other hard objects, slapping his face with his hands, punching his face and head with his fists, hitting his shoulder with his chin, and kicking himself. Infrequently he would also pinch, bite, and scratch others.

At age 8, bilateral cataracts, a complete detachment of the left retina, and partial detachment of the right retina were discovered. An ophthalmologist has suggested that the cataracts were probably congenital but were not noticed until they matured and that the retinal detachments were likely caused by head-banging. The cataract in the right eye was removed soon after its discovery, leaving Sam with some light-dark vision and possibly some movement perception.

Upon arrival at Murdoch Center, Sam was assigned a room in the infirmary and drugs were immediately discontinued. Casual observations were made for the first two weeks while he was adapting to his new environment. Following the adaptation period, eighteen 30-min daily observation periods were conducted during which a female research assistant held Sam, tried to interest him in games, and ignored all SIRs. These observations yielded a median daily average

SIR rate of 2.3/min (range: 0.9-7.9/min). A second type of observation consisted of 5-min periods four times a day at random intervals. Over a 26-day period the median daily average SIR rate was 1.7/min (range: 0.3-4.1/min). SIB, therefore, was a frequent form of behavior observed under a wide variety of situations.

Observations also revealed the following: Sam had a firm hemotoma approximately 7 cm in diameter on his forehead—a result of previous head-banging. His speech was limited to jargon and to approximately twenty words usually spoken in a high-pitched, whining manner and often inappropriately used. He was not considered autistic at this time because he obviously enjoyed and sought bodily contact with others. He would cling to people and try to wrap their arms around him, climb into their laps and mold himself to their contours. When left alone and free, he would cry, scream, flail his arms about, and hit himself or bang his head. When fully restrained in bed he was usually calm, but often engaged in head-rolling and hitting his chin against his shoulder.

Study I: Control by Withdrawal and Reinstatement of Human Physical Contact

Early observations of Sam strongly indicated that physical contact with people was reinforcing to him and that being alone, particularly when he was standing or walking, was aversive. Study I was undertaken in an effort to learn if a procedure of withdrawing physical contact when a SIR occurred and reinstating the contact after a brief interval during which no SIRs occurred could be used to control Sam's SIB.

Procedure

Study I began on the fourth day following the end of the 26-day observation period mentioned. During the three weeks preceding the commencement of the study Sam was restrained in his bed except for morning baths given by attendants and for daily walks around the campus and through the infirmary corridors with two female research assistants (Es). During the walks Es held Sam's hands and chatted to him and to each other and ignored SIRs.

Study I consisted of twenty daily 20-minute sessions run at the same time each day by the same Es. There were five control sessions (SIRs were ignored), followed by five experimental sessions (SIRs were punished), five control sessions, and five experimental sessions.

Control sessions consisted of a walk around the campus with the two Es who chatted with Sam and with each other. Sam walked between them, holding onto a hand of each. When he emitted SIRs the Es ignored them.

Experimental sessions were identical to the control sessions except that when Sam hit himself, Es jerked their hands free so that he had no physical contact with them. The TIME-OUT from physical contact lasted three seconds following the last SIR. At the end of three seconds, Es allowed him to grasp their hands and the walk resumed. No comments were made to Sam when a hit occurred—the only responses to the SIR were withdrawal of contact and cessation of talk if Es were talking at the time.

All sessions began when Sam left his room and entered the corridor leading outside the building. The same route around the campus was followed each day. Each session ended while he was outside the building, but the procedure for the particular session was continued until Sam was returned to his room, undressed, placed in bed, and restrained—usually about 12 additional minutes. Records were kept by one E who silently marked the SIRs on a piece of paper during the walks.

Results of Study I

Virtually all of the SIRs made during the sessions were chin-to-shoulder hits. On a few occasions Sam would punch his head with his fist during punishment but he rarely withdrew his hand from an assistant and hit himself.

Figure 50 presents the average SIRs per minute for each day of the study. The median average rate of SIRs for the first five control days was 6.6 responses per minute and sharply declined to a median average of 0.1 responses per minute for the following five experimental days. The response rate recovered somewhat (median average=3.3) during the second five control days and decreased again during the second five experimental days (median average=1.0). The unusually high rate of SIRs on the second day of the second control run was associated with a temper tantrum which lasted about 15 minutes.

On the experimental days an interesting change in Sam's behavior occurred which was noticed by both Es and the authors. On control days Sam typically whined, cried, hesitated often in his walk, and seemed unresponsive to the environment in general. His behav-

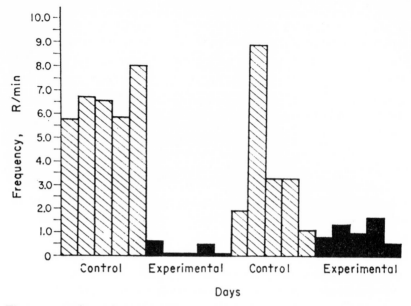

Figure 50. Effect of the punishment procedure of Study I on the daily average frequency of SIRs. On experimental days SIRs were followed by withdrawal of human physical contact and reinstatement of contact after a minimum interval of 3 sec. On control days the SIRs were ignored.

ior on experimental days was completely different—he appeared to attend more to environmental stimuli, including the Es; there was no crying or whining, and he often smiled. A brief discussion on this change in behavior appears at the end of the paper.

The results of this study indicate that the relatively simple procedure of controlling the contingencies of this chronic SIB produced a dramatic reduction in its frequency. Of interest also are the relative effects of punishing the SIR and ignoring it. These results do not, of course, mean that long-term effects would be the same.

During the first 90-minute contingent shock period a total of only five SIRs were emitted (average rate=0.06 responses per minute). The shocks produced a startle reaction in Sam and avoidance movements, but no cries. The authors talked to him, praised virtually all non-injurious responses, and generally behaved pleasantly. When led from the bed to the rocking chair, he immediately began crying and flailing his arms. A SIR was promptly followed by a shock and he became calm. A few seconds later he was sitting in the chair and smiling with apparent pleasure. At the end of the 90-minute period Sam was returned to his bed and left in it free while being observed over closed-circuit television. Throughout the second 90-minute observation period he remained quietly in bed posturing with his hands. Four SIRs were emitted and were followed by delayed shocks. The SIR rate had decreased from 2.0/minute in the last minutes of the free responding period to 0.4/minute. At the end of the period a meal was offered which he refused. He was then restrained for the night.

The following day Sam was free from 9:00 a.m. until 2:30 p.m. All of this time was spent in bed with toys except for one hour in the afternoon during which the authors encouraged him to rock in a rocking chair and walk around his room. Twenty SIRs of light intensity occurred during the five and one-half hour period (average rate=0.06 responses per minute). Four of these were followed by immediate shock and the other 16 by delayed shock.

On the second day following the commencement of shock Sam was free from 8:00 a.m. until 4:30 p.m. There were only fifteen SIRs during the entire day (average rate=0.03/minute) but most at night because of limited personnel available to check him. He was out of bed about three hours being rocked, walked, and entertained with toys.

In the ensuing days Sam's daily activities were gradually increased until he remained out of bed nine hours a day. He was still restrained at night because of limited personnel available to check him. He began attending physical therapy classes for the severely retarded three hours a day where he was encouraged to play with a variety of toys. He now apparently enjoys walks, playground equipment, and playing "games" involving following directions and making discriminations, for example, various objects (ball, book, music box, etc.) are put on a table across the room and he is asked to bring a specific one to E. He is more spontaneous in his activities than he was when he arrived and he is now capable of walking and running alone without clinging to people.

Punishment of SIRs with shock was continued and the decline in rate progressed. Since the beginning of shock 167 days have elapsed. The last observed SIR was emitted on day 147.

Other Changes in Behavior

Sam's intake of food and liquids had undergone an overall decrease since his admission although there were wide day-to-day fluctuations. Three months after his admission (five days before the use of shock), his weight had decreased by 14 pounds (20 per cent). On days when he ate nothing he usually held great quantities of saliva in his mouth for hours—emptying his mouth only by accident or when forced to. In the 36 hours preceding the commencement of shock, Sam ate only a small portion of one meal and drank only 400 ml of liquids. Supper was refused on the day shock was first administered. The following day he drank a small quantity of milk and ate some cereal for breakfast, but all other liquids and food were refused during the day—he had started saving saliva again. In addition he was posturing with his hands most of the day (posturing had been observed before any treatment began).

On the second day following the commencement of shock he refused food during the morning. At 2:00 p.m., he was again offered juice which he refused. He was then told firmly to drink but he would not open his mouth. It was then discovered that a firm command followed by the buzz of the shock prod (but no shock delivered), would cause him to open his mouth and take the juice, but he then held it in his mouth without swallowing. Again, a command and a buzz produced swallowing. The sequence of "Drink," and "Swallow," was repeated until he had consumed all of the juice. Verbal praise and affectionate pats were used to reinforce each desirable response. With this procedure, command-buzz-reinforcement, he also drank a glass of milk and ate some ice cream. This was the most food he had consumed in four days. Only one shock was actually administered—buzzing of the prod was sufficient the other times. This procedure was continued for the evening meal and the following day. On the third day he began eating spontaneously and has continued, although there are still occasions when he has to be prompted. In the following 15 days he gained 10 pounds and his weight continues to increase, but at a normal rate.

The posturing was stopped in similar fashion. When, for example, Sam held his hands up instead of down by his sides, he was told firmly to put his hands down, and if he did not, the buzzing of the prod was presented. The act of holding saliva in his mouth was stopped by telling him firmly to swallow and sounding the prod if he did not obey. The same procedure was effective in reducing his clinging to people.

Discussion

Both punishment procedures effectively reduced SIB in this psychotic boy. Aversive control by withdrawal of physical contact was immediately effective both times it was used.

Aversive control by painful electric shock also reduced the SIB immediately and has remained effective over a six-month period. In addition, it was found that eating behavior could be reinstated, posturing could be stopped, and saliva-saving and clinging could be terminated by firm commands followed by the sound of the shock apparatus if there was no compliance, and followed by social reinforcement if compliance occurred. Over the six-month period since the inception of shock, its use has decreased. Part of the beneficial effects of punishment by shock obviously were derived from the more stimulating environment provided him following the initial treatment—an environment which could not have been provided had the SIR rate not been suppressed to avoid injury. A secondary gain was probably derived from the marked positive change in behavior of attendants and nurses toward Sam. It should also be noted that punishment by electric shock prevented accidental reinforcement of SIRs. Before any treatment began it was sometimes necessary to interfere with SIRs by holding Sam's arms, a procedure which may have been reinforcing to him. No deleterious effects of the shock were observed.

An intriguing area of speculation is how to account for the complete change in behavior observed on experimental days of Study I and observed often after shock was delivered in Study II. One plausible explanation for the difference in behavior is that the whining, crying, and SIB belong to the same response class and the suppression of SIB also suppresses these other behaviors. Once the undesirable behaviors are suppressed the more desirable ones, e.g. smiling, listening, attending to the environment, and cooperating with others can occur.

Another conjecture is that both types of punishment produce a general arousal in the central nervous system which results in increased attention (Hebb, 1955). Attention to the external environment could account for the cooperative behavior, smiling and apparent listening. This idea is further supported by the immediacy of the punishment effect—not only did SIB, whining, crying, and negativistic behavior cease abruptly, but within seconds the more desirable behaviors emerged.

Acknowledgments—The authors would like to thank Mrs. Beth Maxwell and Mrs. Gail Spruill for their invaluable assistance in carrying out these studies, and Mrs. Rose Boyd for typing the manuscript.

References

Ball, T. S.: Personal communication, 1965.

Cain, A. C.: The presuperego turning inward of aggression. *Psychoanal Q 30,* 171-208, 1961.

Dollard, J., Doob, L. W., Miller, N. E., Mowrer, O. H. and Sears, R. R.: *Frustration and Aggression.* Yale University Press, New Haven, 1939.

Freud, A.: Problems of infantile neurosis: a discussion. In *The Psychoanalytic Study of the Child,* Vol. IX. International Universities Press, New York, 1954.

Goldfarb, W.: Psychological privation in infancy. *Am J Orthopsychiat 15,* 247-255, 1945.

Greenacre, P.: Problems of infantile neurosis: a discussion. In *The Psychoanalytic Study of the Child,* Vol. IX. International Universities Press, New York, 1954.

Hartmann, H., Kris, E. and Loewenstein, R. M.: Notes on the theory of aggression. In *The Psychoanalytic Study of the Child.* Vols. III-IV. International Universities Press, New York, 1949.

Hebb, D. O.: Drives and the C.N.S. (conceptual nervous system). *Psychol Rev 62,* 243-254, 1955.

Lovaas, O. I., Freitag, G., Kinder, M. I., Rubenstein, D. B., Schaeffer, B. and Simmons, J. B.: *Experimental Studies in Childhood Schizophrenia. Developing Social Behavior Using Electric Shock.* Paper read at American Psychological Association Annual Convention, Los Angeles, California, 1964.

Sandler, J.: Masochism: an empirical analysis. *Psychol Bull 62,* 197-204, 1964.

Chapter 3

BEHAVIOR MODIFICATION OF AN AUTISTIC CHILD*

ELEANOR R. BRAWLEY, FLORENCE R. HARRIS,
K. EILEEN ALLEN, ROBERT S. FLEMING, *and*
ROBERT F. PETERSON

THE CHILD WHO SUFFERS from early infantile autism presents one of the most difficult treatment cases. He may display few appropriate behaviors and a host of inappropriate behaviors. Infantile autism was first proposed as a separate diagnostic entity in 1943 by Rimland (1964). He listed as characteristic of the disease (1) onset before the second year of life, (2) profound withdrawal from contact with people, (3) either mutism or uncommunicative speech as echolalia, (4) stereotyped preoccupation with certain inanimate objects, and (5) evidence of potential intelligence. Tantrum and self-destructive behaviors may also be evidenced.

Traditional forms of psychotherapy have had little success in dealing with these problems. Kanner (1949) has pointed out that autistic children who received intensive psychiatric treatment have not improved as much as those who received little or no treatment. In recent years, however, techniques derived from operant learning principles have had some success in treating the autistic child. It has been possible to enlarge the range of the child's behaviors (Ferster and DeMyer, 1962), to decrease tantrums and self-injurious behaviors (Wolf, Risley, and Mees, 1964), and to teach reading (Hewett, 1965).

*From *Behavioral Science*, 1969, 14, pp. 87-97. Reprinted by permission of the Journal and the author.

The present study was designed to further explore and extend operant learning techniques as a form of therapy for an autistic child. Social reinforcement in the form of adult attention was the primary therapeutic tool, although food was also used. These reinforcers were given contingent upon all desirable behaviors and withheld during and for 15 seconds following inappropriate responses. In addition, the authors attempted to demonstrate the importance and function of the reinforcers by reversing their effects for a short time.

Subject

The subject, Steve, was a slender, seven-year-old boy with blonde hair and brown eyes. At two-and-one-half he had been diagnosed by a pediatrician as suffering from early infantile autism. At five years he was admitted to the Children's Psychiatric Day Care Unit of a hospital, where psychiatrists confirmed the earlier diagnosis. At the time of the present study, he had been attending the Day Care Unit daily for 17 months. An *EEG* and an *LP* taken during that time were both normal.

Steve was the seventh of eight children who ranged in age from five to 20 years. The other children were apparently normal; the child a year older than Steve was enrolled in an accelerated school program. Both parents were college graduates, the father a professional man, and both seemed to be warm, responsive people.

The parents reported that, while the pregnancy and the birth were apparently normal, Steve had from his earliest days behaved in a "different" fashion, not responding to affection and cuddling as the other children had. He walked at 16 months and was toilet-trained by two. He spoke a few words at that time and could verbally indicate some of his desires. By his second birthday, the parents were concerned about his development, thinking that he was retarded.

At the time the present study began, the parents reported that Steve was exceedingly difficult to handle in the home. He did not play with toys, had frequent severe tantrums and crying episodes, rarely spoke a word, generally ignored the parents and family members, and did not seem to discriminate one member of the family from another.

Observations of Steve's behavior on the ward showed that he was extremely withdrawn. Steve rarely used speech and spent long periods lying on couches staring at the wall. He handled materials and toys infrequently. At irregular intervals he would repeatedly slap himself forcefully about the face and head, crying loudly while doing so. He also displayed bizarre body and hand movements, as well as spitting, and licking the wall.

Procedure

Steve was seen by the therapist three times a week, each session lasting an hour. Sessions were conducted in a room off the main hospital ward. The room was pleasant, with windows across one end, and was large enough for active play. It was furnished with a table, two chairs, a sink, and a variety of materials used in the therapy sessions.

In addition to modification of Steve's behaviors in the experimental sessions, an attempt was made to GENERALIZE his behaviors by involving other ward personnel in the reinforcement procedures during the rest of the day. This staff included a teacher, a psychiatrist, two nurses, and an occupational therapist. This group met weekly with the authors to discuss the child's treatment program.

The study began with a selection of behaviors which were to be either strengthened or weakened. They were defined as follows:

Appropriate behaviors

(*a*) Appropriate verbalization—the enunciation of a comprehensible word or words.
(*b*) Appropriate use of materials—use of materials as they were intended to be used, for example, riding a tricycle, looking at a book, building with blocks and so on.
(*c*) Compliance—the following of a request or command.

Inappropriate behaviors

(*a*) Self-hitting—striking, slapping, or patting any part of the body.
(*b*) Junk verbalizations—the emission of sounds or combinations of sounds that are not standard words, such as spitting and hissing sounds.
(*c*) Withdrawal—lying facing the wall or staring, with no other activity; sitting, standing, or staring with no other activity.
(*d*) Tantrum—self-hitting plus any one or more of the following: loud crying, kicking, or throwing himself or objects about.

Since social reinforcement was given in the form of adult attention, it was defined as one or more of the following:

(a) Touching the child.

(b) Being within two feet of and facing the child.

(c) Talking to, touching, assisting, or going to the child.

Recording

The behaviors of both child and adult were observed, coded and recorded during successive 10-second intervals of each session. The observer sat in the room in an unobtrusive position where she could both see and hear well. The recording system has been previously described by Allen, Hart, Buell, Harris, and Wolf (1964), and in greater detail in Sloane and MacAulay (1968). In order to secure reliability measures, two independent observers recorded behaviors during nine sessions spaced throughout the study. The percentage of agreement of records, interval by interval, ranged from 70 per cent to 98 per cent, with an average of 85 per cent.

The study was conducted over a three-month period and was divided into four phases, a baseline and first reinforcement period, followed by the reversal and second reinforcement periods.

Baseline period

During this portion of the study, the behaviors of both child and staff were observed and recorded while they were interacting on the ward. This continued over a period of seven one-hour sessions. The observations were taken during free play sessions at the same hour of each day.

First reinforcement period

This phase consisted of 21 sessions conducted over a 10-week interval. During the first few sessions the therapist checked the potential reinforcing effectiveness of a number of FOODS such as potato chips, ice cream, candy, and so on, by noting which Steve preferred. Potato chips seemed most desired. The therapist thereafter PRESENT-ED PRAISE and a potato chip simultaneously following desired responses. In subsequent sessions praise was used CONTINUOUSLY while food was delivered on a variable basis. However, during a new task or whenever the child's response appeared to be particularly appropriate, such as, spontaneous speech regarding materials, the child received both food and praise. Concurrently, the therapist turned away from Steve and did not look at or speak to him whenever and so long as he emitted behavior defined as inappropriate. When appropriate behavior again recurred, the therapist looked up and without comment continued the activity from where it had been interrupted.

An effort was made to elicit as much speech as possible from Steve throughout the entire session. To begin with, every time he uttered a comprehensible word the therapist presented him with a potato chip, smiled and said, "That's right, Steve; I heard you; good for you," or some similar approving statement.

Because Steve evidenced some interest in music, the first session began with the therapist singing and playing an autoharp. This activity continued as long as Steve appeared to attend to it. If he engaged in bizarre behaviors the singing stopped and the therapist turned away. Singing was resumed when the inappropriate behavior terminated. Later in the session the therapist engaged Steve in a number of concrete tasks such as blowing soap bubbles, tracing shapes, and clapping hands. In each case the therapist MODELED the response, helped the child perform it, and praised him and gave him food for doing so. After 20 minutes of these activities Steve was taken back to the ward.

During the second session Steve was presented with a notebook which contained the teaching materials to be used at the table during the first half of the session. During the latter half of the session, play materials were again presented and play skills emphasized. Gradually, the time spent in the experimental room was increased until by the sixth session Steve remained for one hour, spending the first half hour seated at the table across from the therapist and working on the language and reading materials and the second half hour working on gross motor play activities. All subsequent sessions followed this pattern.

Language and reading procedures

To stimulate verbal responses, the therapist worked first to develop attending and IMITATING BEHAVIORS. Each day she presented a range of selected actions to imitate (actions like slapping or rapping on the table and making letter and word sounds) and materials to respond to (such as familiar objects, pictures of objects, activities, colors, and shapes). Presentations were programmed from SIMPLE IMITATION AND THE GROSS ACTIONS DEMONSTRATED BY THE THERA-

PIST TO MIMICKING SOUNDS AND THEN WORDS SHE ENUNCIATED. Soon Steve was able to mimic names of objects and pictures, names for colors and shapes, and finally phrases and sentences about items presented. Steve's speech repertoire soon included immediate and correct identification of primary and secondary colors, circles, squares, triangles, rectangles, and ovals. He then progressed to sorting colors or shapes, verbalizing each name as he did so.

In describing pictures, Steve was first asked to mimic one or two word combinations. Gradually these were expanded into complete sentences about the pictures. Finally, the whole sentence was mimicked before the response was reinforced. Then PROGRESSIVELY THE THERAPIST SHORTENED THE CUE until Steve could give the entire sentence in response to an appropriate but dissimilar verbal or visual cue. For example:

The therapist: "My name is Steve."
The child: "My name is Steve."
The therapist: "My name is ————."
The child: "My name is Steve."
The therapist: "My name —— ————."
The child: "My name is Steve."
The therapist: "My ——— —— ————."
The child: "My name is Steve."
The therapist: "What is your name?
   My ——— —— ————."
The child: "My name is Steve."
The therapist: "What is your name?"
The child: "My name is Steve."

These techniques were based in part on the earlier work of Risley (1966), the general procedure being to increase the difficulty of tasks as Steve became more competent.

Similar procedures were used in teaching the child a variety of conversational responses such as where he lived, his age, and descriptions of his play activities.

Because Steve responded to music, singing was part of each session. It was useful in building imitative behaviors as well as for using complete sentences and sustained speech. Voice inflection also seemed responsive to singing. Steve was soon able to sing several folk songs and asked for favorites at the beginning of each session.

Steve responded so well to the visual discrimination tasks such as sorting and matching shapes and pictures that letters were presented for matching. Since he readily performed this task, the therapist introduced the complete alphabet. The phonic sound and name of each letter were presented. Sandpaper letters were used so that Steve could trace with his finger in preparation for writing. Within two-and-one-half weeks Steve could name without error both the upper- and lower-case letters of the alphabet. "Letter *D*, *D* makes the duh sound," was the form of his response.

Pictures of things beginning with *D* were then presented for naming. On several occasions he named other words that began with the sound, without receiving a visual cue from the therapist. After Steve had mastered the picture cards, the printed words were presented without the accompanying picture. Word matching, sorting, and matching word to picture were all activities that were used.

Finally, Steve was reading short sentences which the therapist put into book form, each day adding one or two new words to be read in sentences. The words used were ones which came out of Steve's experiences. For instance, the day after he had a tooth pulled, the word "tooth" was traced, sorted from other known words and then read in a sentence. He did this readily. Writing with a crayon and pencil were worked on in later sessions. Since Steve had hardly held a crayon in his hand before, he needed considerable practice in this area. He became able to draw a human figure and a house when asked.

Use of materials

During the second half of the session, Steve was directed to engage in gross motor activities such as situps, hopping, skipping, running, throwing a ball, walking a balance beam, and turning somersaults. Next Steve was instructed in the use of creative materials including fingerpaint, clay, crayons, and cutting and pasting. The therapist demonstrated, made suggestions, and reinforced Steve for the appropriate use of each material, for example, "Let's make a big circle in the finger-paint (holding Steve's hand). Now make one yourself." Each attempt by the child was followed by social and (at this time) food reinforcement. Other activities such as block building, car and truck play, bead stringing, and water play were also included.

Even though the latter half of the session involved play activities, it was also oriented toward the use of receptive language and speech. The therapist required some verbal approximation before she would initiate certain activities—such as, "water on," "open door," "swing me"—before she turned on the tap, opened the closet door, or gave the child a swing around the room.

If Steve engaged in tantrum behaviors during a session, he was isolated in a nearby empty room until he was quiet for a two-minute period. He was then allowed to return to the experimental session.

Reversal period

In order to determine whether the reinforcement operations were a significant factor in the development of Steve's newly acquired verbal and motor responses, a four-day partial REVERSAL of the reinforcement contingency was carried out. It was deemed undesirable to reverse all of his new behaviors because of the severity of Steve's problems. Therefore, appropriate use of material continued to receive social and food reinforcement as before, except when accompanied by appropriate verbalizations. Appropriate verbalizations, however, were given no reinforcement. Inappropriate behaviors were now reinforced.

Thus, the therapist talked to Steve and presented the same cues for speech as before, but when he responded verbally, the therapist withdrew her attention and did not look at him or comment on his verbal behavior. Instead she focused on "busy work" beside the table. When Steve hit himself the therapist verbalized solicitous concern: "You don't have to hit yourself, Steve. Do you feel angry with yourself? Was that (task) too hard?" In addition, the therapist attempted to keep the amount of reinforcement per session, the variety of materials presented, the program format, and the gradient of presentation of new work the same as that of the first reinforcement period.

Second reinforcement period

Continuous social and intermittent primary reinforcement was again instituted for comprehensible verbal behavior and appropriate use of materials. All contingencies were identical to those of the first reinforcement period. The second reinforcement period continued for five sessions.

Results

Figure 51 shows total appropriate behaviors and total inappropriate behaviors emitted by Steve during the baseline and initial reinforcement period. The per cent of adult attention directed to each class is also represented.

Total appropriate behavior was derived by adding the 10-second intervals in which one or more appropriate behaviors and no inappropriate behaviors occurred. Total inappropriate behavior was the sum of the 10-second intervals in which one or more inappropriate behaviors occurred. If both appropriate and inappropriate behaviors occurred in a given interval, that interval was counted as an interval of inappropriate behavior. Because of slight variation in the total number of intervals recorded per session, data were compiled as percentages. The percentages were derived by dividing the total intervals in which a given behavior occurred by the total intervals per session. During the seven sessions of baseline, total appropriate behavior (filled circles) averaged 28 per cent of each session, and total inappropriate behavior (open circles) averaged 46 per cent. The data also indicate that inappropriate behavior received, on the average, approximately twice as much attention as appropriate behavior, since each class received attention about half the time.

On the first day (Session 8) of reinforcement procedures, total appropriate behavior rose abruptly to 68 per cent, an increase of 46 per cent over the last day of baseline. Total appropriate behaviors ranged between 50 per cent and 80 per cent throughout the reinforcement period, averaging 70 per cent. Almost all appropriate behavior received attention throughout the period. After the first few experimental sessions, inappropriate behavior was attended to less than 1 per cent (on the average) of the time.

Figure 52 shows total appropriate verbalization in relation to the total appropriate behavior throughout the study. During baseline, total appropriate verbalization averaged two per cent. There was an immediate increase to 10 per cent on the first day of reinforcement, followed by a jump to 40 per cent on the sixth day (Session 13). The percentage of appropriate verbalization continued to increase averaging 46 per cent per session in the eight sessions prior to reversal. While the data show a steady quantitative increase in appropriate verbalization, qualitative improvement, although present, was not measured. Thus, one word spoken during a 10-second interval of an early session was given the same score as two compound sentences

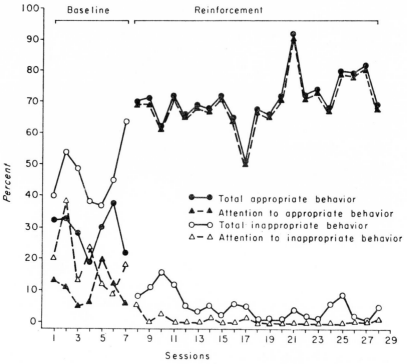

Figure 51. Total appropriate and inappropriate behaviors and the attention given to each.

recorded during the final session. Both the therapist and observer noted, however, a rapid sequential development of more complex verbal skills. Steve progressed from the naming of simple objects to the mimicking of short phrases and sentences. He was able to describe pictures, ask as well as answer questions, read words, phrases, and finally groups of sentences. In a short time he exhibited surprising skills in performing word-discrimination and memory tasks, often requesting this kind of activity. These results sharply contrast with Kanner and Eisenberg's (1955) findings which indicate that autistic children who have not acquired speech by the age of four are unlikely to do so.

On the first day of reversal (Session 29) appropriate verbalization immediately decreased to 20 per cent of the session. It dropped to 16 per cent on the fourth and last session. When reinforcement was resumed (Session 33), the percentage rose immediately to its former

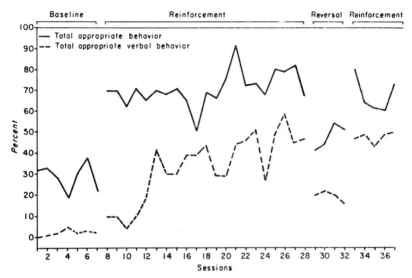

Figure 52. Total appropriate behaviors (appropriate use of materials plus appropriate verbalizations) compared with appropriate verbalizations.

level of 47 per cent, with an average of 47 per cent during the second reinforcement period.

The rate of appropriate verbalization tended to recover between each reversal session. This is shown in Figure 53. This graph compares verbalization rates during the first 35 minutes of four pre-reversal, four reversal, and the four post-reversal sessions. The data indicate that during the first five minutes of each reversal session, Steve's rate of comprehensible speech was similar to that of pre- and post-reversal sessions, even though it was receiving no attention. In the second five minutes, the rate during reversal dropped sharply as contrasted with the rates during the reinforcement periods. Although the data are expressed in averages for five-minute blocks of time of the several days, the same phenomenon occurred daily during each reversal session. The graph also shows the decrease in rate following the first 25 minutes of the session. This decrease coincided with the transition from table work to large motor activities.

The EXTINCTION of three inappropriate behaviors, withdrawal, self-hitting, and junk garble (verbalizations), is displayed in Figure 54. During the baseline period, withdrawn behavior occurred an average of 25 per cent of the time, with a high of 36 per cent during the last session. With the inauguration of extinction procedures, withdrawn behavior immediately dropped to less than one per cent (dur-

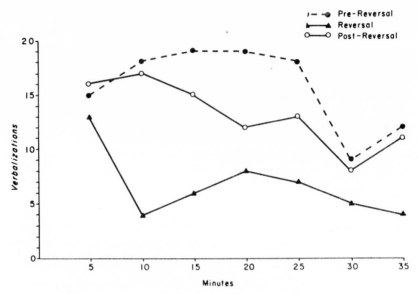

Figure 53. Frequency of verbalizations during successive five minute intervals of four pre-reversal, reversal, and post-reversal sessions.

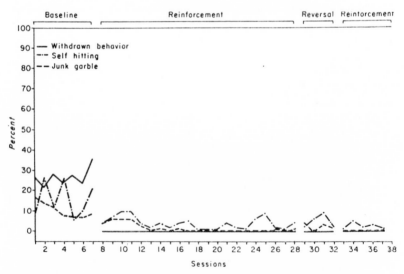

Figure 54. Per cent of inappropriate behavior during baseline, extinction, and reversal.

ing the first session) and did not occur again.

Steve's rate of self-hitting averaged 15 per cent during baseline, with highs of 20 per cent in two sessions. Self-hitting was subsequently reduced during the extinction procedures to an average of three per cent. During the reversal period when self-hitting was again followed by attention, it averaged about five per cent with one high of 10 per cent. In the second extinction period, it averaged three per cent, varying between zero and five per cent. During the course of the study, the topography of self-hitting also changed. The intensity of self-slapping diminished considerably; often they were no more than gentle pats.

Junk verbal responses averaged 10 per cent during baseline and did not show the erratic variability of the self-hitting behavior. Like the others, junk verbal behavior also dropped on the first day of reinforcement. By the sixth day of reinforcement (Session 13), it had decreased to less than one per cent and it remained stable thereafter. It increased slightly during reversal on three out of four days, but dropped out immediately with the return of the extinction procedures.

Tantrum behaviors are not represented in the graphs since they occurred only once during reinforcement sessions. During baseline they averaged three per cent. These behaviors did not reappear during the treatment sessions and were reported to occur less frequently when Steve was on the ward.

Follow-up data were obtained in a three-month period following this study. During this time the therapist continued working with Steve to expand his newly acquired behaviors and to increase his interaction with other children. Post checks taken during eight sessions showed that appropriate verbal behavior remained in the 40 to 50 percentiles, with total appropriate behavior in the 60 to 70 percentiles. Inappropriate behaviors remained under five per cent. Following this period Steve was discharged from the hospital to a special school where he has remained in attendance.

Further Follow-up Details

To extend Steve's social behaviors to other children, the therapist first included another child in his training sessions. The child selected for this special training had well developed verbal and play skills and could provide a good model for Steve. Adult attention was given to

Steve as an immediate consequence of his approaching to within three feet of the other child and playing beside him, as well as for verbalizing to him. Verbalizations of greeting and of suggestions for play were at first CUED by the teacher and reinforcement delivered for his imitation, as had been done in the individual situations. Gradually the cue was diminished and Steve's words became more spontaneous. Concurrently, he was given attention on the ward for use of these phrases with any other child. The nurses were also encouraged to cue his use of the phrases with other children. The records indicated steady increase in his verbal interactions with other children, as well as increasing social play.

During this same follow-up period the therapist worked twice a week with the mother and Steve. The therapist first discussed and demonstrated the methods being used to elicit and reinforce speech and language. With guidance from the therapist, who observed through a one-way screen, the mother then conducted learning sessions with Steve. The mother readily learned to maintain appropriate contingencies. Indeed, so improved was Steve's general behavior as a consequence of the reinforcement guidance that the mother communicated her learnings to the whole family.

That the mother had successfully carried effective attending procedures into the home was evident to the therapist when she accepted an invitation to dinner. At the table Steve suddenly emitted the bizarre behavior of vigorously shaking both hands and his head. As one person, all members of the family immediately turned away from him. When shortly he stopped, they turned back and resumed their usual interactions, giving attention to any appropriate comment he made and to other appropriate behaviors. When dessert was served, Steve grabbed for a piece of pie. The mother withheld it, asking, "What do you want, Steve?" "I want a piece of brown and white chocolate pudding pie," he responded, and was given the pie he so accurately described. He interacted with various family members, and looked toward or went to those whose names were used.

By the close of the follow-up period, Steve not only accepted but gave affectionate greetings and responses to the therapist, his nurses, and members of his family. Occasionally he cried when his mother left in the morning. He always ran to greet her when she came for him in the afternoon.

Reports from the special school, which motivates the acquisition of study behaviors and basic academic skills through control of environmental consequences, indicate that Steve is progressing well. His speech is reported to be appropriate and functional though not extensive. He reads, does arithmetic, and writes and spells at primary levels. Although he is not yet "a normal child," he continues to expand his repertoire of "normal" behaviors.

Discussion

The results of this study indicate that the systematic application of reinforcement procedures along with a carefully sequenced program of materials can bring about striking changes in an autistic child. In addition to the increase in verbal and academic skills, Steve also displayed an increased tendency to seek attention from others in his environment. He often ran to greet the therapist and was observed to give and receive affection from the hospital staff and members of his family. It should be noted that an important element in effecting such behavioral changes is the establishment of the therapist as a social reinforcer. For this reason FOOD was paired with the social responses of the therapist during the initial portion of the study, in an attempt to strengthen the reinforcing properties of her behavior. However, the therapist must do more than simply function as a social reinforcer. Data from the reversal period suggest that she must apply reinforcers in a selective fashion. Figures 52 and 54 show the effects of withdrawing reinforcement from one set of behaviors and applying them to another. Even though the total amount of reinforcement (about 70 per cent of the session) remained the same, appropriate verbal responses weakened while inappropriate behaviors began to increase. Thus, what is apparently most important in effecting behavior modification is not the amount of reinforcement but its delivery contingent upon certain behaviors. This finding concurs with those of Johnston, Kelley, Harris, and Wolf (1966) and Hart, Reynolds, Brawley, Harris, and Baer (1968).

The operation of some reinforcement contingencies may, however, interfere with the effectiveness of others. Thus, the failure of inappropriate behaviors to return to baseline levels during reversal may have been due to the reinforcement Steve was receiving for the use of materials. To a large degree, USING MATERIALS APPROPRIATE-LY IS INCOMPATIBLE WITH BIZARRE BEHAVIORS in that the child cannot engage in both simultaneously. Reinforcement for using materials may also have been responsible for the sharp declines in inappropriate behaviors during the first reinforcement period.

The effectiveness of a reinforcement procedure may also depend upon the current strength of a given behavior in the child's REPERTOIRE. One should distinguish between those behaviors where the child lacks most of the basic components of the response and behaviors where basic response components are present. In either case the behavior may occur at a low rate. With Steve, appropriate verbal behavior provides a good case of the former while appropriate use of materials exemplifies the latter. Figure 52 shows that almost no appropriate verbalizations were observed during baseline. Those that were observed were extremely primitive. Only after considerable training was it possible to develop the basic verbal components and then expand them into more complicated behaviors. In contrast, use of materials required less training and increased sharply as soon as reinforcement was instituted. This result suggests that Steve was previously capable of such behaviors but that the behaviors were not being adequately reinforced.

Observations of staff behaviors indicate that although episodes of withdrawal and self-hitting often brought adult attention in the form of cuddling, reassurance and restraint, appropriate behaviors tended to receive considerably less notice (Figure 51). This finding may indicate one reason why certain forms of intensive psychiatric treatment do not improve the autistic child (Kanner and Eisenberg). Such a finding also raises questions about psychotherapeutic methods which involve encouraging, "working through," or interpreting to the child his undesirable behaviors. If this procedure involves attending to psychotic behavior, the therapist may inadvertently strengthen undesirable responses and at the same time weaken appropriate behaviors.

References

Allen, K. Eileen, Hart, Betty M., Buell, Joan S., Harris, Florence R. and Wolf, M. M.: Effects of social reinforcement on isolate behavior of a nursery school child. *Child Dev 35*, 511-518, 1964.

Ferster, C. B. and DeMeyer, Marian K.: A method for the experimental analysis of the behavior of autistic children. *Am J Orthopsychiat 32*, 89-98, 1962.

Hart, Betty M., Reynolds, Nancy J., Brawley, Eleanor R., Harris, Florence R. and Baer, D. M.: Effects of contingent and non-contingent social reinforcement or the isolate behavior of a nursery school girl. *J Appl Behav Anal 1*, 73-76, 1968.

Hewett, F. M.: Teaching speech to an autistic child through operant conditioning. *Am J Orthopsychiat 35*, 927-936, 1965.

Johnston, Margaret K., Kelley, C. Susan, Harris, Florence R. and Wolf, M. M.: An application of reinforcement principles to development of motor skills of a young child. *Child Devel 37*, 379-388, 1966.

Kanner, L.: Problems of nosology and psychodynamics of early infantile autism. *Am J Orthopsychiat 19*, 416-426, 1949.

Kanner, L. and Eisenberg, L.: *Psychotherapy of childhood.* New York, Grove & Stratton, 1955.

Rimland, B.: *Infantile autism.* New York, Appleton-Century-Crofts, 1964.

Risley, T.: The establishment of verbal behavior in deviant children. Unpublished doctoral dissertation, University of Washington, 1966.

Sloane, H. and MacAulay, B. (Eds.): *Operant procedures in remedial speech and language training.* New York, Houghton Mifflin, 1968, Chap. 3.

Wolf, M. M., Risley, T. and Mees, H.: Application of operant conditioning procedures to the behavior problems of an autistic child. *Behav Res Therapy 1*, 305-312, 1964.

Chapter 4

USE OF PAIN AND PUNISHMENT AS TREATMENT TECHNIQUES WITH CHILDHOOD SCHIZOPHRENICS*

JAMES Q. SIMMONS, III, M.D. *and* O. IVAR LOVAAS, Ph.D.

Introduction

IN RECENT YEARS, considerable attention has been directed toward the use of reinforcement therapy with children who fall within the broad category of disorders called childhood schizophrenia. For the most part, this approach has utilized positive reinforcement in the form of providing food, social approbation, or pleasurable activities for acceptable behaviors.[1-6] However, the reinforcement paradigm provides another set of alternatives which has been minimally explored—the use of negative reinforcers or aversive stimuli to suppress unacceptable behaviors through punishment, and to facilitate the learning of acceptable behaviors through an ESCAPE or AVOIDANCE situation.

According to Church,[7] there are basically three reasons why the use of punishment finds considerable opposition among psychologists: "(a) It is less effective than some of the alternatives; (b) It produces undesirable side-effects other than the reduction of the

*From the *American Journal of Psychotherapy*, 1969, 23, 23-36. Reprinted by permission of the Journal.

strength of the response, and (c) it is unkind to the individual." These objections are, in part, supported by experimental evidence in which punishment results in response facilitation. This will be referred to later in the discussion. Perhaps the most serious objections result from commentaries such as those of Bandura,[8] that punishment as a behavorial control device provides a model for aggressive behavior and may either augment the very response which the treatment was designed to control or lead to the establishment of other undesirable behaviors. For the most part, this statement is made in the context that punishment is primarily used to manage aggression.

The history of psychiatry offers much anecdotal evidence of the failure of punitive techniques to modify abnormal behavior. This type of evidence, combined with the comment by Szasz[9] in *Pain and Pleasure*, that medicine is "a socially structured defense against pain," makes it unacceptable on a social or ethical level to consider using pain as a tool to facilitate treatment. In addition to objections of a social or ethical nature, numerous theoretical formulations have postulated pain as a major factor in the etiology of psychopathology. For example, Freud,[10] in *Beyond the Pleasure Principle*, noted, "The specific unpleasure of physical pain is probably the result of the protective shield having been broken through in a limited area. There is then a continuous stream of excitation—an anti-cathexis on a grand scale is set up—all the other physical systems are impoverished" (p. 36). Further, Freud states, "We describe as traumatic any excitations from outside which are painful enough to break through the protective shield," and "such an event as external trauma is bound to provoke a disturbance in a large scale in the functioning—and to set in motion every possible defensive measure" (p. 35).

Despite these theoretical and social objections, some findings seem to indicate that PAIN, WHEN USED AS PUNISHMENT, may serve some useful function in the modification of behavior. From an experimental point of view, the reviews of Solomon,[11] Church,[7] and Azrin and Holz,[12] would support this contention. Without attempting to do justice to these exhaustive surveys of punishment—and the experimental literature on punishment is extensive—one can draw the following conclusions: (1) In general, punishment tends to alter behavior by suppressing responsiveness. The greater the intensity of the painful stimulus, the more effective it is in response suppression. (2)

If punishment is given on a RESPONSE CONTINGENT BASIS, there is greater suppression of the specific response being punished and less suppression of responses not being punished. Under these conditions there is less generalization of the emotional response to the painful stimulus. (3) In a situation where the individual has more than one response available, punishment for a "wrong" response facilitates RESPONSE DIFFERENTIATION. (4) There is an inverse relationship between the amount of response reduction and the time interval between response and punishment; the shorter the interval, the more response reduction.

Despite this evidence, the use of punishment to modify deviant human behavior has been quite restricted. Perhaps this comes about because much of these data are based on animal research. However, the use of punishment in the society at large can be fairly well judged by Will Durant's comments in his *History of Civilization*.[13] Durant quotes an early Egyptian manuscript as follows: "The youth has a back and attends when he is beaten, for the ears of the young are placed on the back," and a former student who wrote to his teacher saying—"Thou did'st beat my back and thy instructions went in my ear." Over the several thousand years since these observations were made, we are still faced with the fact that punishment is fairly commonly used. This is exemplified by the results of the survey of Sears, *et al.*[14] on child rearing. The bulk of the mothers surveyed utilized physical punishment on their children at one time or another (p. 325), and the majority reported that it helped in rearing children. Despite this long history of usage, actual studies on punishment with human beings have been somewhat limited. The possible use of punishment as a treatment technique has been almost completely ignored.

Some studies have been done on the use of painful stimuli in the classical (respondent) conditioning situation, in such problems as alcoholism[15] and the sexual perversions.[16] These are basically extensions of the wellknown studies using chemical substances as aversive stimuli, particularly in alcoholism (alcohol paired with noxious stimuli in an attempt to make alcohol elicit the same aversive reaction as the noxious stimuli). Less known are the uses of punishment in an operant conditioning paradigm, which is at times difficult to distinguish from the respondent paradigm. The case reported by Boardman[17] in 1957 represents one of the few examples of the operant approach appearing in the scientific literature. In this instance, the author utilized spanking, administered contingent upon aggressive behavior, in an attempt to control that behavior. The investigator also attempted to arrange desirable behavioral alternatives to aggression. The spanking was carried out by the child's parent. Although the behavior was brought under control, it was unclear that punishment was the decisive variable.

Recently, there has been increased interest in the possible use of punishment with children.[18, 6, 19, 20] Risley presented a case of a six-year-old child with the diagnosis of autism where one of the major behavioral problems centered on climbing into high places, which could have injured the child. Various experimental manipulations suggested that the behavior was intrinsically reinforcing. For example, it did not seem to be maintained by the parents' concern for its presence or absence. Mild but painful electric shock|| was delivered contingent upon the recurrence of self-destruction, and the rate of the dangerous behavior was reduced to zero. Even though the experimenter administered the punishment, he apparently did not become aversive, at least as measured by the increase and persistence of eye-to-face contact the child made with him subsequent to the procedure. Perhaps this came about because the experimenter also fed and otherwise cared for the child. Risley also established a negative secondary reinforcer of sitting in a particular chair and was able to use that event as punishment, thus reducing the use of shock.

The study by Lovaas, Schaeffer, and Simmons[20] involved the use of aversive stimuli in the form of an electrified floor grid to manipulate various behaviors in a pair of five-year-old autistic twins. The results of this study were fairly clear-cut and can be summarized as follows: first, stereotyped behavior (autoeroticism) could be suppressed by the application of painful stimuli contingent upon the appearance of the behavior. Secondly, the children developed a specific kind of relationship to those people who manipulated the pain (that is, presented pain contingent upon undesirable behavior and withdrew it contingent upon acceptable conduct). This relationship could best be described as affectionate. The children would hug and smile while sitting in the safe haven of the adult's lap. This type of response on the part of a child was maintained for considerable

|| 300 to 400 volts at very low amperage.

periods of time with minimal shock application. It also generalized from the laboratory setting and the experimental staff to the children's ward and the nursing staff. It was demonstrated in the study that such words as "no" acquired punishment properties when paired with painful stimuli, which allowed the adults to delete shock in much subsequent work with the children.

On the basis of similar evidence from animal work and the Lovaas and Risley studies, painful stimuli have been used in experimental treatment of nine children at the Neuropsychiatric Institute, UCLA, and it is judged useful to summarize and discuss these findings and their implications for treatment.

Subjects

The group of nine children used in these studies consisted of eight boys and one girl between the ages of four and ten. All of these children had been diagnosed as childhood schizophrenics in the broad sense defined by Blau,[21] Goldfarb,[22] or Menolascino.[23] The children were characterized behaviorally by (1) abnormalities in speech manifested by mutism or echolalia; (2) failure to develop the usual social behaviors such as habit patterns (toilet training, table manners, and so forth) and the social amenities; (3) failure to develop appropriate play; (4) the presence of repetitive stereotyped bodily movements; (5) failure to develop social responsiveness, and (6) abnormalities of attention frequently manifested by absence of startle response, peculiarities in orienting and habituation to external events,[24] and at times the reverse, with intense preoccupation with a limited source of certain external events, such as staring at a light or listening to a ventilation duct. Historically, the children showed a somewhat diverse picture, but generally, indicators of the disorder developed within the first year of life.

For the most part, the decision to use painful stimuli was made when (1) it was found that the child consistently failed to attend cues from his environment, namely, consistently "drifted," was grossly inattentive during school-like training offered him, or (2) showed a high incidence of repetitive stereotyped movements which interfered with the establishment of other behaviors, and (3) if he engaged in self-destructive behavior to the extent of endangering his own health. Even with these characteristics present, more evidence was required before the decision to use shock was made. Specifically,

(a) the judgment that extinction procedures would be too protracted and thus harmful to the patient; (b) the child remained unresponsive after three to four months of treatment (not using shock), and (c) extensive staff discussion of the problem. When the decision was finally made to utilize this approach, it was discussed with the parents, and their written consent was obtained to carry out the program.

Application of Painful Stimuli

The aversive stimuli utilized in our laboratory can be ranked in degree of aversion from a loud "no" to a slap on the hand or bottom, to mild but painful electric shock. The child's responsivity to any of these stimuli determined the level employed, that is, we did not employ electric shock if a slap would suffice.

The electric stimulus was delivered in one of three ways: (1) an electrified grid was placed on the floor of the lab consisting of an adhesive tape coated on one surface with a conducting substance. The grid was connected to an electric source consisting of a six-volt battery and a Harvard inductorium. The child was placed in the room with his shoes and socks off. The painful stimulus was delivered for a brief period of time through the feet, and it was impossible for the child to tell who delivered the stimulus; (2) a remote control device, the Lee Lectronic Trainer* which delivered a signal from a hand-held device to a cigarette-sized receiver taped to the child's waist. The shock was delivered to the buttocks through two copper electrodes fastened there. Again, the electric stimulus (which was of the same order of magnitude as the "shock stick") was brief and the child did not know who was delivering the stimulus; (3) the so-called "shock-stick" was the most useful device. It is commercially available and is a battery powered instrument in which a painful shock could be delivered by touching two electrodes at the top of the stick to the child's leg. In contrast to the other two methods of delivery, it was clearly apparent to the child who was delivering the painful application.

Slapping the child was carried out by striking him either on the buttocks or the extremities. It is not too difficult to see that this popular social technique was fraught with difficulties. These included quantification of the stimulus and physical injury to the child.

*Lee Supply Company, Tucson, Arizona.

All of the above stimuli can be called PRIMARY REINFORCERS, and as such, are used sparingly. Whenever they are used, they are coupled with a number of verbal and nonverbal actions on the part of the attending adult. These actions include verbal admonitions such as "no," "don't do that," "stop that," and nonverbal gestures such as a stern visage or a threatening move. By association, these actions take on some of the aversive characteristics of the primary stimuli and become established as SECONDARY NEGATIVE (PUNISHING) REINFORCERS. The obvious result is that there can be a reduction in the use of primary aversive stimuli and increased reliance on more common social behavioral controls such as disapproval.

Four Clinical Cases

In order to best exemplify the clinical usefulness of punishment, a description of four situations will be undertaken. The first relates to the study by Lovaas, Schaeffer, and Simmons,[20] involving a pair of five-year-old autistic twins. The main characteristics of these twins were aloofness toward any other human being, failure to respond to social direction of any sort, and a high percentage of time engaging in repetitive stereotyped motor behavior. Electric shock was used to intervene in each of these areas, but the one to be focused upon here is the alteration of the aloofness directed toward human beings. Initially, the children were placed in the laboratory with two adults who asked them to "come here"—gesturing with outstretched arms. There was no observable response. Shock was applied and remained on until the child went to one or the other adult, thus establishing escape from shock. The child was physically prompted to approach the adult if he failed to engage in the escape behavior. The child learned rather quickly to avoid the shock altogether by approaching the attending adult. Once these behaviors were learned, they were very durable, lasting almost a year. When the responses extinguished, they could be reinstated with a single shock. Since pain was reduced by the child's approach to the adults, it was reasoned that the adult would be discriminate for pain reduction and, thus, take on positive reinforcing characteristics. This was clearly demonstrated in the RESISTANCE TO EXTINCTION of a new response to receive a view of the experimenter's face.

The response to human beings developed in the laboratory generalized to the nonlaboratory situation and has been maintained in part for a three-year period. Currently, one of the twins remains in the hospital and, at the age of nine, shows positive affectionate responses to adults in his environment which appear to be a continuation of the behaviors established in the original experimental situation.

The second clinical situation involved a nine-year-old girl, Pamela, one of identical twins, with a history of delayed motor development, poor socialization, and a high incidence of self-stimulatory behavior. Within the first two years she developed bizarre repetitive movements, hyperactivity, and temper tantrums. Speech development was delayed and when it was established, consisted mainly of echolalia. The child was treated fairly intensively over a six-year period both as an outpatient and on an inpatient basis with little modification of the total picture. She was seen in our research program for approximately 15 months, during which time it became obvious that the repetitive stereotyped movements which she displayed for considerable periods of time were interfering with attempts to gain her attention and alter her general behavior pattern. Initially, her attention and task performance could be maintained using primary reinforcers such as food, but she would not respond to social reinforcement. Instead, she spent quite lengthy periods of time staring into space, flapping her hands in front of her eyes, grimacing, and laughing. Apparently, these behaviors were more reinforcing than the social rewards, and, consequently, it was decided to apply a painful stimulus to suppress this type of behavior and permit the establishment of potentially more useful behaviors maintained by social reinforcement.

In the training session, slaps and the word "no" were delivered contingent upon the appearance of unacceptable interfering behaviors. Within a brief period of time these behaviors diminished in number and could soon be suppressed using the words "no" and "stop that," without the physical intervention. As soon as these behaviors were under control, the child was directed to an activity such as identification of colors or naming of objects, which she was able to perform and for which she would be generously rewarded with praise. In this situation, the defined acceptable behaviors increased to an expected criterion and interfering behaviors diminished to zero (Figure 55). The original regressive behaviors were recaptured if a person associated only with positive reinforcement was trying to work with her; the repetitive behaviors returned and the socially use-

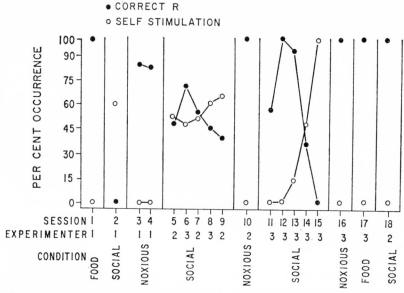

Figure 55. Per cent occurrence of correct responses versus self-stimulatory behaviors in Pamela, comparing food reinforcement with social reinforcement, both before and after shock.

ful behaviors again dropped out. Despite the fact that certain behaviors were modified and maintained over a period of time, the over-all picture remained unchanged. The continual restraint. After transfer to the Neuropsychiatric Institute, the child was removed from restraints and observed in order to establish a base rate of self-hitting. While isolated in a bare room, the rate decreased slightly. However, because of the possibility of serious injury during prolonged extinction it was felt that isolation and simple nonreinforcement was not an appropriate alternative. An effort was made to suppress the self-hitting by establishing competing behaviors such as feeding, which when performed would not permit the motor activity of hitting, but the rate of hitting remained unchanged. Therefore, it was decided to use negative reinforcement in the form of painful stimuli contingent upon the self-hitting behavior. The painful stimuli included both slapping and electric stimuli. Each acted to reduce the self-hitting behavior to zero within a period of eight days. This reduction in hitting was maintained in a variety of situations outside the laboratory for several weeks (Figure 56). The child has been returned to the

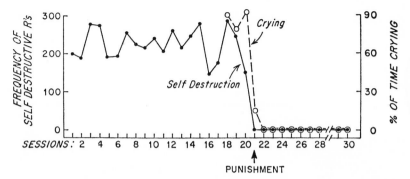

Figure 56. Baseline frequency of John's self-destructive behavior and the response to contingent shock. Note the parallel decrease in crying behavior.

State Hospital where it has been possible to maintain the suppression of self-hitting if the conditions under which it was suppressed are maintained.

Discussion

Any general consideration of punishment should be prefaced by a brief discussion of evidence cited against its use. Perhaps the outstanding criticism is a moral and humanitarian one which is of great moment. However, Church[7] dismissed this in his comment that "whenever the alternative to punishment involved deprivation or extinction, the relative moral values are difficult to assess." A second criticism centers on the general idea that punishment does no good. This contention frequently arises out of experience with the use of punishment in general to deter certain behaviors, such as criminal behavior or insanity. Examination of these social conditions reveals that punishment which has been utilized to manage the abnormal behavior was probably given on a noncontingent basis for such global activity as being "crazy" or being "bad." In this type of situation the chances of gaining an expected outcome are minimal, since cardinal principles of behavior modification are completely ignored. These principles are basically that (a) the punishment was probably not given contingent upon a clearly specified behavior; (b) the time relationship between behavior and punishment was probably of long and variable length, making the relationships between the two quite uncertain, and (c) it may have been that no clear-cut escape behaviors within the functional capacity of the individual were offered.

Experimental findings on paradoxical effects of punishment in facilitating an index response have often been invoked as good reasons for not using it. Church[7] has delineated a series of four hypotheses under which punishment may facilitate the appearance of a punished response. The first was the discrimination hypothesis in which the negative reinforcement reinstated a condition of training for that particular response, namely, the situation in which punishment followed a given response was similar to the situation in which positive reinforcement was used. Therefore, it could be postulated that the likelihood of a clear-cut discrimination would be decreased. The second hypothesis concerned the fear response, in which fear itself, with whatever concomitants existed, simply facilitated the punished response. The competing response hypothesis was established to account for those instances where a skeletal response to the painful stimulus was similar to the punished response. Lastly, the escape hypothesis was postulated in which the punished response was similar to the response occurring at the time of termination of the painful stimulus.

In the third clinical situation of the series described above, a punished response (whining and fussing) was increased merely by the sight of the instrument used, and also initially by the sight of the individuals who had utilized it. This probably represented an instance where a fear response was the same as the punished response. However, despite these objections it seems apparent that if the contingencies are clear concerning which behaviors will result in punishment, and if the escape responses are unique and within the performance capabilities of the individuals, no response facilitation should take place.

On the basis of information derived from our experimental work, several possible uses of punishment seem worthy of comment. Perhaps the most interesting possibility is the use of punishment developing out of the effects in the first clinical situation. This involves a person taking on secondary positive reinforcing qualities by being associated with pain reduction. The situation in which a child is placed in a noxious environment modified only by the appearance or endeavors of a particular person offers something perhaps analogous to one aspect of the role of a mother in normal infant rearing. In the particular patient group we are dealing with, one of the most characteristic problems relates to the failure to develop positive relationships with the parents and other people. Irrespective of the particular theoretical view one might hold (behavioral, dynamic, biologic), it is possible to conclude that this particular technique might be useful.

From the strictly behavioral point of view, Lovaas, Schaffer, and Simmons[20] demonstrated that the adults did acquire reinforcing properties. From a dynamic point of view, it could be reasoned that these children have experienced abnormal transactions between themselves and significant others during infancy. Consequently, the introduction of threatening situations which can be altered, diminished, or alleviated by people could be rationalized as a recreation of one aspect of a much earlier human condition, and, thus, by repeatedly rescuing the child, that person would become significant to him.

When considering punishment, it is essential to focus on the significance of escape or avoidance behaviors. Punishment is more effective if the individual is provided an alternative as opposed to the situation where suppression alone is being attempted. This is particularly apparent if the behavior being punished is one which is intrinsically reinforcing. This was clear from Risley's study[18] and could also account for the difficulty we have encountered in the children described in the first two clinical situations. In both instances an effort was made to suppress stereotyped repetitive behaviors. Although these could be suppressed, they tended to reappear if punishment was discontinued. Consequently, the children were taught incompatible behaviors, such as ball play, for which they were positively rewarded and which could be substituted for the punished response. Even in instances where the punished behavior was not necessarily intrinsically reinforcing, it was also more effective to offer an alternative which was positively reinforced. This alternative could explain why in the third clinical situation the child overcame an initial aversive response both to the shock and to the attending adult, and was able to develop positive affectionate behaviors which were subsequently almost uniformly reinforced.

Perhaps the most clear-cut situation in which punishment can be used is the fourth clinical example. For anyone who has worked with a self-destructive, retarded, or schizophrenic child who requires periodic or almost constant restraint, the use of pain to suppress this behavior appears justified. Although it is possible that the self-injurious behavior is an operant which can be extinguished through the removal of reinforcers, it takes a strong will to endure the results of the first few moments or longer of the extinction period during which the rate goes up. This is particularly difficult if a hematoma appears or actual tissue destruction takes place. It is in these specific situations that the care-taking personnel rescue the child and reward the behavior, thus insuring its continued presence. In view of the results in the fourth case, it is clear that punishment offers an acceptable alternative.

It is necessary to keep in mind that punishment is utilized purely to restrict certain unacceptable behaviors, but not to suppress behavior in general. To avoid the latter, the application of pain must have certain limitations in intensity and total usage, and the concurrent positive reinforcement of acceptable behaviors must be maintained. The intensity of pain must be titrated to where it is bothersome, but not overwhelming. The total usage must be limited both by the reinforcement ratio which is reduced as soon as possible, and also by pairing painful stimuli with the usual words used in this general context to modify behavior. These could include "no," "stop that," and so on, which have been shown to take on significant secondary reinforcing powers in this type of situation, thus decreasing the need for shock.

Careful attention must be paid to the comment about restricting behavior. In all of the clinical situations, the major focus was on the reduction of unacceptable behaviors utilizing pain. The establishment of new behaviors in almost all instances was carried out by using a positive reinforcement approach once attention could be gained. The building of a social type of behavior in the escape or avoidance situation is the only situation where a new behavior was established utilizing punishment.

Some evidence from our laboratory suggests that where attempts were made to teach a child new speech or social behaviors with negative reinforcement for nonperformance, the over-all function of the child deteriorated.

Finally, the use of pain is extremely unsettling to the personnel involved in the procedures. One must always carefully avoid the use of punishment because of irritation with the performance of the child or out of some other personal motive wherein the contingencies, for the child, become less clear. Obviously, the use of techniques such as this by care-taking personnel are contrary to the basic concepts of care-taking and, thus, make it impossible for some people to utilize it, since it presents a considerable conflict. This conflict alone, however, should not be the determining factor in whether pain is or is not used; rather, one should rely on the experimental evidence which shows the uses and limitations of the technique.

Summary and Conclusions

Painful stimuli were used in behavioral control with nine children diagnosed as suffering from childhood schizophrenia and moderately severe retardation. Indications for use of this technique were: (1) failure of the child to attend and respond to cues from his environment; (2) the presence of repetitive stereotyped behaviors which have interfered with learning; and (3) self-destructive behavior which presents a significant problem. Four clinical situations were presented to illustrate these principles. Painful stimuli were administered, using electric shock and slapping, both of which were always paired with admonitory words. These words took on reinforcing powers and soon replaced the primary stimuli as control techniques.

Evidence was reviewed relating to actual experimental results following the use of negative reinforcement which might prove useful. These include: (1) Punishment tends to alter behavior by suppressing responsiveness. (2) If it is given on a contingent basis, the suppression is more specific. (3) In a two-choice situation, the punishment for a wrong response facilitates learning the correct response; and (4) There is an inverse relationship between response strength and the interval between response and punishment.

In clinical situations, punishment seems to have possible application. The applications which seem most apparent at this time are: (1) the establishment of people as positive and significant reinforcers by being paired with pain reduction; (2) the use of pain to suppress self-destructive behaviors in patients otherwise requiring continual control; and (3) the establishment of certain acceptable behaviors through escape or avoidance.

References

1. Ferster, C. B.: Positive reinforcement and behavioral deficits of autistic children. *Child Dev 32*:437, 1961.

2. DeMeyer, M. K. and Ferster, C. B.: Teaching new social behavior to schizophrenic children. *J Am Acad Child Psychiat* 1:443, 1962.

3. Weiland, I. H. and Rudnik, R.: Consideration of the development and treatment of autistic childhood psychosis. *Psychoanal Study Child* 16:549, 1961.

4. Lovaas, O. I., Freitag, G., Kinder, M. I., Rubenstein, B. D., Schaeffer, B., and Simmons, J. Q.: Establishment of social reinforcers in two schizophrenic children on the basis of food. *J Exp Child Psychol* 4:109, 1966.

5. Lavaas, O. I., Berberich, J. P., Perloff, B. F. and Schaeffer, B.: Acquisition of imitative speech by schizophrenic children. *Science* 151:705, 1966.

6. Lovaas, O. I.: *A Behavior Theory Approach to the Treatment of Childhood Schizophrenia.* University of Minnesota Press, Minneapolis, 1967.

7. Church, R. M.: The varied effects of punishment on behavior. *Psychol Rev* 70:369, 1963.

8. Bandura, A.: Punishment revisited. *J Consult Psychol* 26:297, 1962.

9. Szasz, T.: *Pain and Pleasure.* Basic Books, New York, 1957.

10. Freud, S.: *Beyond the Pleasure Principle.* Liveright, New York, 1950.

11. Solomon, R. L.: Punishment. *Am Psychol* 19: 239, 1964.

12. Azrin, N. H. and Holz, W. C.: Punishment in Operant Behavior. In *Operant Behavior. Areas of Research and Application.* Honig, W. K., (Ed.) Appleton-Century-Crofts, New York, 1966.

13. Durant, W.: *The History of Civilization. Our Oriental Heritage.* Simon and Schuster, New York, 1936.

14. Sears, R. R., Maccoby, E. and Levin, H.: *Patterns of Child Rearing.* Row Peterson & Co., Evanston, Ill., 1957

15. Sanderson, R. E., Campbell, D. and Laverty, S. D.: An Investigation of a New Aversive Conditioning Treatment of Alcoholism. In *Conditioning Techniques in Clinical Practice and Research.* Franks, C. M., Ed. Springer Publ. Co., New York, 1964.

16. McGuire, R. J. and Vallance, M.: Aversion Therapy by Electric Shock: A Simple Technique. In *Conditioning Techniques in Clinical Practice and Research.* Franks, C. M., Ed. Springer Publ. Co., New York, 1964.

17. Boardman, W. R.: Rusty: A brief behavior disorder. *J. Consult Psychol* 26:293, 1962.

18. Risley, T.: The effects and "side-effects" of the use of punishment with an autistic child. *J Appl Behav Anal* (in press).

19. Lovaas, O. I., Freitag, G., Gold, V. J. and Kassorla, I. C.: Experimental studies in childhood schizophrenia: analysis of self-destructive behavior. *J Exp Child Psychol* 2:67, 1965.

20. Lovaas, O. I., Schaeffer, B. and Simmons, J. Q.: Experimental studies in

childhood schizophrenia: building social behavior in autistic children by use of electric shock. *J Exp Res Pers 1*:99, 1965.

21. Blau, A.: The nature of childhood schizophrenia: a dynamic neuropsychiatric view. *J Child Psychiat 1*:225, 1962.

22. Goldfarb, G.: *Childhood Schizophrenia.* Harvard University Press, Cambridge, Mass., 1961.

23. Menolascino, F. J.: Autistic reactions in early childhood: differential diagnostic considerations. *J Child Phychol Psychiat 6*:203, 1965.

24. Bernal, M.: GSR Studies of Autistic Children. Presented at the annual meeting of the American Psychological Association, Chicago, Ill., 1965.

ANNOTATED BIBLIOGRAPHY

The references listed below are those which the authors recommend as additional examples of recent work in behavior therapy. It is not an exhaustive bibliography; instead, the citations were carefully selected for quality and relevance to the topic categories by which this book was organized. The articles are classified below according to the chapter which most nearly matches their contents.

CHAPTER 2

Bernal, M. E.: Behavioral treatment of a child's eating problem. *Journal of Behavior Therapy and Experimental Psychology*, 3:43, 1972.
    The problem-eating behaviors of a four-year-old girl who refused to feed herself or eat table foods were modified using a gradual shaping procedure. The girl's mother was trained in behavior shaping and acted as the reinforcing agent.

Clement, P. W.: Elimination of sleepwalking in a seven-year-old boy. *Journal of Consulting and Clinical Psychology*, 34:22, 1970.
    A conditioning model, similar to those used in behavior therapy of enuretics, brought about changes in the sleepwalking behavior of a seven-year-old boy.

Edelman, R. I.: Operant conditioning treatment of encopresis. *Journal of Behavior Therapy and Experimental Psychiatry*, 2:71, 1971.
    A twelve-year-old encopretic girl was treated in the home situation by a combined procedure involving punishment for soiling behavior and being allowed to avoid an unpleasant task when she did not soil.

Garvey, W. P. and Hegrenes, J. R.: Desensitization techniques in the treatment of a phobia. *American Journal of Orthopsychiatry*, 36:147, 1966.
    Fear of attending school was eliminated in a ten-year-old boy by having him approach the school accompanied by a behavior therapist. School related stimulus situations were ordered from the least anxiety-provoking to the most fearful. The child and therapist proceeded through this series of graded steps for 20 consecutive days until the boy was able to resume normal school attendance. A two-year follow-up showed no return of symptoms.

Kaufmann, L. M. and Wagner, B. R.: Barb: a systematic treatment technology for temper control disorders. *Behavior Therapy*, 3:84, 1972.

Lack of temper control following an aversive stimulus was successfully eliminated in a fourteen-year-old boy through a systematic treatment technique labelled "the barb". This technique is an individualized programming procedure involving a systematic representation of provoking stimuli, response specification, and reinforcement for responding in a required manner to the provoking stimuli.

Miller, A. L.: Treatment of a child with Giles de la Tourette's syndrome using behavior modification techniques. *Journal of Behavior Therapy and Experimental Psychiatry, 1*:319, 1970.

Rewarding the non-performance of undesirable behavior removed the symptoms of Giles de la Tourette's Syndrome in a five-year-old boy. The boy's mother and teacher were both involved in the therapy under professional supervision.

Wahler, R. G., Sperling, K. A., Thomas, M. R., Teeter, N. C., and Luper, H. L.: The modification of childhood stuttering: some response-response relationships. *Journal of Experimental Child Psychology, 9*:411, 1970.

Two boys, whose presenting problem was stuttering, were observed and treated in clinic and home settings. As a consequence of the application of contingency management procedures to secondary behavior problems both the secondary problems and the stuttering were reduced.

Wetzel, R.: Use of behavioral techniques in a case of compulsive stealing. *Journal of Consulting Psychology, 30*:367, 1966.

The compulsive stealing behavior of a ten-year-old boy was eliminated over a three and one-half month period. This study illustrates the use of nonprofessionals in a field situation in the modification of disturbing behavior.

Williams, C. D.: The elimination of tantrum behavior by extinction procedures. *Journal of Abnormal and Social Psychology, 59*:269, 1959.

Tantrum behavior was successfully extinguished in a 21-month-old baby.

CHAPTER 3

Brooks, R. B. and Snow, D. L.: Two case illustrations of the use of behavior-modification techniques in the school setting. *Behavior Therapy, 3*:100, 1972.

Two cases illustrate effective behavioral techniques for classroom use; positive reinforcement was used to increase academic performance and group contingencies were utilized to decrease deviant behavior.

Coleman, R.: A conditioning technique applicable to elementary school classrooms. *Journal of Applied Behavior Analysis, 3*:293, 1970.

A procedure was described for use in the classroom in which only one child in the room needs modification of appropriate behavior. Reinforcers were contingent upon appropriate behavior by the target child and were distributed to the entire class.

Ferritor, D. E., Buckholdt, D., Hamblin, R. L., and Smith, L: The noneffects of contingent reinforcement for attending behavior on work accomplished. *Journal of Applied Behavior Analysis, 5*:7, 1972.

Behavioral contingencies in two elementary classrooms improved attending behavior and decreased disruptive behavior, but did not improve performance. Performance contingencies increased academic performance, but disruptive and non-attending behavior increased. Combined contingencies increased both performance and attending.

Hall, R. V., Panyan, M., Rabon, D., Broden, M.: Instructing beginning teachers in reinforcement procedures which improve classroom control. *Journal of Applied Behavior Analysis, 1*:315, 1968.

Increased study rates and reduction of disruptive behavior were observed during an experimental period in which systematic reinforcement contingencies were in effect. A brief reversal period during which teachers provided almost no reinforcement for study behavior produced low rates of study. Reinstatement of the experimental contingencies resulted once again in marked increases in study behaviors.

Kirby, F. D. and Toler, H. C., Jr.: Modification of preschool isolate behavior: a case study. *Journal of Applied Behavior Analysis, 3*:309, 1970.

Interaction with preschool classmates was markedly increased in a five year-old boy during periods of time when he passed out candy to them in the classroom.

McClain, W. A.: The modification of aggressive classroom behavior through reinforcement, inhibition and relationship therapy. *Training School Bulletin, 65*(4):122, 1969.

An individualized training program, based on the principles of operant conditioning and relationship therapy was used to modify the aggressive acting-out classroom behavior of a ten year-old boy. A team approach involving a classroom teacher and a behavioral therapist was utilized.

Nolen, P. S., Kunzelmann, H. P. and Haring, N. G.: Behavior modification in a junior-high learning-disabilities classroom. *Exceptional Children, 34*:163, 1967.

Eight junior high school students with serious learning and behavior disorders made significant academic gains over a teaching period of 100 days while under individually programmed behavioral contingencies.

O'Leary, K. D. and Becker, W. C.: Behavior modification of an adjustment class: a token reinforcement program. *Exceptional Children, 33*:637, 1967.

A token reinforcement program was instituted in a third grade adjustment class in which teacher's ratings were exchanged for reinforcers. Deviant behavior was greatly reduced even when delay of reinforcement was increased to four days.

Ramp, E., Ulrich, R., and Dulaney, Sylvia.: Delayed timeout as a procedure for reducing disruptive classroom behavior: a case study. *Journal of Applied Behavior Analysis, 4*:235, 1971.

The disruptive behavior of a nine year-old boy was eliminated by a delayed time out from reinforcement procedure. Contingencies were removed and disruptive behavior returned to its baseline level.

Ward, M. H. and Baker, B. L.: *Journal of Applied Behavior Analysis,* *1*:323, 1968.

Three teachers were instructed in the use of immediate attention and praise contingent upon the child's exhibiting target behavior in the classroom. Observation measures showed a significant reduction in deviant behavior and a significant increase in task-relevant behavior from baseline to treatment in a group of four first-grade children identified as behavior problems. No significant changes for same-class controls were observed.

CHAPTER 5

Phillips, E. L., Phillips, E. A., Fixsen, D. L., and Wolf, M. M.: Achievement place: modification of the behaviors of pre-delinquent boys within a token economy. *Journal of Applied Behavior Analysis, 4*:45, 1971.

A token reinforcement system produced reliable modification in "pre-delinquent behaviors" in six boys at a community based, family-style center for pre-delinquent and delinquent boys.

Staats, A. W. and Butterfield, W. H.: Treatment of nonreading in a culturally deprived juvenile delinquent: an application of reinforcement principles. *Child Development, 36*:925, 1965.

A fourteen year-old delinquent boy was given forty hours of reading training which extended over 4½ months using a token reinforcement program. Subsequently, attention was at a high level, new words had been acquired and retained, reading achievement vastly improved, grades improved, and misbehaviors at school were eliminated.

Schwitzgebel, R. L.: Short-term operant conditioning of adolescent offenders on socially relevant variables. *Journal of Abnormal Psychology, 72*:134, 1967.

In both a laboratory and natural setting two classes of positive operants were increased when followed by positive consequences. Punishment of negative operants had no significant effect.

CHAPTER 6

Conger, J. C.: The treatment of encopresis by the management of social consequences. *Behavior Therapy, 1*:386, 1970.

Contingent withdrawal of maternal attention and physical contact totally eliminated soiling behavior of four-years duration in a nine year-old boy.

Hawkins, R. P., Peterson, R. F., Schweid, E. and Bijou, S. W.: Behavior therapy in the home: amelioration of parent-child relations with the parent in a therapeutic role. *Journal of Experimental Child Psychology, 4*:99, 1966.

Modification of objectionable behaviors in a four year-old boy was observed following a behavioral treatment program implemented in the home with the boy's mother as therapist.

Salzinger, K., Feldman, R. S., and Portnoy, S.: Training parents of brain-injured children in the use of operant conditioning procedures. *Behavior Therapy, 1*:4, 1970.

Parents of brain-injured children were taught to carry out behavior modification programs for their own children. All parents who carried out the programs succeeded in altering undesirable behavior. Some parents did not attempt to carry out the programs and some did not keep required records.

Wahler, R. G.: Oppositional children: a quest for parental reinforcement control. *Journal of Applied Behavior Analysis, 2*:159, 1969.

Subjects were two boys reported by their parents to be highly oppositional to parental control. The parents were trained in the use of a combination timeout and differential-attention program, following which they were able to implement these treatment procedures to greatly reduce oppositional behavior. Parental reinforcement value was higher during the treatment period than during a baseline period.

Wahler, R. G., Winkel, G. H., Peterson, R. F. and Morrison, D. C.: Mothers as behavior therapists for their own children. *Behavior Research and Therapy, 3*:113, 1965.

This study demonstrated that systematic modifications of maternal reactions to specific classes of deviant behavior in their children produced marked changes in those behaviors.

Zeilberger, J., Sampen, S. E. and Sloane, H. N., Jr.: Modification of a child's problem behaviors in the home with the mother as therapist. *Journal of Applied Behavior Analysis, 1*:47, 1968.

Aggressive behavior was increased and obedience increased in a four year-old boy by means of differential reinforcement contingencies programmed by his mother in the home.

CHAPTER 7

Jensen, G. D. and Womack, M. G.: Operant conditioning techniques applied in the treatment of an autistic child. *American Journal of Orthopsychiatry, 37*(1):30, 1967.

Application of operant conditioning procedures to a clinical ward treatment program of an autistic child resulted in a decrease in temper tantrums, improved language functioning and better peer interaction.

Leff, Robert: Behavior modification and the psychoses of childhood: a review. *Psychological Bulletin, 69*:396, 1968.

The use of operant training procedures with psychotic children was reviewed. The evidence was interpreted as supportive of a social-learning model of severely pathological behavior and an operant-training model of therapy.

Lovaas, O. I., Berberich, J. P., Perloff, B. F. and Schaeffer, B.: Acquisition of imitative speech by schizophrenic children. *Science, 151*:705, 1966.

Two mute schizophrenic children were taught imitative speech by operant conditioning procedures. Reward was contingent upon closer and closer imitations of the attending adults' speech.

Ney, P. G., Palvesky, A. E., and Markely, J.: Relative effectiveness of operant conditioning and play therapy in childhood schizophrenic. *Journal of Autism and Childhood Schizophrenic,* 1:337, 1971.

An experimental study showed that both play therapy and operant conditioning were effective in increasing the mental ages and language functioning of schizophrenic boys. A comparison showed that after several months of treatment there was significantly greater improvement following operant conditioning than subsequent to play therapy.

Risley, T. R.: The effects and side effects of punishing the autistic behavior of a deviant child. *Journal of Applied Behavior Analysis,* 1:21, 1968.

Punishment with electric shock was used to greatly reduce dangerous climbing behavior in a severely deviant child, first in the laboratory and later in the home. Autistic rocking was also eliminated by a punishment technique. Side effects of the punishment procedures were monitored and were, for the most part, found to be desirable.

Risley, T. and Wolf, M.: Establishing functional speech in echolalic children. *Behavior Research and Therapy,* 5:73, 1967.

Procedures used to develop speech behavior in echolalic children is summarized. These procedures are based upon shaping, imitation training, extinction, time-out from reinforcement, and differential reinforcement.

Ross, R. R., Meichenbaum, D. H. and Humphrey, Carol: Treatment of nocturnal headbanging by behavior modification techniques: a case report. *Behavior Research and Therapy,* 9:151, 1971.

Nocturnal headbanging was eliminated in a sixteen year-old institutionalized girl. The treatment program involved the use of desensitization to dream content and removal of consequent events.

Wetzel, R. J., Baker, J., Roney, M. and Martin, M.: *Behavior Research and Therapy,* 4:169, 1966.

The behavior of a six year-old autistic boy was significantly changed after three months of intensive out-patient behavior therapy. The boy's parents were trained in shaping and maintaining new behaviors.